TOTAL ENGAGEMENT

The Healthcare Practitioner's Guide to Heal Yourself, Your Patients & Your Practice

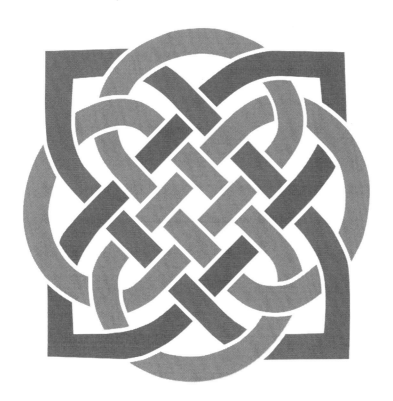

Mimi Guarneri, MD & Mark J. Tager, MD

Copyright © 2014 by Mimi Guarneri, MD, and Mark J. Tager, MD

All rights reserved. In accordance with the U.S. Copyright Act of 1976, the scanning, uploading, and electronic sharing of any part of this book without the permission of the publisher constitute unlawful piracy and theft of the author's intellectual property. If you would like to use material from the book (other than for review purposes), prior written permission must be obtained by contacting the publisher at info@changewell.com. Thank you for your support of the author's rights.

Published by

ChangeWell Inc.

PO Box 7303

Rancho Santa Fe, CA 92067

www.changewell.com

First Edition: October 2014

ISBN 978-0-99716250-3-7

To order additional copies or to learn about Total Engagement workshops or training programs, please contact us.

info@changewell.com
1-858-756-1491

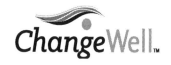

Acknowledgements

If you want to get something done in an efficient manner, you can't beat a hub and spoke model. The hub of *Total Engagement* was Alexandra Hazzard, a millennial who has convinced us that some major problems in the world might get solved if we place more faith in these spiritually and digitally gifted young people. From research to layout and illustrations, to keeping track of all the citations, through countless revisions, Alexandra did it all with unfailing grace while operating under tremendous time pressures.

Nancy Van Allen has designed all eight of Mark's books and from the Dara Knot concept—which she came up with—to its execution through more than two dozen revisions, she continues to amaze. We had to lure her away from concentrating on her fine arts and get her in the commercial ring one more time.

We recruited James Tager, the newly minted Harvard trained Human Rights lawyer to return to his earlier roots as a medical writer to help with some of the interviews and research. Marissa Tager did an early read on the manuscript and added some practical insights.

We are grateful to Ellen Stiefler, an attorney who manages talent and intellectual property rights, for clearing the way to allow *Total Engagement* to be made available to the physician marketplace.

A shout out to an old colleague of Mark's: Barry Taylor, ND, who was kind enough to provide some early guidance on the manuscript. We have also benefited tremendously from the editorial guidance of Erik Goldman, co-founder and editor in chief of *Holistic Primary Care*. He was kind enough to share some of their survey data with us.

Three groups are truly worth of our gratitude. Thanks to our colleagues at AIHM, many of whom have graciously shared their most intimate stories with us. You will find these narratives sprinkled throughout the book. We hope that they will be a source of personal inspiration for you. We deeply appreciate the contributions of our colleagues at Atlantic Health System, especially Vice President Linda Reed, whose tireless dedication continues to help guide this innovative organization. And finally, the great team at Pacific Pearl La Jolla, especially Rauni Prittinen King, who continued the noble work of healing while we sat typing words on a screen.

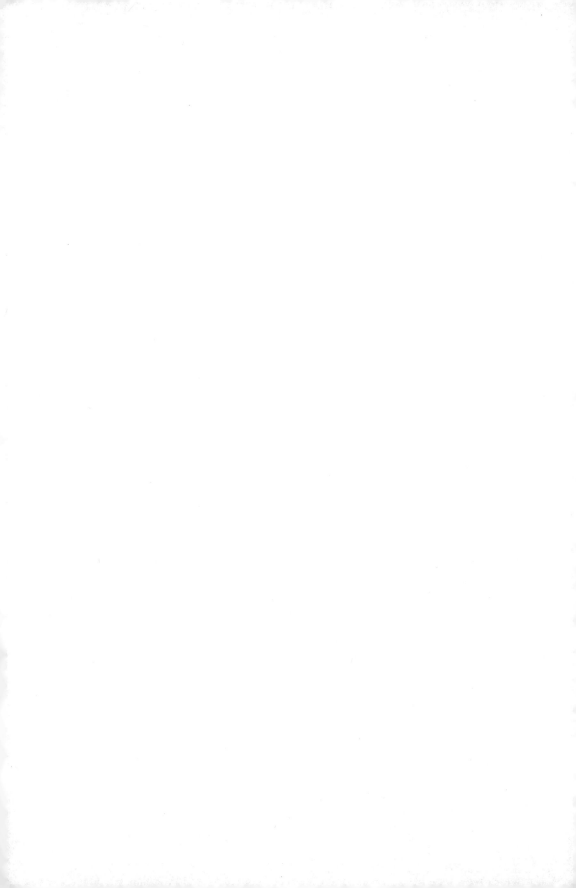

Contents

Introduction
From Grumpy to Great   2

Part One: Heal Yourself
Chapter 1: The Clinician's Chief Complaint   24
Chapter 2: Physician Happy Thyself   44
Chapter 3: Should I Stay or Should I Go?   72
Chapter 4: The Courage to Change   96

Part Two: Heal Your Patients
Chapter 5: The Art and Science of Patient Healing   122
Chapter 6: The Lifestyle Paradigm   148
Chapter 7: The Functional Medicine Paradigm   178
Chapter 8: The Holistic Paradigm   202

Part Three: Heal Your Practice
Chapter 9: Apply Tinctures of Time & Passion   232
Chapter 10: Ingredients of a Successful Practice   264
Chapter 11: Life Beyond Clinical Practice   294

Appendix   322
Bibliography   328
Index   341
About the Authors   352

INTRODUCTION

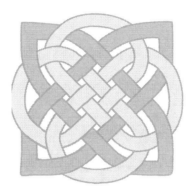

The Dara Knot

The Dara knot shown on the cover is a Celtic symbol that originates from the Irish word *doire*, for oak tree. These types of unbroken and interconnected knots were first used in the 7th century. The Dara knot, in its many forms thoughout this book, always represents the roots of the oak.

The Celts considered oak trees to be sacred. In times of challenge and hardship, they would evoke the spirit of the oak to increase their internal strength and fortitude. The Dara knot has been associated with other traits such as wisdom, power, endurance, perseverance and leadership.

From Grumpy to Great

This is a book about transformation. And like every story of change, it begins with discomfort.

In working with hundreds of clinicians, we have found that many healthcare professionals are suffering from the same wellness-related issues that affect their patients. Our observations are supported by ample surveys and literature.

Many clinicians today are looking very much like the patients they counsel: overweight, depressed, under-exercised, over-stressed, and fatigued by the rigors of work. They are increasingly subjected to the ravages of systemic inflammation, neurotransmitter depletion, metabolic syndrome, sleep deprivation, musculoskeletal tension, and chronic pain syndromes.

Health problems are pervasive throughout the conventional healthcare system whether you are a primary care physician, a specialist, a surgeon, or a non-physician member of the care team—a nurse, PA, NP, or mental health professional, odds are you're feeling less than optimally healthy these days.

Healthcare practitioners work hard and sacrifice each day for their noble profession, only to find that the rules keep shifting, and the giving-getting compromise seems out of balance: too much giving, not enough getting.

Only, physicians have a unique additional burden; each carries heavy self- and patient-centered expectations to help and heal. While other types of healthcare practitioners may take issue, physicians are currently positioned at the center of the health-care system, with all the obligations, responsibilities and potential liabilities that such a position entails. Plus, no physician can fall back on an 'ignorance is bliss' excuse and claim that 'lack of knowledge' is preventing us from being healthy.

The transformational process outlined in this book can benefit all

INTRODUCTION

disciplines of healthcare professionals. We have included personal accounts from nurses, mental health professionals, and complementary practitioners in *Total Engagement*. But, as physicians ourselves, and for the reasons outlined above, we will be focusing the majority of our attention on medical physicians.

If you're feeling grumpy, it is probably for good reason. You are giving, caring, and worrying about your patients all day long—and part of the night—and when you get home, you are drained and have little left for those you love. You are frustrated by a system that provides little time and few tools to help patients make the lifestyle changes they need to get well. When you look out on the horizon, you notice that things don't seem like they are going to get better. There will be more of the same, and given the changes in the healthcare system, things could easily become worse.

We meet more and more physicians and other practitioners who are looking for a change. At medical reunions and meetings, we are constantly interacting with medical peers who say things like, "You got out; how can I get out?" It's evident that many of our colleagues do not see a clear path to fulfillment and satisfaction. They know that they are not happy, but don't know what they can do to feel better.

We wrote this book to help our fellow clinicians who are struggling with these issues. But, to start, we should establish that each individual practitioner's motivations for change are unique and so, too, are the paths for wellbeing. Although we cannot show you the path forward, we hope to guide you onto a path that will lead you in the right direction.

We are not going to spend much time on the negative aspects of the healthcare system and its stressors; you are already an expert in this realm. Rather, we will help you answer these, and other questions that may be on your mind:

- How can I make my present practice more enjoyable, meaningful and profitable?
- What alternative paths are available? For myself and for my patients?
- What options and choices do I have?
- Which are the ones that work best for me? My practice? My family?
- Which are consistent with my values and beliefs?

- What skills do I have that can transfer to a new model of care?
- What new skills should I learn? And where should I go to gain them?
- Where will I find the most joy and fulfillment?
- Which paths will diminish my anxiety and provide me with enough income to find joy and fulfillment elsewhere?
- What are the barriers and fears that accompany my desire to change, and how can I overcome them?
- Who can help support me through the change process?

The Four Elements

If you always do what you've always done, you'll always get what you've always got.

Given the wide range of personal and professional interests and activities that make up our lives, the notion of making meaningful change can be bewildering. Where to start? Do I try to improve my current situation incrementally or make a complete break and start something new? Should I be learning a new therapeutic modality or sharpening my practice management skills? Do I go it alone or try to team up with others? Am I better off as an employee or as an independent?

Many people stick with their existing circumstances—however negative they may be—because they feel overwhelmed by all the different questions that come into play when considering a change.

In the pages ahead we will attempt to help you sort this out by presenting options that touch on four elements of change. (Figure 1) The options are defined by their scope (incremental versus major) and whether the changes are focused primarily on yourself personally, on your practice or a combination of both. We also note that some physicians may elect to use their health and medical knowledge outside of clinical practice; some physicians leave medicine entirely and use their non-healthcare related skills in other endeavors. We'll begin our discussion with the incremental steps.

INTRODUCTION

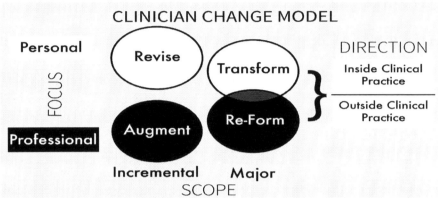

Figure 1: The Clinician Change Model

Start Small: Create V2.0 You

You will find our concern for physician wellbeing reflected throughout the pages of *Total Engagement*. You will also find our recommendations for initiating, achieving and maintaining meaningful health behavior change for yourself as well as for your patients.

Just as we advise patients to set short-term, realistic, bite sized goals to experience early success with lifestyle changes, so too can physicians avail themselves of these same techniques. Simple changes could include taking up yoga or meditation, working one day less per week, spending more time with family or loved ones, or finally tackling some of your own stress-related issues. It could involve making the changes to your diet that your scientific mind knows you should have made years ago, or joining a gym. Maybe it means finally giving in to that secret wish you've always had to learn how to play the guitar. These are the types of changes that may yield incremental improvement in your emotions, thoughts and behaviors.

Focusing on personal health improvement also serves an important psychological role, namely to narrow the gap between values and actions. This gap is often reflected in the clinician's advice to patients to improve their diet, exercise more and manage stress better, when the clinician personally does not engage in these practices. In addition to the personal benefits you receive, the net effect of "walking the talk" provides you with greater authenticity and personal power to affect change in others.

Start Small by Augmenting Your Practice

Small changes are indicated if you are generally satisfied with your medical practice but want to tweak it for greater efficiency, productivity and profit. For physicians whose primary stressor is financial, there are many opportunities to augment their practice. One approach involves adding a direct-pay product or service component. Examples include medical weight loss, in-office diagnostic tests, nutraceuticals, cosmeceuticals, or aesthetic services such as lasers, injectables or skin care into your practice.

First of all, know that you are not alone in seeking to increase your practice revenue—the majority of clinicians are looking for new cash streams. According to a 2014 survey of more than 600 primary care clinicians by *Holistic Primary Care,* 63% of respondents say they are actively seeking new revenue options, and this is especially true among practice owners, 71% of whom are looking for fresh revenue streams.

Other revenue options being considered by cash-strapped primary care clinicians include: creation of educational products such as books, DVDs and webinars (50%); instituting group visits (41%); offering teleconsults (39%); advanced diagnostic procedures (33%); aesthetic procedures (15%), and spa services (14%).[1]

Another recent survey indicates that 23% of all primary care practices now sell products to bring in ancillary revenue. One out of every three orthopedic practices provides direct patient pay products and service.[2]

We believe there is tremendous opportunity in the rapidly growing field of telehealth. InMedica, a medical market research group, predicts a 600% increase in the number of telehealth patients in the United States between 2012 and 2017. That will mean a base of over one million patients within the next few years.[3] With this growth comes the need for physicians and other practitioners at the other end of the phones and screens.

This need will only grow as e-devices and online platforms become more prevalent, as pressure for cost efficiency continues to bear down, and as patients continue to reach out for second opinions or for health counseling.

One intriguing thing about telehealth is that it opens opportunities for stay-at-home or retired physicians, or for conventional insurance-based

INTRODUCTION

physicians seeking supplemental income. Telehealth also offers an additional way of connecting with patients.

Aesthetic procedures such as hair removal, laser and IPL skin rejuvenation, non-invasive body contouring and skin tightening that were once the province of specialists like plastic surgeons and dermatologists are increasingly being adopted by clinicians who are neither.

Cosmetic service adoption by non-aesthetic specialty physicians had been growing steadily from early 2000 on, but became derailed during the economic crisis of 2008-2010 when financing became all but impossible for non-specialists to obtain. As the economy has rebounded, so too has the growth of medical spas, owned or overseen by physicians. The field has benefited from improved training, safer equipment and better protocols.

Keep in mind that the needs and expectations of aesthetic patients differ greatly from conventional medical patients. Depending upon the treatments you offer, you will need to clearly establish reasonable expectations for hair removal; wrinkle, pigment and redness improvement; skin tightening; and face and body shaping and always err on the side of conservatism. You must also be on the look out and avoid treating patients with body dysmorphic disorder.[4]

Beyond aesthetics, many other modalities like home sleep monitoring, retinal exams, carotid intima media thickness measurement (CIMT), or treadmill testing have moved out of their original specialties and into other areas of clinical practice. All of these can create new cash streams whether it be through cash-pay or reimbursment by insurance.

In most states, physicians can legally delegate aesthetic procedures to non-MD ancillary personnel under supervision. Vendors of CIMT and treadmill testing will often staff the procedures with their certified personnel. This can create strong revenue opportunities without creating further demands on physician time.

There are many ways to learn the ins and outs of things like aesthetic procedures, nutritional testing, dispensing supplements and cosmeceuticals, and medical weight loss. There are dozens of conferences, seminars, and books. There are packaged 'turn-key' programs you can easily incorporate into your existing practice. Be aware that some of these products and programs have a strong evidence-base; many do not.

In this book we will focus more on the context for incorporating new clinical tools and new revenue streams into practice rather than on the tools themselves.

These incremental changes can lead to ample reward if your needs are primarily financial. The new service offerings can also become interesting in their own right. We have profiled a number of physicians who started out dabbling in aesthetics, advanced cardiovascular testing, or nutrition supplementation only to find that the exploration awakened their passion and changed the emphasis of their practice.

There are other ways to augment your practice. You could improve the workflow by integrating new online practice management tools, trying new marketing practices, or even giving the clinic an appearance makeover. As with any other process of improvement, vendor selection becomes critical, so choose wisely.

Structure Changes Function: Re-Form Your Practice

While few clinicians these days are happy with the general state of reimbursement, for many the real pain is related to lack of time—especially time to spend with patients.

The norm in a conventional medical practice is a 15-minute visit. For a good portion of that time, the physician is glued to an EHR.[5] Thorough diagnosis and meaningful therapeutic interventions require far more time than most visits allow.

One of the greatest problems in our current healthcare system is that physicians are paid so little for their time and the cognitive aspects of practice. The unfortunate reality is that time is money. For patients who want greater attention from their physicians, and for clinicians who want to provide more thorough and attentive care, it will be necessary to restructure the practice to provide some form of direct pay.

A growing number of physicians are moving toward hybrid models of care in which they provide both insurance-reimbursable and direct pay care. According to *Holistic Primary Care's* 2014 survey, 20% of primary care practitioners consider their practice models to be 'mixed.' It is interesting to note that 47% of the survey respondents said they were considering making a significant change to their practice models within the next 2-3 years.

INTRODUCTION

The hybrid model is gaining traction with clinicians interested in lifestyle, holistic, integrative and functional medicine.

In this model, the physician takes commercial insurance or Medicare for a portion of their patients who get the customary 15-minute visits. For additional fees, usually ranging from $25-$100 per month, patients can obtain greater access including longer visits, 24/7 cell phone access, and additional concierge type services. Patients may also pay directly for non-covered products and services. The direct pay component can help streamline administration and smooth out cash flow.

A small but clearly growing number of doctors have opted to totally eliminate third party payment and have either adopted a total membership or a direct pay-for-service model.

The total membership model is gaining prominence in both integrative care, and in conventional medical care, where it is often referred to as 'concierge care.'

Concierge medicine involves providing comprehensive services for a limited patient population of 150-600 patients who pay a fixed annual fee to be members of the practice. In many cases, these patients are drawn from a physician's existing base of 2,000-4,000 patients. Many physicians enlist the help of consultants to help them make the transition into direct-pay. Others join concierge groups such as MDVIP or Paradigm.

Some practitioners—and patients—find the term 'concierge' off-putting, as it has a connotation of elitism. In actuality, membership practices need not be limited exclusively to the wealthy. There are practices all over the nation that are proving that direct-pay and membership models can work in less than affluent communities.

Supporters of the membership or concierge model contend that the real issues are choices and priorities. They point out that annual fees to join good membership-based practices are equivalent to the aggregate cost of one daily specialty coffee drink for the year.

According to Michael Tetreault, Editor of *Concierge Medicine Today* and *The Direct Primary Care Journal*, "There are slightly less than 4,000 physicians who are verifiably, actively practicing concierge medicine or direct primary care across the United States, with probably another 8,000 practicing under the radar."[6]

The annual membership model, however, is on the minds of physicians across the country. A 2012 survey of US physicians by Merritt Hawkins, a national physician-recruitment company, revealed that almost 7 percent of doctors are considering the switch to a concierge-type model.[7] *Holistic Primary Care's* 2014 survey indicates that 22% of primary care clinicians are looking at the concierge/membership model, and 32% are considering a switch to a straight-up cash-pay practice.

There is no doubt that physicians who have successfully transitioned to direct-pay or membership models are enjoying a higher quality of life and providing more satisfying care for their limited patient populations. These practice models give clinicians the freedom to connect and communicate more deeply with their patients. Practitioners become more intimately familiar with their patients' histories and can help guide them toward improved lifestyle, self-care and medical decision-making. Concierge physicians can act as, or in conjunction with, a hospitalist to provide continuity of care and support if a patient requires hospitalization.

Direct-pay, membership and hybrid practice models are essentially changes in fiscal transactions and financing mechanism. They address the 'how' of care, but not the 'what' of care. If your main dissatisfactions are related to limitations of time and money, then they are certainly worth considering.

However, a conventionally-trained clinician who ports his or her existing clinical skills over to the membership model may still struggle with the limitations of standard medical care. Confronting these limits—the 'what' of care—will require a broad discussion.

Transform Yourself & Your Practice

In this book, we will be focusing much of our attention on the transformational path that is known as Integrative Medicine (IM) and the necessary steps for moving yourself and your practice in this direction.

First, a definition: *Integrative Medicine (IM) is the practice of medicine that reaffirms the relationship between practitioner and patient, focuses on the whole person, is informed by evidence, and makes use of all appropriate therapeutic approaches, healthcare professionals and disciplines to facilitate optimal health and healing.*

INTRODUCTION

IM is rooted in the belief that happiness, health and fulfillment occur when body, mind and spirit are in alignment. When these three elements are in sync, a person operates out of a place of calmness and focus. If you, as a healthcare professional, can cultivate this kind of alignment, you can share this state with patients and inspire them to make meaningful changes in their own lives.

An IM practitioner acknowledges both the advantages and limitations of our current healthcare system. Our conventional treatment model excels for the patients with acute conditions, trauma or infectious diseases who require a thorough diagnostic workup, trauma or acute care, infectious disease treatment or pharmaceutical or surgical interventions. The advances of conventional medicine are often life saving.

Allopathic medicine is not nearly as effective in addressing lifestyle related-conditions and the growing epidemics of obesity, cardiovascular disease, and metabolic diseases. Despite spending $2.8 trillion, or $8,915 per person in 2012,[8] the United States is only ranked 37th in the world in health outcomes.[9]

Our healthcare system is structured in ways that create major impediments to improving overall health status. Physicians operate in silos of 'ologies' such as cardiology, pulmonology, neurology, nephrology, etc. In this model, each individual becomes a distinct entity unto him/herself; each organ system becomes a protected fiefdom isolated from the others; and each symptom is matched to a pharmaceutical solution.

Thus, gastroesophageal reflux disease calls for an H2 blocker, depression an SSRI; migraines engender a prescription for triptans; for irritable bowel syndrome there are anticholinergics. The result of such care is an ever-mounting list of prescriptions that rises steadily with patient age. A Kaiser Permanente study showed that the annual per capita number of retail prescriptions filled at pharmacies expanded from 4.1 for ages 0-18; to 11.9 for ages 19-64; to 28.0 in people 65 years and older.[10]

For those of us who have cared for patients whose list of prescription medications comes perilously close to, or even exceeds, the number of days in a month, it becomes clear that somehow, we are missing the forest for the trees.

Even if you recognize that lifestyle is the major determinant of health (Figure 2 below), you are likely beset by the frustration that your current knowledge base, experience, existing clinical tools, and practice structure can not provide do not allow you to provide your patients with what they really need to heal themselves.

Most physicians are woefully unprepared to guide patients through even the basics of lifestyle modifications including diet, exercise, and stress management, let alone help them with emotional, spiritual, interpersonal, or mental wellbeing issues. In conventional medicine, we are ignoring the whole person and focusing instead on their parts.

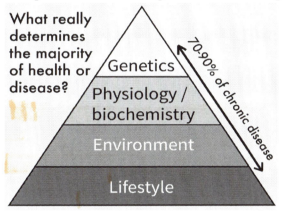

Figure 2: The Health Determination Pyramid

IM practitioners, regardless of their initial specialty training or the healthcare disciplines from which they come, share a philosophy of whole person care. It is important to understand that conventional medicine is based in a reductionist way of looking at things: we seek the source of a problem in the component parts that is comprised of the 'diseased' organ or organ system.

So, for example in cardiovascular disease we look for the 'source' of the myocardial infarction in the arteries of the heart, or more precisely in the walls of those arteries. Or still more precisely, in the various types of lipids that make up the plaques in those arteries. Ultimately, we end up treating MIs by removing or bypassing the vascular obstructions, and then use highly targeted drug therapies that modulate lipid metabolism in the hopes of preventing further plaque formation.

Sometimes it works, but all too often it does not.

The holistic viewpoint looks at a problem in terms of its broader context. Using our cardiovascular example, heart disease is not really a disease of the heart, it is a complex combination of systemic inflammation,

INTRODUCTION

out-of-control stress responses, poor mismatch between diet and genetics, the contributions of a sedentary lifestyle and dysfunctional eating patterns, and psychosocial distress that happen to manifest as an MI in a particular individual.

Many people view the holistic approach as antithetical to or somehow 'against' conventional medicine. This need not be the case. The holistic and the reductionist modes of seeing should ideally balance each other. Using the reductionist mind, we examine Humpty Dumpty's broken bits and pieces; using the holistic mind, we remember that those parts are somehow supposed to fit back together into a beautiful egg-shaped whole.

Rooted in the philosophy of IM are the following principles:

■ **A recognition of the multi-factorial nature of illness.** In assessing patients, IM practitioners take into account macro- and micro-nutrition, the quality of air and water, levels of physical activity and structural harmony, sleep and restorative functions, balance in the energy system, emotional and mental status, stress resilience, and the social and spiritual aspects of a person's life.

■ **A personalized and predictive strategy.** This includes tailoring a patient's health strategy based on a personalized map of health risks accompanied by the measurement of both conventional and novel biomarkers. Examples of novel biomarkers include tests to detect and monitor vascular inflammation, hormonal fluctuations, and levels of potentially toxic substances. Assessment of the genome and the microbiome are increasingly important parts of clinical assessment. While genomic testing may include the identification of single nucleotide polymorphisms (SNPs), the focus is on epigenetics and how genetic expression may be modified by lifestyle.

■ **A balanced patient-physician partnership.** IM physicians take comfort in the fact that they don't need to have all the answers. More of the responsibility for restoring health is shifted to the patients. This changes the practitioner's role from 'care provider' to educator, coach, and trainer. The emphasis shifts from a reactive focus to a proactive one, from illness to wellness, and from disease treatment to functional enhancement. Within this partnership comes the opportunity for transformational education in which both parties–the patient and physician– learn from one another.

■ **The creation of healing communities.** It has long been recognized that cultural support is critical for maintaining any type of healthy behavior change. Healing communities emphasize maintaining patient dignity. They also embrace global traditions of healing. In this context, the physician's office becomes a center of learning, rather than a place for episodic care.

■ **An appreciation for mind-body-spirit connections.** IM places emphasis on mindfulness, the day-to-day, minute-to-minute awareness of thoughts, breathing, and attentiveness to others. Spiritual aspects of health are embraced, along with the recognition that love, gratitude and forgiveness are powerful adjuncts to care.

■ **The use of complementary techniques.** IM practices increasingly incorporate the services of a cadre of professionals from disparate backgrounds, demonstrating a growing recognition that multiple modalities are often necessary to enable the patient to heal herself. These include professionals who perform services such as exercise counseling, massage therapy, chiropractic, naturopathic, classical Chinese medicine, health coaching, meditation training, yoga, energy medicine, cognitive behavioral therapy, and nutrition.

Complementary Medicine on the Rise

Unfortunately, in an effort to assess and track the use of these disparate treatments, government agencies have lumped them together with the term CAM (Complementary and Alternative Medicine). CAM treatments share two criteria: firstly, they are outside the scope of conventional medicine, and secondly, the evidence for their effectiveness has not been well demonstrated. Complementary treatments may precede, coincide with, or occur after appropriate conventional care, and are increasingly viewed by healthcare practitioners and the public as important adjuncts to healing. Controversy arises with inappropriate inclusion of the word, 'alternative' in the CAM designation. IM is not alternative, it combines the best of both conventional and complementary treatments.

The growing popularity of CAM techniques is reinforced by data from the National Health Interview Survey (NHIS) conducted by the National Center for Health Statistics (NCHS), part the Centers for Disease Control and Prevention. The survey is conducted every five years. Most of the available compiled data are from 2007; selected data from 2012 are just being released.

The 2007 NHIS survey revealed that 38 percent of American adults and 12 percent of children had used at least one CAM therapy in the previous 12 months. The top three therapies were 'natural products,' deep breathing and meditation. The 2012 survey reported that the most common complementary health approaches used by Americans were non-vitamin, non-mineral dietary supplements (17.9%), practitioner-based chiropractic or osteopathic manipulation (8.5%), yoga with deep breathing or meditation (8.4%), and massage therapy (6.8%).

Americans use complementary and alternative treatments to care for a variety of ailments such as back pain, arthritis, colds and flu, headaches, elevated lipids, fatigue and mood disorders. It is estimated Americans spent $34 billion on CAM therapies in 2007 (the latest year in which these figures have been reported)—roughly one in every 10 dollars spent out-of-pocket on health care.[11] This amount still pales when measured against the cost of chronic disease.

And while one cannot ignore the business ramifications of CAM, perhaps what is most important—in an era in which quality of care includes meeting and exceeding patient expectations—are how millions of patients are taking a more proactive approach to their own health, bringing a new, alternative and complementary language to their interaction with clinicians.

IM: Making Inroads into the Healthcare System

While CAM has its critics—the most vocal of them being Paul Offit, MD, chief of the infectious diseases division at Children's Hospital of Philadelphia, and author of *Do You Believe in Magic? The Sense and Nonsense of Alternative Medicine* (Harper)—it appears that the tides of skepticism are rapidly receding, in large part due to a growing body of data attesting to the efficacy of IM treatments.

A recent NCBI PubMed query on "evidence-based complementary and alternative medicine" turned up more than 3,400 publications. This, coupled with the recognition of patient expectations around holistic treatment, has moved conventional medicine toward greater adoption of IM approaches.

- The Veterans Administration (VA) is treating soldiers who suffer from posttraumatic stress disorder with therapies such as acupuncture and meditation.[12]
- The American Medical Association (AMA), which represents mainstream physicians, has recognized the popularity of CAM. In 2006, the organization passed a resolution to raise "awareness among medical students and physicians of the wide use of complementary and alternative medicine, including its benefits, risks, and evidence of efficacy or lack thereof."[13]
- The Affordable Care Act has embraced CAM by protecting licensed CAM practitioners from discrimination by insurers and health plans.
- The venerable Cleveland Clinic opened a Chinese Herbal Therapy Clinic, becoming one of the first hospital-based herbal clinics in the U.S. The clinic is designed to "provide supplementary options for patients seeking a holistic, natural approach to their care."[14] They have also just opened a Center for Functional Medicine and recruited noted functional medicine physician Mark Hyman, MD as the director.[15]
- A Department of Defense review of 120 military treatment facilities identified a total of 275 complementary and alternative medicine programs. The most visits were for chiropractic care (73%) with the remaining 27% distributed among acupuncture, clinical nutrition therapy, meditation, yoga, massage, cognitive behavioral therapy, biofeedback, breath-based practices, naturopathic medicine and spiritual prayer based practices. Active duty military members used 213,515 CAM visits in 2012.[16]
- Integrative health techniques are finding their way into corporate America. A pilot stress management program was conducted for 800 employees of Aetna, the third largest insurance company in the United States. The program involved teaching yoga philosophy—how we should treat others and how we should be treated—along with postures, meditation and heart rate variability monitoring. The pilot resulted in a 7.5% decrease in health care costs and 69 minutes more productivity per employee as well as in quality of life improvements. The program has been expanded and now includes 6,000 employees nationwide.[17]

Perhaps the most telling sign of integration is to be found at academic

INTRODUCTION

medical centers, many of which now have IM clinics and substantial integrative medical training for students and residents.

The evolution of programs in IM at the nation's medical schools and residency programs has been fostered in part by The Bravewell Collaborative, an initiative dedicated to promoting a more holistic and humanistic approach to healthcare. Founded by philanthropists Christy Mack and Penny George in 2002, Bravewell's effort spanned more than a decade and produced the first report on how IM is being practiced in clinical centers across the United States.

The report, entitled *Integrative Medicine in America*, presented data on 29 physician-directed centers that were in operation for at least three years, had significant patient volume, and offered both conventional and IM. Data was collected through structured surveys and site visits by the study team. Twenty-five of the twenty-nine centers were affiliated with a medical school. The survey revealed the inclusiveness of different types of practitioners in the healthcare team as shown in Table 1 below.

Percentage of Centers Employing the Following Practitioners Either Full or Part Time			
Practitioner	**Percentage**	**Practitioner**	**Percentage**
Physician	96%	Hypnotherapist	41%
Massage Therapist	86%	Holistic Nurse	38%
Meditation Instructor	83%	Chiropractor	38%
Acupuncturist, Lac	79%	Pain Specialist	34%
MBSR Instructor	79%	Psychiatrist	34%
Dietitian/Nutritionist	69%	Naturopath	28%
TCM Practitioner	62%	Physical Therapist	28%
Yoga Instructor	62%	Exercise Physiologist	24%
Psychologist	59%	Physician Assistant	21%
Healing Touch/Reiki Practitioner	55%	Health Coach	21%
Nurse Practitioner	55%	Osteopath	21%
Acupuncturist, MD	48%	Ayurvedic Practitioner	17%
Biofeedback Practitioner	45%	Homeopathy Practitioner	17%

Table 1: IM Practitioners in Major Teaching Centers.

The study also documented the congruence of treatment algorithms for a handful of conditions—evidence that a best practice methodology and consensus is beginning to develop in key treatment areas. This congruence is shown in Table 2 below.

The Conditions That were Treated the Most Similarly are:	
Heart and Hypertension	.973
Heart and Diabetes	.946
Hypertension and Diabetes	.944
Pre-Op and Post-Op	.939
Fatigue/Sleep and Depression/Anxiety	.938
Stress and Depression/Anxiety	.936
Stress and Fatigue/Sleep	.925

Table 2: Concensus IM Treatments.

"With chronic health issues costing the U.S. economy more than $1 trillion a year, it's essential to find the most effective ways to treat and prevent the most prevalent conditions," said Donald Abrams, MD, co-author of the report and professor of clinical medicine at the University of California, San Francisco.[18] To this end, the centers agreed on the types of chronic conditions for which integrative treatments held the greatest likelihood of improvement. These are shown in Figure 3 below.

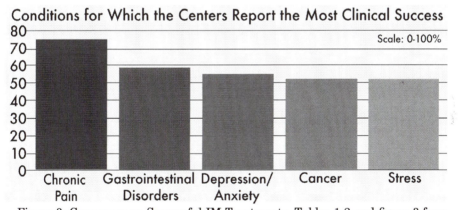

Figure 3: Concensus on Successful IM Treatments. Tables 1-2 and figure 3 from Integrative medicine in America: How integrative medicine is being practiced in clinical centers across the United States. (2012). Encinitas, CA: The Bravewell Collaboration. Reprinted with permission.

On the Path To Wholeness

The path toward IM begins with you. It starts with healing yourself. To paraphrase Gandhi, "You have to be the change you wish to see." You

INTRODUCTION

then incorporate the same principles and practices you have adopted for yourself and apply them to the recommendations and treatments you prescribe for your patients.

The path of becoming an IM doctor involves some hard work and personal investment in the change process. It requires mental flexibility. You embark on this path by challenging your assumptions, examining your perceptions, and clarifying your values and beliefs. You take inventory of your strengths and weaknesses and then you gain clarity by crafting a vision of what is possible. You figure out what you really want to be doing in medicine.

For the grumpy, wounded physician, this is the surest road to self-healing.

In the course of writing this book, we have interviewed nearly one hundred physicians who decided to take this path of deeper and broader engagement. You will find their personal narratives woven throughout the book. We also conducted a survey of the approximately 200 physicians who belong to the American Board of Integrative Holistic Medicine and the American Holistic Medical Association. We asked why and how they made the leap to a more integrated model of care. You will find their responses in Chapter 1.

Going the Non-Clinical Route

For the physician who seeks change, it is also possible to orient personal revision and professional restructuring in another direction, namely outside of clinical practice. You have a high-degree of training with tremendously valuable knowledge and a range of skillsets, some of which you might not even realize you had. In today's world there are ample opportunities for clinicians to parlay their skills and their knowledge into new career options.

If you are involved in a medical practice, you are already a businessperson, whether you recognize that or not. With some focus and skills acquisition, you may be able to move into consulting, or to find positions in industry: pharma, biotech, medical device or natural products. Physician expertise is needed in private equity and venture capital.

You could also pursue the dream of entrepreneurship. This passion is shared by the thousands of members of the Society of Physician

Entrepreneurs (www.sopenet.org), and is a secret flame burning in countless others. The path of the medical entrepreneur can be greatly rewarding if you can navigate the hairpin curves of obtaining financing, recruiting and building a team, anticipating and responding to market and regulatory challenges, and ultimately leading a company to success.

You could apply your medical knowledge to utilization review, independent medical exams, corporate wellness, or become an expert medical witness.

There are many ways to make use of your communication skills outside the clinic: as an author, seminar leader, or keynote speaker. You might even leverage your network of contacts and become a physician recruiter.

You may decide to reenter the healthcare system in a new form as an administrator or a teacher. And if you feel that you have personally mastered the stresses and challenges of medical practice, you could coach and counsel our wounded colleagues.

Or you may decide to write the great American novel, paint or sculpt the next masterpiece, or join a rock band.

There is a bottom line that goes beyond business and is the common denominator to finding happiness in life and work: you have to identify your passion and then have the courage to pursue it with persistence.

How This Book is Organized

In the pages that follow, we will attempt to guide you in identifying your passion. Our recommendations are organized in three sections:

Part One: *Heal Yourself,* begins by examining the phenomenon of physician burnout. We'll help you answer the crucial question: "Should I stay or should I go?" Is it reasonable and feasible to remain in your current practice situation and to implement a few incremental changes? Or, do you need to make a complete break and find a new path? We'll cover models of personal change and provide lessons from physicians who have successfully made transitions, both large and small. We'll also share our own stories of change.

In Part Two: *Heal Your Patients*, we'll revisit IM and its potential to transform both your personal and professional life. We will broadly

INTRODUCTION

describe concepts and modalities from the interconnected disciplines of lifestyle, functional and holistic medicine that can help you better serve your patients. Many of these are skills that you can begin to implement in your current practice; others may require more dedicated resources or significant changes in your practice structure. We'll explore the options on both ends.

In Part Three: *Heal Your Practice*, we'll revisit how physicians have structured their professional lives to find greater satisfaction and fulfillment. We will concentrate on new approaches to attract the types of patients you will most enjoy treating. We will look more closely at private pay options, the important role of physician leadership, and how to create an atmosphere and culture that engenders health and prosperity.

Throughout these sections, this book will guide you through a journey of deepening engagement: with your life, with your patients, and with your work. Above all, we hope it helps you to deepen your engagement with that great mission we've all taken upon ourselves: the mission of healing others. Before we move on, please take a moment and answer our CME question below:

What is Total Engagement?

A. The moment the fetal head or presenting part enters into the upper opening of the female pelvis.

B. An agreement to be married; statistically 80% follow through. [19]

C. Surveys by Gallup indicating degree of motivation to perform work; worldwide, only 13% of employees meet this criterion. [20]

D. A term used to describe alignment in values and incentives between hospitals and physician groups, and the biggest issue facing hospitals that have acquired physician practices.

E. A rekindling of the spirit and the inherent joys in the practice of medicine in which passion is in great evidence, time flies, and meaning and purpose prevail.

PART ONE
HEAL YOURSELF

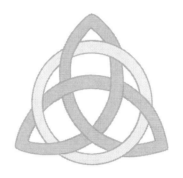

Pain always seems to push us until vision starts to pull us.

—Lee Lipsenthal, MD

1
The Clinician's Chief Complaint

Pain. It is one of the most common chief complaints patients bring to our offices. As a health care practitioner, you are no doubt very familiar with its many manifestations. An entire medical lexicon has been developed to categorize the perception of pain: sharp, dull, throbbing, radiating, made worse with food, movement, pressure? How much pain? Pick a number from 1-10.

But there's more than just physical pain driving the $600 billion spent on pain relief in the US each year.[21] There's psychological distress; the somatization of unease, tension and anxiety. The American Institute of Stress estimates that 60 to 90 percent of all visits to primary care physicians are for complaints and conditions that are related to stress.[22] Each week, 112 million people take some form of medication to ease stress-related symptoms.[23]

Increasingly, as the pressures of practice mount and satisfaction drops, clinicians are finding themselves among the ranks of those seeking relief from this type of pain.

What's behind this growing dissatisfaction among physicians and other healthcare professionals? Feel free to check the issues that apply to you; add others as you see fit:

- The ever-growing mountain of seemingly meaningless work and box-checking
- Continuous aggravations of hospital politics, made worse by the recent uptick in hospitals buying medical practices
- Decreasing reimbursement coupled with increasing labor and operating costs
- The sense that government and other third-parties are increasingly coming between you and your patient, preventing quality care

- An inability to keep up with the burgeoning peer-reviewed literature in your field
- Liability/defensive medicine pressures
- An EHR that literally stands between you and your patients, demands time for data entry, requires frustrating template-generated notes, and lacks interoperability with outside systems
- Serious concerns about income and making ends meet while paying off loans or investing in family and personal needs.

In a recent study of 13,575 US physicians, more than 80% cited 'patient relationships' as the #1 most satisfying part of their jobs, yet this is the aspect that is suffering most under the burdens of healthcare bureaucracy. That's a big part of why an overwhelming majority—77%—reported that they are pessimistic about the future of medicine. Eighty-two percent believe they have little ability to change the healthcare system. More than 84% feel that the medical profession is in decline and nearly 58% were reluctant to recommend medicine as a career to their children.[7]

For the logic-oriented physician, there is a pervasive frustration that things in healthcare just don't make sense. For example:

- Your staff waits on hold for 10 minutes to get a routine precertification for an MRI. 99% of the time it is approved. That's 10 minutes of staff time that could have been utilized attending to patients.
- You have 15 minutes to spend with a patient with metabolic syndrome, mild depression, low back pain and fatigue. You are tired of hearing yourself say, twenty five times a day, "Get more exercise, eat a low-fat diet, lose weight, manage your stress, and take the medications as prescribed."
- You know you can improve your patient-scored quality rating by loosening up on prescriptions for pain medications and antibiotics for viral infections, though you know this is not good medicine.
- In the last days or weeks of a patient's life, family members press you for heroics, to exhaust every option to gain days, or hours, regardless of the quality of that time, or the wishes of the patient.
- Medicare pays more for the identical medical services delivered in a hospital versus a physician office.

- New acronyms crop up each day, none of which are really designed to strengthen the patient-practitioner relationship: DRG, ACO, SGR, PCORI, IPAB, etc.
- Your ongoing fight to collect insurance payment threatens to worsen with an impending change from ICD-9 to ICD-10. This new coding system will increase the number of classifications from the current 13,000 to 68,000! Believe it or not, ICD-10 now includes "V96.03 Balloon collision injuring occupant," "35.XXXA Exposure to volcanic eruption," "W56.21 Bitten by orca," and of course, the very common: "V97.33XD Getting sucked into a jet engine."

Feeling the pressures of burnout, many physicians are throwing in the towel. Over the next one to three years, more than 50% of physicians will cut back on patients seen, will begin work ing part-time, switch to concierge medicine, retire, or take other steps to reduce their workloads.[7]

Without a substantial increase in the number of new physicians, this will, of course, reduce patient access. It is estimated that if these patterns continue, 44,250 full-time-equivalent (FTE) physicians will be lost from the workforce in the next four years. In addition, if the predicted 100,000 physicians transition from practice-owner to employed status over the next four years, there could be 91 million fewer patient encounters.[24]

This comes at a time when the Affordable Care Act could conceivably bring an additional 30 million formerly uninsured patients into the healthcare system.

Those physicians who choose to stay within the status quo models of care need to reconcile themselves with a new reality: fewer doctors having to do even more work. Expect more pain ahead from a system and a process that no longer seems within your control.

Slicing the Salami: The Dwindling Economics of Practice

And then of course, there's the money. If you are one of the dwindling breed of clinicians who is independent and runs a small business, either in partnership or in solo-practice, you cannot help but be affected by sluggish Medicare payment, insurance company constraints, Medicaid payment cuts, and the ever-increasing pressures of managed care. These are the thin cuts of the salami, with each eating away at your livelihood.

The changes that are foisted upon you—and over which you have no control—take money out of your pocket. During a recent meeting, a family physician in a two-doctor practice lamented that she and her partner were only taking home $125,000 each, and that the $80,000 she needed to invest for an EHR would cut significantly into her compensation.

Amitabh Chandra, an economist at Harvard Kennedy School of Government, led a team of researchers in an analysis of twenty years of data related to health care professionals' pay. The study compared how physicians, physician assistants, dentists, nurses, pharmacists, and health and insurance executives have fared over the decade from 2000 to 2010. Chandra showed that physician earnings grew less than those of all the other health professionals. Annual earnings rose significantly for PAs and pharmacists but decreased for physicians.[25]

Many physicians take great umbrage at the enormous jump in health insurance CEO salaries in 2013. Compensation for CEOs at the nine largest insurers ranged from $7 million to $30 million. This occured at a time when physicians were being constantly cut back.[26]

Multiple surveys confirm that the desire for a steady income is the number one reason physicians leave independent practice to join integrated healthcare systems. According to the 2013 MedSynergies Physician-Hospital Alignment Survey other reasons include declining reimbursement, escalating practice expenses, enhanced lifestyle and fear of patient loss from payer's closed networks."[27]

Why Selling Out is No Panacea

Over the last decade, hospitals first focused on acquiring the larger procedure-focused specialty clinics. According to the *Wall Street Journal*, nearly 25% of specialists who saw inpatients are now employed by hospitals. This represents a fivefold increase from the 5% in 2000.[28] Now hospitals are increasingly turning their attention to the acquisition of primary care practices. This has resulted in a near-doubling of hospital-employed primary care physicians over the last ten years.[29]

If you are contemplating the sale of your practice, be forewarned: this course of action may not be the windfall you had hoped for.

Federal regulations constrain hospitals from offering more than fair market value for your practice. The acquisition price usually includes payment for hard assets such as equipment, fixtures, cash, and an allowance for accounts receivables. However, hospitals rarely pay for goodwill unless the physician is a key opinion leader and adds marquee value to the hospital.

Signing bonuses are usually modest and are often designed to cover the tail on malpractice claims. What's more, small practices are often not worth acquiring; the process is too expensive and time-consuming for the hospitals.

While cash in hand and a guarantee of income in the short term may seem attractive, the shifting landscape of healthcare financing will always be beneath your feet. Physicians who sell typically get a 2 to 3 year compensation guarantee that is often tied to previous earnings. After that period they usually have to meet a minimum number of relative value units (RVUs) to maintain their base salaries. Some find themselves unemployed after completing the term of their initial agreements.

Is the grass greener? The data is mixed. Life as an employed physician is fraught with limited autonomy, more paperwork and for the most part, a lower take home pay, all of which contribute to decreased satisfaction.[30] One noted exception is the Permanente Medical Group, which employs more than 6,000 physicians. According to Robert Pearl, MD, executive director and CEO, the majority of Permanente's physicians are happy. Comparing the Permanente Medical Group's physician satisfaction with that of a Harris Interactive report on community medicine, Pearl notes that Permanente physicians score twenty points higher.[31]

Pearl goes on to explain that quality of professional life is as important, perhaps even more so than competitive salaries. Physicians working within Kaiser Permanente have a fair amount of autonomy. There is no insurer standing in the way of the physicians obtaining authorization and approval for testing, procedures, admissions or referrals.

Productivity and Stress Go Hand in Hand

The healthcare environment is one of increasing complexity and change. Similar to any workplace that strives for productivity and efficiencies, healthcare organizations place stress on all healthcare professionals and support staff. This stress is a natural component of work and life.

Hans Selye, MD, the so called father of stress management, noted that when stress enhances an individual's functioning it may be considered eustress, or 'good stress.'[32] High demand environments can generate heightened arousal, which increases attention and focus.[33] This heightened awareness can keep you sharp. However, too much arousal can be problematic.

This relationship between stress and performance was first elucidated by psychologists Robert M. Yerkes and John Dillingham Dodson in 1908. Their curved data plot showed how performance increases with physiological or mental arousal, but only up to a certain point. When levels of arousal, or stress, become too high, performance decreases. A variation of the curve, the Hebbian version (Figure 5), looks at the relationship of the variables in the performance of more complex tasks.[34]

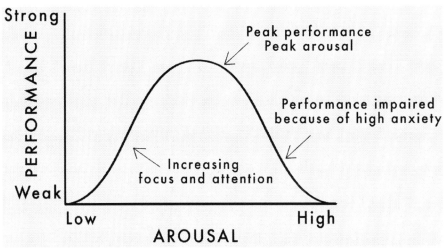

Figure 4: The Hebbian Curve Modified. Diamond, D. M., et. al. (2007). The temporal dynamics model of emotional memory processing: A synthesis on the neurobiological basis of stress-induced amnesia, flashbulb and traumatic memories, and the Yerkes-Dodson law. Neural Plasticity, 2007, 1-33. Reprinted with permission.

In this model, the positive aspects of stress turn into distress, a "process that arises where work demands of various types and combinations exceed the person's capacity and capability to cope."[35] Once you begin to travel down the slope, the powerful manifestations of excess catecholamine and cortisol exert their physiological effects. The cardiovascular and metabolic consequences of unmitigated stress are profound and include the following:

- Coronary vasoconstriction and increased platelet stickiness that promote clot formation.[36]
- Increased homocysteine, CRP and fibrinogen, all of which are associated with increased risk for CHD.[37]
- Deep abdominal fat deposits that secrete inflammatory cytokines that promote insulin resistance and the cardiovascular complications of metabolic syndrome.[38]
- Atrial fibrillation and ventricular fibrillation, the leading cause of sudden death.[39]
- Takotsubo cardiomyopathy, also referred to as "Broken Heart Syndrome."[40]
- Increases in the standard Framingham risk factors (cholesterol levels, smoking, hypertension), as well as diabetes and obesity.[41]
- Precipitating and/or worsening of congestive heart failure.[42]
- Reduced heart rate variability, an accurate and sensitive measure of coronary disease and a powerful predictor of sudden death.[43]
- Decreased resistance to infections that can incite inflammation and destabilize arterial plaques.[44]
- Increased incidence of myocardial infarction in the absence of significant atherosclerosis.[45]

For physicians, there's another important variable that impacts the stress-performance relationship; it is known as compassion fatigue. It was first defined as "deep physical, emotional and spiritual exhaustion that can result from working day-to-day in a caregiving environment."[46] Another term for compassion fatigue is burnout, a mental state that can be assessed with the widely used Maslach Burnout Inventory (MBI). The MBI evaluates three variables:

- Emotional exhaustion: losing enthusiasm for work.
- Depersonalization: treating people as if they were objects.
- Low personal accomplishment: having the sense that work is no longer meaningful.

A 2012 Mayo Clinic/AMA survey of 7,288 physicians indicated that nearly half of US physicians report at least one symptom of burnout.[47] According to the survey:

- 45.8% of doctors experienced at least one symptom of work-related burnout.
- 37.9% had high emotional exhaustion.
- 29.4% had high depersonalization.
- 12.4% had a low sense of personal accomplishment.

The conclusion of the survey was that U.S. doctors are burning out "at an alarming level," with primary care physicians being particularly vulnerable.

The disparate toll that burnout is exacting on primary care physicians is not unique to those practicing in the United Sates. A survey of 564 general practitioners in Essex, England revealed that 46% had high levels of emotional exhaustion, 42% had depersonalization characteristics, and 32% had low levels of personal accomplishment. An aging population that demands more medical care is fueling the flames of burnout.[48]

There is ample evidence that common sequelae of burnout such as depression, suicide, and substance abuse disorders are more prevalent among physicians than the general population.[49] Each year 400 physicians commit suicide.[50] One study reported that 9.4 percent of fourth-year medical students and first-year residents have entertained suicidal thoughts.[51] Female physicians have a two-fold greater suicide rate over the general population.[52] In addition to the personal health consequences of stress, physician fatigue can also diminish the quality of care, compromise patient safety and treatment outcomes, reduce patient satisfaction, erode staff morale, and increase nurse turnover.

The stresses on physicians engender negative emotions that impact health. The role of psychological factors and their contribution to CAD has been well elucidated. Emotions such as anger, hostility, cynicism, distrust, anxiety and depression are all linked to CAD.[53]

Negative emotions such as fear, anxiety, anger and sadness affect our immune system and ability to fight infections. In one study, researchers measured salivary IgA levels after students watched an emotionally charged film on Mother Teresa's activity ministering to the sick and poor. Salivary IgA increased in 92% of the subjects, and decreased in 8%. The students were then shown a photo of a couple on a park bench and were asked to write a story about the couple. The students whose stories showed themes of distrust, manipulation or abandonment had lower IgA responses to the Mother Teresa film. Those same students had had significantly more illness during the previous year.[54] Negative emotions also narrow our perception. They prevent us from seeing the big picture and gaining perspective on what is taking place in our lives.[55]

Fear Based Training

Danielle Ofri, MD, PhD, author of *What Doctors Feel* (Beacon Press) traces the behavioral roots of physician distress back to medical school and the early training. She believes it is, "the natural outcome of putting smart, competitive perfectionistic people in a high stress system with myriads of ever-changing tasks for which they feel responsibility, coupled with sleep deprivation and the granite-hard fact of only twenty-four hours in a day."[56] Ofri makes the case that medical school and residency training rob us of empathy and encourage desensitization. This is evidenced by the culture of medical slang, which on the surface may appear merely callous, but in actuality, derives from fear. She writes:

> "Some of the states in which our patients live—or die—are downright terrifying. To empathize with these patients, to put yourself in their shoes, may be a bit too existentially disconcerting. And so doctors unconsciously try to protect themselves by widening the moat between their own good health and their patients' dauntingly mortal conditions. Hence an elderly, demented, incontinent, babbling patient from a nursing home is a 'gomer' or is 'gorked out'. A dying patient is 'circling the drain.'"[56]

It is the rare physician who makes it through training without stigmatizing patients in an effort to gain distance from disease and death, or to fit in better with colleagues. Many of us can vividly recall moments of humiliation or embarrassment suffered in the process of 'pimping,' the commonly employed pedagogical style whereby attending physicians or senior residents ask junior colleagues a series of probing questions. Some argue that these highly charged emotive states promote learning. To this day, each of us can vividly recall these incidents.[57, 58] Collectively these experiences may impart information we will never forget, but they also contribute to the erosion of humanism in medicine.

It is reasonable to wonder whether this fear becomes ingrained in the white coat that was designed to set us apart from our patients, and whether fear still remains as a major driver behind physician distress. To maintain homeostasis in the face of a stressor—either real or perceived—the body activates a complex range of endocrine, nervous and immune reactions, which Selye described as the General Adaptation System.[59] He noted three stages: an alarm stage, a resistance stage and an exhaustion stage characterized by different physiological reactions. Selye was among the first to describe how the stress response is mediated by the hypothalamic-pituitary-adrenal (HPA) axis.

The HPA establishes the well recognized fight or flight response characterized by enhanced alertness, increased cardiovascular tone and respiration rate, shunting of blood from the gut to the muscles, and bracing of the neck with elevation of the shoulder muscles. The HPA is regulated by corticotropin releasing factor (CRF), which initiates the cascade of events that result in a glucocorticoid response from the adrenals. Among the initiators of HPA stimulation is the limbic system, the reptilian brain that houses the primal emotion of fear.

Chronic stress can cause constant cortisol exposure that can trigger the accumulation of body fat,[60] exacerbate complications of type 2 diabetes,[61] trigger depression in patients with COPD,[62] and alter immune function.[63]

Fear and all its many variants—anxiety, defensiveness, dismissiveness, etc—is pervasive in medical training and medical culture. It is amplified by the economic pressures of today's healthcare environment and by the constant threat of lawsuits. We know that physiologically it can be highly detrimental to us as practitioners, and it is none-too-healthy for the patients we treat.

Bouncing Back from Burnout

No one single factor 'causes' burnout. The stresses of life and work, the negative emotions that we create, the lack of introspection and inability to focus on the bigger picture of happiness, all combine to rob our energy and health. All of us know previously joyful colleagues who have been brought down by the demands of the profession; some of us have experienced this personally.

The good news is, none of this is inevitable or irreversible. As illustrated in the story below, the sequelae of unmitigated stress can be surmounted by introspection and a willingness to change.

By training, Romila Mushtaq, MD, or Romie as she prefers, is a neurologist who completed her residency at The Medical University of South Carolina, a neurophysiology fellowship at University of Pittsburgh Medical Center and an epilepsy fellowship at the University of Michigan. Mushtaq was passionate about and primed for a career in academic medicine until burnout took its toll on her health.

> "I was sleep deprived for almost 15 years of my career. I never went a complete week without being woken up in the middle of the night. The sleep deprivation began very early on in my neurology residency training and, looking back, I can see that it was crippling me. This was in 1999, before we had the data we have today about how sleep deprivation affects memory, mood and physical health. As a woman I was already a minority and when lack of sleep started to change my personality, I really internalized it and started to feel like a failure.
>
> We are taught that we are soldiers in the war of medicine and that you are a failure if you can't move forward. So, as a practicing academic neurologist, I stuck it out. Between the sleep deprivation and carbohydrate cravings, in a four-year period I gained 30 pounds. I was unhappy and not in shape.
>
> My wake up call came when I started to have severe chest pains initially diagnosed as reflux. I was put on proton pump inhibitors for several years without much relief. My pain continued to progress. I was not only waking up in the middle of the night because of my pager going off, but I was also waking up choking on my own vomit and saliva. As a 35 year old, I was getting frequent pneumonia. Finally I was diagnosed with achalasia and by this time, my condition was so severe, I needed urgent surgery.
>
> When we are trying to get off the hamster wheel, many of us think 'Oh, if we just change the scenery, we'll get better.' So I left academic medicine and went into community medicine. But I found that while the stressors were different, the demands on my time were the same. I had already gone through surgery and I found myself in the same patterns of

60, 80, 100 hour work weeks. The chest pains began again. I knew that a repeat surgery for my condition would likely end in permanent disability.

This time around I finally got it: The thing that had to change was me. So I took a sabbatical, a year to find out who I was and what I wanted to do. I rekindled a joy in practicing yoga and meditation. I used to think it was a hobby until I went into my initial surgery. I noticed that when I was meditating or practicing yoga my sadness would dispel and I would actually feel happy. During these times, my chest pain would go away and for several hours afterwards I was chest pain-free and not vomiting.

I also reconnected to my childhood dream, which was my love of speaking and writing. Growing up in Danville, Illinois, my middle school English teacher transformed my love of sharing stories into knowledge of public speaking. I won my first state speech competition in the 7th grade, and by high school the speech team was my after-school sport. I realized that, throughout my entire medical career, I derived enjoyment from speaking to large audiences—both doctors and patients. If I was meant to survive what I survived, then speaking and writing had to be part of my mission. I made this transition into the world of being a physician entrepreneur."

Today, Mushtaq spends three-quarters of her time working with patients one-on-one on mind-body medicine teaching mindfulness techniques to heal from stress-based illnesses such as insomnia, headaches, anxiety and depression. The other quarter of her time is spent conducting seminars and workshops for consumers and corporations, all the while making certain to get seven to eight hours of sleep a night.

When Life Gangs Up On Us

In the mid-sixties, Thomas Holmes, MD, and Richard Rahe, MD, of the University of Washington School of Medicine attempted to quantify the effect of life changes, both good and bad, on our health. They developed the Social Readjustment Rating Scale (SRE), which assigned impact points to forty-three life events. Big events such as the "death of a spouse" received 100 points, divorce, 73, marital separation, 65. Smaller events such as "trouble with boss" were assigned 23 points, "change to a different line of work."[64]

Interestingly, the original scales only measured socially acceptable traumas and did not include other traumatic events such rape, sexual affairs, or involvement in actions that caused the death of another person.[65] The SRE also did not take into account the typical stresses of the 'sandwich generation' in which individuals care for both older parents and younger children.

Glynis Ablon, MD, a 48-year old dermatologist in Manhattan Beach, has her practice life working for her. A solo dermatologist and Associate Clinical Professor at UCLA, she has practiced aesthetics and general dermatology for 18 years in the affluent community of Manhattan Beach, California. She has control over the nature and pace of her work, and takes great pride in her hands-on approach to beauty.

Ablon's life situation, on the other hand, attests to the validity of the Holmes Rahe scale, showing how cumulative life stressors can predispose anyone to illness.

In addition to being a single mother of two children, 12 and 18, Ablon is also the primary caretaker for her elderly parents, a happily married couple for 60 years, who live 5 minutes from her. With three generations almost under the same roof, meeting everyone's needs is a juggling act, which, Ablon usually handled well—until her mother came down with bacterial meningitis and was hospitalized for 11 days in the ICU in a coma.

For those eleven days, Ablon lived in the chair by her mother's side, bathing her, turning her, and telling her that she needed to fight and that those who loved her needed her. While at her mother's bedside, she functioned both as a supportive daughter and an overseeing physician-advocate, all the while reassuring her father and younger sister, and even having to choose her DNR status. In fact, Ablon had to forgo her practice until the miraculous moment when her mother woke up—just as her children and her sister's children came to say goodbye.

Her mother recovered and came home, and for a little while things returned to normal. But the respite was short-lived. Her mother went on to have a perforated bowel, sepsis, aspiration pneumonia, and surgical replacement for a broken hip.

CHAPTER ONE

It was when her mother was finally stabilized that Ablon woke up with a weird sensation around her mouth and terrible piercing ear pain. She jumped to the mirror and found she couldn't move the entire right side of her face, including closing her eye, and since "even my forehead didn't move, I knew it was Bell's palsy and not a stroke. That was the only good part!" All through the Bell's palsy, Ablon continued to see patients, although on one occasion her condition did affect her relationship with a patient. "I recommended neuromodulators for this one woman to address her facial wrinkles only to have her pause and comment, 'That's okay, I just don't want to come out looking like you,'" said Ablon. Fortunately after four weeks time, the palsy remitted without sequelae.

The Bell's palsy episode provided the impetus for Ablon to step back and reconsider her philosophy on life, stress, and the pursuit of beauty. Her synthesis can be found in a consumer book entitled *What's Stressing Your Face?* (Basic Health Publications, Inc.) to be released spring 2015.

Research is continuing to document how the stressors of life are affecting both quality and longevity of life. Work done by Elissa Epel, PhD, at the University of California, San Francisco sheds much light on the ways in which stress adversely affects caregivers' health. Epel's 2004 study examined telomere length in women who cared for critically ill children versus controls. Telomere length is a measure of cellular aging; shorter telomeres are indicative of increased cellular turnover and decreased longevity. The leukocyte telomeres in the caregiver group were shorter than those in controls, the length discrepancy equating to at least one decade of additional aging as compared to the lower stress group.[66]

In a subsequent study, Epel, along with her colleague Nobel Prize winner Elizabeth Blackburn, PhD, examined twenty-three post-menopausal women divided into a group who cared for partners with dementia versus age- and BMI-matched non-caregivers. The researchers collected salivary cortisol samples at waking, 30 min after waking, and bedtime, and a 12-hour overnight urine collection. All of the women were subjected to the modified Trier Social Stress Test[67] consisting of four 5-minute stressful periods, that included having to prepare and give a speech and have it videotaped while addressing two evaluative, non-responsive audience members. Those with greater cortisol responses to the acute stressor had shorter telomeres.[68]

Stress underlies much of the illness we see in our patients, and if we count ourselves among their ranks, in ourselves as well. The warning messages are easy to recognize: physical signs and symptoms, negative thoughts and feelings, and altered behaviors. It is all too common for physicians to unconsciously eat the high glycemic index foods that are ubiquitous in the healthcare setting, to forgo exercise for alcoholic beverages, or to spend inordinate time with colleagues grousing about the state of medicine. It is too easy to lose our inner focus on health. Even when we seem to have our work life in relative balance, as we see in Ablon's case, stressors can come from out of left field.

The physician's chief complaint requires a work up. Diagnostics include an examination of the quantity and magnitude of your stressors and whether you can affect them, modify them, or prevent them from affecting you. Physical findings will reveal the extent to which stress is impacting your thoughts, emotions, behaviors and altering your physiology. 'Imaging studies' consist of a healthy dose of introspection. Ultimately, you can determine whether an operative procedure on your lifestyle and/or your workstyle is required.

The Drivers of Change

Physicians make changes in their lives and their practice patterns for many reasons. The greatest drivers of change are often the most deeply personal. In our survey of 3,000 physician members of the American Board of Integrative Holistic Medicine and the American Holistic Medical Association, the most common reason physicians provided for either including integrative techniques into their conventional practices, or leaving conventional practice structures was personal interest in the emerging field of IM.

This is a healthy sign! Physicians and other healthcare professionals should never lose our inherent curiosity in the processes of healing, and the fascinating ways in which the human body works. Ideally, this curiosity coupled with the desire to expand our knowledge and our skills, and the wish to help others should be driving our personal and professional decisions.

That said, the desire to mitigate stressors also played a prominent role in respondents' transformations. Dissatisfaction with conventional practice, personal burn out, health problems, and lack of time for family or things of personal importance were also important drivers of change.

CHAPTER ONE

Roughly one quarter of the respondents cited a personal or family health crisis that pushed them up against the limitations of conventional medicine. The survey question results are shown below.

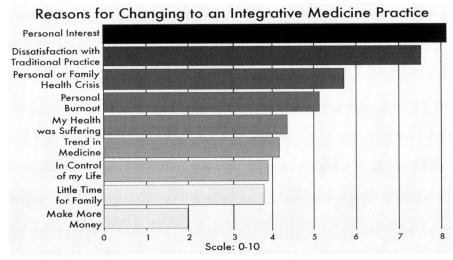

Figure 5: ABIHM/AHMA 2014 Practice Satisfaction Survey

Equally revealing were the online answers to the open-ended invitation to briefly describe their reasons for change. Here are a few examples:

> "Increasingly frustrated with the fragmentation of medicine and the erosion of my interaction with patients across the continuum of care (loss of local ER and hospital, new management focused on RVU's and "payor-centered care" rather than patient-centered care), I have found new ways to connect with patients. Integrative techniques (of which I am a master of none but a student of many -- functional medicine, nutritional medicine, herbology, biofeedback) offer an additional toolbox for approaching patient care, particularly chronic care, which is increasingly the domain of outpatient primary care. I weary of worshiping the false gods of so called quality metrics and seek healing relationships that honor patient autonomy while offering education and patient empowerment. I feel I am still very near the beginning of my journey but it is one of the few aspects of modern medicine that gives me hope for myself and for humanity."

> "Dissatisfaction with being a glorified secretary. The ill-to-pill approach. Probably had postpartum depression 2 to burn out. Spirituality,

yoga, mind-body medicine interest me. Found deep satisfaction in practicing them. Better patient relationship. Took a life long commitment to learn more and manage stress in my own life and give tools for patients. Chronic stress is Number one health risk. This realization was very important and actually took lot of time to learn."

"Family medicine was much more frustrating than I'd ever dreamed; patients wanted to get better, but not take pills, and diet and exercise were difficult to sell. A large chunk of patients had ill-defined symptoms that conventional medicine had no way to address or evaluate. I was at a conference and a speaker got up and mentioned alternative medicine. I had enjoyed her presentation up to that point, but then I turned my brain off and wrote her off as a crackpot. She then gave the most interesting example and evidence to back it up, and I thought, "Maybe I don't know everything I think I know." I decided to research alternative medicine, but I was torn as I didn't want to let go of the good things in conventional medicine. I stumbled across the Scripps conference and ended up having a long talk with my husband about switching gears and learning more about this. We attended the conference, and I felt like I had a whole new way to look at a patient. Going to that first conference was probably the best thing I've ever done in my professional life. My patient's satisfaction grew, I felt fully present in patient interviews for the first time in years. I had a whole new set of tools to use for those vague, ill-treatable symptoms. Patients re-engaged, I re-engaged, and life got so much better...a large portion of my new patients are expressing interest in integrative modalities when they find I don't shudder when they mention fish oil. I keep hearing "I'm so glad you listened to me/don't think it's in my head/aren't putting me on another pill." The public is starving for this approach. My biggest issue now is getting specialists within my very large group to meet with me long enough for me to show them I'm not a crazy crackpot, which is a surprisingly hard challenge."

"Gradual disillusionment with not having med school or residency training in appropriate skills to be responsive to patient with acute and chronic pain, weight gain, depression and mood issues, work stress, and innumerable issues affecting their well-being."

CHAPTER ONE

"I was a conventional pediatrician who developed FM and IBS. I was referred to an acupuncturist by a massage therapist and that visit changed my life. I realized that there were things I had not learned in medical school, so I started to study and learn to help myself and others. I was finally able to leave conventional pediatrics, move to another state, and start practicing with an integrated dentist and other holistic practitioners. It wasn't easy at first, and I took many trainings including a Naturopathic M.D. degree and learned various techniques including Autonomic Response Testing. I incorporate various energy healing modalities as well as Homeopathic drainage remedies, supplements, probiotics, etc."

"I've always been interested in alternative and complementary medicine. I became jaded in med school when I realized that the hospital is a place where we try to make people well. Yet, it's one of the sickest places to be, and the very people taking care of the sick were ironically part of an institution that did not seem to promote well-being or health. I came to realize that there is so much more to health than what we are taught in med school and residency, and there is so much more we can do for patients. I feel that though conventional medicine has its place, it can be limited and short-sighted. It seems to further the cycle of victimizing the patient and taking away hope. I decided that I want to empower others in a deeper way to health and well-being. Practicing integrative medicine has allowed me to practice in the spirit that aligns with my philosophy. Through it, I've found a community of like-minded individuals who are trying to change the current system. I am currently transitioning to practice more as an integrative health coach, rather than a physician, so that I can help others along their journey as well."

--Hansie Wong, MD

There is a common theme in these personal narratives: these clinicians chose the path of Integrative Medicine. But there are many other choices and options for change. Whatever direction you ultimately choose, self-diagnosis is the first step. Begin by identifying your present pain and observing the ways in which it is causing you to be detached from your passion and how chronic stress is affecting your health.

Ask yourself whether you can spend another five, ten, fifteen, or twenty years going down the road you are now traveling. Then see if you can decipher what combination of attitudes, thoughts, and behaviors can help you relieve your stress, remove your pain, revitalize your practice and ultimately make you happier.

Take inventory of your personal health and resilience by asking yourself some key questions:

- What specifically do I love most about my current practice?
- What do I most dislike about my practice?
- What would I like more of in my professional life?
- What do I need more of in my personal life?
- What's my chief complaint?
- As I look at how I respond to stress and change, what patterns emerge?
- Which of the stressors are controllable? Which do I need to just accept?
- How resilient would I be in the face of a sudden, unexpected stressor? (in other words, how close is my camel's back from breaking?)

Now that we have covered the first half of Lipsenthal's driving forces for change—pain, let's turn to the second component—vision. In this case, a vision built upon happiness.

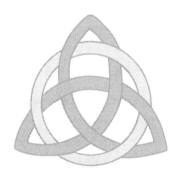

In many shamanic societies, if you came to a medicine person complaining of being disheatened, dispirited or depressed, they would ask one of four questions. When did you stop dancing? When did you stop singing? When did you stop being enchanted by stories? When did you stop finding comfort in the sweet territory of silence?

— Gabrielle Roth

2
Physician Happy Thyself

Just as the Maslach Burnout Inventory identifies the three dimensions of burnout, psychologists use three opposite dimensions to define happiness: frequent positive affect, high life satisfaction, and infrequent negative affect. These elements provide a measure of subjective well-being.[69]

Crossing the great divide from burnout to better and from grumpy to great can be done. It does, however, require the stepping-stones of positive affect and satisfaction that line the path to happiness. We'll be discussing these two elements, and the skills needed to achieve them in this chapter.

There's a lot to recommend about happiness! It has multiple benefits, among them:

- Social rewards: higher likelihood of marriage and lower rate of divorce, more friends, stronger social support, and richer social interactions[69]
- Superior work outcomes: greater creativity, increased productivity, higher quality of work, and higher income[70]
- More activity, energy, and flow[71]
- Greater self-control, self-regulatory and coping abilities[72]
- Enhanced immune system[73]
- Longevity[74]
- More cooperative, pro-social, charitable, and other-centered activity[75]

What is happiness? Where does it come from? How do I get more of it? To understand happiness, it is important to separate it from the pursuit of wealth and material possessions. In fact, just because people are wealthy, it does not mean they are happy. Having great wealth does not guarantee that people have health-promoting belief systems, strong values, or positive relationships.

CHAPTER TWO

In completing her doctorate in social psychology, Elizabeth Dunn, PhD, co-author (with Michael Dunn) of *Happy Money: the Science of Smarter Spending* (Simon & Schuster), surveyed the literature on the relationship between money and happiness. Dunn found that the approximately 17,000 articles pointed to one conclusion: additional income, beyond a certain point, provides surprisingly little happiness. This correlation runs counter to most Americans' belief system, namely that more money equates to more happiness.

A national survey of Americans tested people's belief that, if their income were doubled, from $25,000 to $55,000, happiness would be doubled as well. The data revealed that those people making $55,000 per year were only nine percent more satisfied with their lives than those making $25,000 per year. Yet most Americans still believe that winning the lottery will miraculously transform their lives for the better.[76]

Studies of people who have won lotteries reveal that, after the initial elation settles down, winners are no happier than a control group of average people. Any gains in happiness are fleeting because people adapt so quickly to change and the once-novel pleasures become the expected norm and previous pleasures seem dull by comparison.[77] Many lottery winners lose much of the joy that they once got from small daily pleasures. They also don't keep their wealth. A Florida study showed that the bankruptcy rate for lottery winners is twice that of the general population.[78]

Psychologist Dan Baker, PhD, has been studying the art and science of happiness for three decades. Baker has authored a series of books on what happy people—and happy companies—know. When he counseled financially successful guests at the Life Enhancement Center at Canyon Ranch Health Resort in Tucson, he observed that private planes, expensive cars, fancy clothes, and jewelry cannot fill a sense of personal emptiness, or address the primal fear that resides inside all of us.

According to Baker, the yearning for money comes from an innate sense of scarcity. It is fear hardwired into our neural circuitry, part of the reptilian brainstem whose critical job was to always be on alert for predators. This is the center of the brain responsible for the classic fight or flight syndrome. Because in our minds money is inextricably linked to survival, many people have a nagging sense that there will never be enough of it.

Learning happiness skills can help stave off two hardwired fears that humans face: the fear of not having enough and the fear of not being enough.

The search for happiness begins by understanding the architecture behind it. Research has shown that 50% of happiness relates to genetics. Our genes determine a certain range or set point in happiness level. "The set point likely reflects relatively immutable intrapersonal, temperamental, and affective personality traits, such as extraversion, arousability, and negative affectivity, that are rooted in neurobiology."[79]

Life events and circumstances together account for another 10% of the happiness equation: income, health, religion, status and job security, traumatic life events. That leaves approximately 40% within individual control that can be influenced by intentional physical activities, habits, attitudes, practices, and presence.

Intentional activities are discrete actions or practices that are undertaken voluntarily and that require some degree of effort. For the physician who wants to be happier, it takes effort to act on the demanding circumstances of medical practice, and to develop intentional habits to sustain well-being. The following story sheds light on both.

Edward (Lev) Linkner, MD, ABIHM, is an internist and family medicine practitioner in solo practice in Ann Arbor, Michigan. Linkner has been taking care of patients in the same town for 37 years and has a lot of older patients in his practice. He accepts Medicare, Blue Cross PPO, Visa and Mastercard. He keeps his prices low. If his patients want to use their insurance, and their HMO doctor needs to submit a blood test, he writes a letter to the HMO physician.

He has practiced holistic medicine since he began his practice, and has integrated a wide variety of holistic techniques so that, "I could have a bigger toolbox to serve people, things like herbs, homeopathy, talk therapy and lifestyle counseling."

Twenty-six years ago he founded a holistic center in two large Victorian houses that he literally moved to their present location. In addition to a very busy practice, Linker admits that his "life is chaos with five kids (2 at home) and twin 6 year old grandkids living at home. After a day at the office, the first thing I hear is, 'Papa, let's shoot some hoops…(or do something).'"

CHAPTER TWO

Linkner's philosophy of care is quite straightforward.

> "If you are sick, you are seen. I'm on call 24/7. People have my email, my pager; they know where I live, and I do not get abused at all. Now, if I did get abused, I would tell the patient that this is doctor abuse and encourage them to see someone else."

Linkner handles the challenges of work and life not merely by controlling his schedule, but by making sure his schedule doesn't control him: he includes time for gratitude, for personal fitness, and for wellness into his own routine. Mental and physical health is a natural consequence of the day's routine. As he explains it:

> "I wake up each morning without an alarm around five am. When I wake up is when I do my gratitude practice. I think about all that I am grateful for and focus in on my family, friends, teachers and others. Sometimes it's longer, sometimes shorter. I then go to the gym and work out for an hour and a half. Many of my patients see me there every morning. By the time I get to work and start my day I'm feeling so high. I have a very busy morning. During my lunch break, I take off time to get out in nature. Until most recently, I was accompanied by my dog Laylah. I usually meditate when I return, and then have a full and exciting afternoon schedule. I live a pretty happy lifestyle. I believe that unconditional love is the biggest healer. I try to focus on compassion, reflection and growth. I just feel that I am a health warrior with loving and positive intention helping to serve others. And that's how I do it every day, and it is a blast!"

What Makes People Happy?

Is Linkner's glass half empty, half full, or is it overflowing? The answer always lies in one's personal perspective, a viewpoint that is shaped by attitudes and emotions. In dealing with stressed-out colleagues and patients, one of our favorite maxims is that "you move toward and become like that which you think about."

If we were to hook a 'thought recorder' up to your brain and obtain a 24 hour printout of your self-dialog, what would it reveal about your inner mental health? Would it be filled with positive emotions such as love, gratitude, forgiveness, joy, and acceptance? Or would the self-destructive emotions of anger, hostility, and cynical distrust predominate?

The positive emotions listed above have been shown to increase longevity,[74] reduce morbidity,[80] increase cognitive flexibility,[81] improve memory,[82] improve decision making,[83] increase creativity and innovative problem solving,[84] improve job performance and achievement[85] and lead to better clinical problem-solving.[86]

While we cannot control many of the stressors in our lives, each of us is always in control of our responses and our emotional perceptions. Medicine affords many of us the daily opportunity to reframe how we look at and interpret situations.

One of our medical colleagues shared an insightful moment with us. During her surgical residency she was on the tail end of a grueling 20-hour day in which she had been on her feet for all but a few minutes. She was complaining to one of the other house staff within earshot of a spinal cord injury patient, who turned to her and remarked, "What I wouldn't give to have your day!"

This story serves as a sharp reminder that the perspective you hold on almost any situation is just one of the many possible perspectives available to you. For those who choose to be happy, adopting the practice of gratitude will always yield a full glass.

Among the researchers who have shaped the science of gratitude are psychologists Robert Emmons, PhD, of the University of California, Davis, and Michael E. McCullough, PhD, of the University of Miami. In one study, they asked three groups of participants to write a few sentences each week.

One group was asked to write about occurrences for which they felt grateful. A second group was instructed to write about daily irritations or things that had displeased them. A third group was instructed to write about neutral events. At the end of 10 weeks, participants who wrote about gratitude were more optimistic and felt better about their lives. To the researchers' surprise the optimistic group exercised more and had fewer medical visits when compared to participants who focused on aggravating events.

But the true power of gratitude really lies in expressing positive feelings to others. This was demonstrated in a study conducted by University of Pennsylvania researcher Martin Seligman, PhD, who popularized the field of positive psychology almost twenty-five years ago. In one of his experiments, Seligman instructed a group to write and personally deliver letters of gratitude to people the participant felt had never been properly thanked for extending a kindness. These thankful participants experienced a significant increase in their happiness scores, with the positive feelings lasting for a month.

The positive effects of gratitude, experienced by both giver and recipient have been found to strengthen relationships both at home and at work. Gratitude helps to reset perspective by refocusing on what individuals have instead of what they are missing. Gratitude can be expressed in quiet ways such as taking a few moments each day to mentally thank someone, to pray for others, or to reflect upon the people who are special in your life. Or it could be more demonstrable: you could write a note of gratitude or keep a journal, each day jotting down the few things that you are grateful for.

One of the most practical and near-at-hand techniques was suggested by Atlanta based oculoplastic surgeon Starla Fitch, MD, creator of lovemedicineagain.com.

Inspired by one of her schoolteacher patients who had adopted the habit of saving notes of acknowledgment from students, parents and administrators, and reviewing them at semester's end, Fitch adopted the practice of saving similar treasures in the bottom right desk drawer.

> "When I get an email from an overwhelmed surgical resident, thanking me for the lifeline one of my blog posts has given her, it goes in the drawer. When one of the doctors I'm coaching has an 'aha moment' and brims with new inspired zest for their practice, a note of that conversation goes in the drawer. When one of my patients reminds me of why I went to medical school, it goes in the drawer."

She encourages physicians to "Pick a drawer. A basket. A box, and to get started right away," she comments. The contents of the drawer can be accessed anytime you need to pause, reflect, and reconnect with meaning and purpose. These messages of gratitude also help to generate some seriously needed self-acknowledgment, "the realization how special you truly are to the world of medicine."

Regain Control of Your Autonomic System

"The great thing then, in all education, is to make our nervous system our ally as opposed to our enemy."

--William James

In and of itself, the process of reflection and gratitude has been shown to stimulate the parasympathetic nervous system reducing the physiological effects of the fight or flight response.[87] Most recently, researchers have found that pairing the gratitude practice with deep rhythmic breathing increases heart rate variability (HRV) and can have synergistic effects on stress control. A calm and centered nervous system is a prerequisite for happiness.

HRV is a measurement of the variation in the cardiac beat-to-beat interval. HRV is related to emotional arousal. As such, heart rate variability is a key indicator of autonomic function. HRV decreases with age. Low HRV correlates to higher cardiac risk. Conversely high HRV indicates lower cardiac risk. Low HRV has been shown to be predictive of myocardial infarct and sudden death.[88] In another study that measured the HRV of 14,672 men and women over a two-year period, low HRV was a strong predictor of CHD and mortality.[89]

Emotional strain, elevated anxiety, daily worries and frustrations all decrease HRV.[90] Positive emotions like love, gratitude, mutual caring and connectedness all increase HRV. This is shown in Figure 6 below.

HRV can be affected by increasing vagal tone through deep and regular breathing. The normal effects of respiratory sinus arrhythmia are readily observable as the heart rate increases with vagal nerve suppression during inhalation, and decreases with the return of parasympathetic tone during exhalation. Many relaxation and stress reduction techniques are based on the parasympathetic enhancing power of deep rhythmic breathing.

Techniques and easy-to-use tracking devices developed by HeartMath LLC based on their emWave technology, have made HRV assessment a highly effective and easily accessive therapeutic tool.

CHAPTER TWO

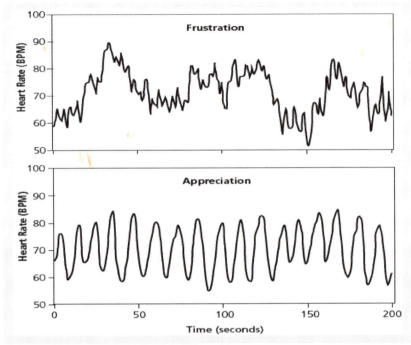

Figure 6: Emotions are reflected in heart rhythm patterns. The heart rhythm patterns shown in the top graph, characterized by its erratic, irregular pattern (incoherence) is typical of negative emotions such as anger or frustration. The bottom graph shows an example of the coherent heart rhythm pattern that is typically observed when an individual is experiencing sustained, modulated positive emotions—in this case, appreciation. Both recordings are from the same individual only a couple of minutes apart. The amount of variability and mean heart rate are the same in both examples, illustrating how the pattern of activity contains information in the absence of changes in physiological activation. McCraty, R. & Zayas, M. (2014). Intuitive intelligence, self-regulation, and lifting consciousness. Global Advances in Health and Medicine, 3(2), 56-65. Reprinted with permission.

Established in 1991, HeartMath's mission is to, "help people bring their physical, mental and emotional systems into balanced alignment with their heart's intuitive guidance." The company offers "effective and scalable methods and technologies to help people self-regulate emotions and behaviors." In addition to devices, HeartMath offers training programs for clinicians based on the powerful effects of coherence on the human body.

When scientists use the term coherence, they are often referring to cross-coherence: two systems vibrating at a coupled frequency. By synching regular breathing with a focus on positive emotions, both the brain and the heart work together to create the calm, focused, intuitive state—coherence—that is central to happiness.

The relationship between the central nervous system and the heart has traditionally been viewed as unidirectional, with the autonomic system exerting complete control over heart rate. However, recent research is showing that the heart is actually in a constant two-way dialog with the brain.

The heart has its own complex nervous system known as the "heart brain." First described by in 1996 by David C. Randall, PhD, a professor at the Department of Physiology, University of Kentucky College of Medicine, it involves interactions between the neurons located in the right atrial ganglionated plexus, an area of the heart that was previously called the pulmonary vein fat pad.

"These 'intrinsic cardiac ganglia' include neuronal types (e.g. sensory and interneurons) other than classic parasympathetic neurites so that the potential exists for intracardiac reflex control of the heart's function."[91] We know that heart-generated signals especially affect the brain centers involved in strategic thinking, reaction times, social awareness and the ability to self-manage.[92]

This dynamic bi-directional system, in fact, was proposed a century earlier by the late 19th century French physiologist Claude Bernard. Writing about Bernard in 1892, Charles Darwin, in *The Expression of the Emotions in Man and Animals*, noted:

> "When the mind is strongly excited, we might expect that it would instantly affect in a direct manner the heart; and this is universally acknowledged and felt to be the case. Claude Bernard also repeatedly insists, and this deserves especial notice, that when the heart is affected it reacts on the brain; and the state of the brain again reacts through the pneumogastric nerve on the heart; so that under any excitement there will be much mutual action and reaction between these, the two most important organs of the body."[93]

How do we interrupt this cycle of heart-brain irritability? By working both sides of the equation to achieve coherence.

Combine deep and regular breathing—a slow five-count inhalation followed by a five-count exhalation—with evocation of positive feelings

Such as love, gratitude, and acceptance, and visualize these feelings coming from the heart. The HeartMath device provides the biofeedback necessary for the user to master the coherence technique.

Positive Stress Management Strategies

Physicians routinely employ many strategies to cope with stress, both positive and negative. Positive strategies include planning and problem-solving, finding humor in the difficulties, and seeking support from colleagues, family and friends. Maladaptive responses include alcohol and drug abuse, both of which have high prevalence among medical professionals.[94-97]

Biofeedback holds great potential as a stress management tool for healthcare practitioners. Many clinicians routinely recommend it to their patients to better manage tension, but surprisingly, there had not been any studies of biofeedback for physician stress management until 2011 when Jane B. LeMaire, MD, clinical professor in the Department of Medicine at the University of Calgary, conducted a biofeedback-based trial with 40 doctors in an urban tertiary care hospital.

The intervention centered around the practice of the 'quick coherence' technique described above, in conjunction with a portable HeartMath device that reads heart rate through a finger or ear lobe sensor and provides reinforcement through visual and audio cues.

Physicians were screened for major depression and those who scored high were sent to a physician wellness support program. Stress levels were assessed with the Global Perception of Stress for Physicians. (Figure 7 below). The treatment group was instructed to use the quick coherence technique three times a day over a 28-day period. Both groups met bi-weekly for retesting.

The HRV intervention group had statistically lower mean stress scores than the control group, and maintained this out to day 56.[98]

The effects of coherence can be profound. Coherence techniques have been shown to improve decision-making; ability to focus, information processing and problem-solving. They increase reaction times and coordination, improve long and short-term memory, and enhance academic performance.[99]

HeartMath programs have been implemented in many US hospitals with positive results. At the Gunderson Health System in La Crosse, WI, participants reported improvements in calmness and ability to stay focused, as well as decreased anxiety and less frustration in the face of day-to-day obstacles. Children's Hospital Colorado, Aurora reported decreases in worry and cynicism, as well as improvements in calm, muscle tension, and rapid heart rates. Fairfield Medical Center in Lancaster, Ohio showed improvements in employee satisfaction and absenteeism as well as a 2:1 savings on healthcare claims.[100]

Stress scale to measure global perceptions of stress

Response set: 0 = never, 1 = almost never, 2 = sometimes, 3 = often, 4 = very often, 5 = always. "R" indicates that the item was reverse-coded. Maximum score 200, where a higher score indicates greater feelings of stress.

Part A: Percieved Stress Scale
In the last month, how often have you...
1. Been upset because of something that happened unexpectedly?
2. Felt that you were unable to control the important things in your life?
3. Felt nervous?
4. Felt "stressed"?
5. Dealt successfully with irritating life hassles? (R)
6. Felt that you were effectively coping with important changes that were occurring in your life? (R)
7. Felt confident about your ability to handle your personal problems? (R)
8. Felt that things were going your way? (R)
9. Found that you could not cope with all the things that happened that were outside of your control?
10. Been able to control irritations in your life? (R)
11. Felt that you were on top of things? (R)
12. Been angered because of things that happened that were outside of your control?
13. Found yourself thinking about things that you have accomplished?
14. Been able to control the way you spend your time? (R)
15. Felt difficulties were piling up so high that you could not overcome them?

Part B: Selected items from the Personal and Organizational Quality Assessment—Revised
Following is a list of words and statements that describe feelings people sometimes have. Please fill in the number which best reflects how frequently you have felt the following during the last month.

Anxiety/anger: resentful; cynical; angry; anxious; annoyed; worried; I am down after I've been upset; uneasy; my sleep is inadequate; calm (R); relaxed (R); peaceful (R)
Physical symptoms: tired; exhausted; fatigued; indigestion, heartburn, or stomach upset; rapid heartbeats; headaches; muscle tension; body aches
Time pressure: I feel there is never enough time; I feel pressed for time; the pace of life is too fast and I can't keep up

Figure 7: Lemaire JB, Wallace JE, Lewin AM, de Grood J, Schaefer JP. The effect of a biofeedback-based stress management tool on physician stress: a randomized controlled clinical trial. Open Med 2011;5(4):e154–e163. Reprinted with permission.

HeartMath has also found its way into military medicine; HRV training has been shown to be an effective intervention for chronic pain in war veterans.[101]

The Focus of a Mantra

Another method for reducing anxiety and promoting harmony can be found in meditation techniques that involve the use of a mantra, a phrase that when repeated silently to oneself over a period of time, usually for 15-20 minutes, induces systemic calmness. During the repetition of the word or phrase, the meditator observes the comings and goings of extraneous thoughts, allowing them to pass through the mind without attachment. Ultimately, this process leads to a state of calmness.

The most well-studied form of meditation has been the Transcendental Meditation® technique promulgated by an international organization founded by the Indian guru Maharishi Mahesh Yogi. Research on the TM technique indicates that it can produce significant reductions in psychological distress,[102] anxiety,[103] depressive symptoms,[104] and emotional distress,[105] as well as improvement in psychological well-being in individuals with chronic illnesses.[106]

TM also has a place in the management of chronic diseases. There are studies showing that the regular practice of TM results in improvements in blood pressure and decreases in insulin resistance in heart disease patients.[107] It can even benefit difficult-to-treat hypertensive populations. In one study, investigators recruited 127 hypertensive African-Americans, aged 55-85. They divided the people into three groups that were then assigned to TM, a progressive muscle relaxation (body scan) practice, or a lifestyle education program.

Meditation reduced systolic pressure by 10.7 mm Hg and diastolic pressure by 6.4 mm Hg, as compared to progressive muscle relaxation that lowered systolic pressure by 4.7 mm Hg and diastolic pressure by 3.3 mm. Lifestyle education had no significant effect.[108]

In a study with implications for burned-out physicians, TM was shown to be highly effective in reducing psychological distress among a group of teachers and support staff at a school for students with severe behavioral problems.[109]

In TM, the meditation teacher prescribes the mantra; however, the use of a self-selected mantra based upon personal values, culture, beliefs and preferences (Figure 8 below), was effective in treating veterans with post-traumatic stress disorder (PTSD).

Jill Bormann, PhD, RN, and colleagues, compared health outcomes of a Mantram Repetition program against outcomes from 'usual care' in a cohort of 136 outpatient combat veterans with PTSD. The mantram group showed significant reductions in PTSD symptom severity; 24% of veterans in the mantram group had a clinically meaningful improvement in PTSD symptoms compared to 12% of controls. As compared to controls, the mantram group had significant improvements in depression, quality of life, and spiritual well-being.[110]

List of Common Mantrams Used in Intervention

Mantram and Pronunciation	Meaning
Buddhist	
Om Mani Padme Hum (ohm Mah-nee Pod-may Hume)	An invocation to the jewel (Self) in the lotus of the heart
Namo Butsaya (Nah-mo boot-sie-yah)	I bow to the Buddha.
Christian	
My God and my all	St. Francis of Assisi's mantra
Maranatha (Mar-uh-nah-tha)	Lord of the heart (Aramaic)
Kyrie Eleison (Kire-ee-ay Ee-lay-ee-sone)	Lord have mercy, or the Lord is risen.
Christe Eleison (Kreest-ay Ee-lay-ee-sone)	Christ have mercy, Christ has risen
Jesus, Jesus or Lord Jesus Christ	Jesus, Son of God
Hail Mary or Ave Maria	Mother of Jesus
Hindu/Indian	
Rama (Rah-mah)	Eternal Joy within. Gandhi's mantra.
Ram Ram Sri Ram (Rahm rahm shree rahm)	(variation on Rama)
Om Namah Shivaya (Ohm Nah-mah Shee-vy-yah)	An invocation to beauty and fearlessness
Om Prema (Ohm Pray-Mah)	A call for universal love
Om Shanti (Ohm Shawn-tee)	In invocation to eternal peace
So Hum (So hum)	I am that Self within
Jewish	
Barukh Atiah Adonoi (Bah-ruk Ah-tah Ah-don-aye)	Blessed are Thou' O Lord
Ribono Shel Olam (Ree-boh-noh Shel Oh-lahm)	Lord of the Universe
Shalom	Peace
Shehenna (Sha Hee-nah)	Feminine aspect of God
Muslim	
Allah	One True God
Bismallah Ir-rahnan Ir-rahim (Beese-mah-iah ir-rah-mun ur-rah-heem)	In the name of Allah, the merciful, the compassionate
Native American	
O Wakan Tanka	Oh, Great Spirit

Figure 8: Common Mantrams Used in Intervention. Adapted from Bormann, J. E. (2005). Efficacy of Frequent Mantram Repetition on Stress, Quality of Life, and Spiritual Well-Being in Veterans: A Pilot Study. Journal of Holistic Nursing, 23(4), 395-414.

One of the values of using a mantra is that it can be incorporated into daily life to provide psychological first aid for times when you feel angry, anxious, upset or afraid. It can be used while you are waiting in lines or stalled in traffic. Repeating a mantra can also help induce sleep. Your mantra can also accompany you on a walk or a jog.

Over the centuries humans have developed many different ways to obtain the benefits obtained with TM and mantra-repetition. A European study showed that mantra use and the repetition of the rosary prayer were both effective in decreasing sympathetic tone, synchronizing respiratory and c-v cycles, and improving HRV.[111]

Bring Mind to Matter

In Western culture, the popularization of mindfulness, one of the key teachings of both Buddhism and Hinduism, can be traced back to Richard Alpert, PhD, who, writing as Ram Dass in 1971, created one of the seminal works on spirituality, yoga and presence. Entitled *Be Here Now* (Hanuman Foundation), the cartoon-like book featured sayings, quotations, and illustrations to provide advice for staying in the present moment. *Be Here Now* inspired the so-called hippie generation; the title has sold more than two million copies.

Herbert Benson, MD, from Harvard Medical School, demystified mind-body practices with a simple formula for the masses. Benson's technique, described in his 1975 book, *The Relaxation Response* (HarperTorch), emphasized pairing regular breathing and silently repeating the word, "one." Benson established mind-science as a legitimate academic pursuit.

The body-mind field experienced its next major advance from the research of molecular biologist Jon Kabat-Zinn, PhD, at the University of Massachusetts Medical School. Kabat-Zinn called his unique synthesis of traditional meditation and awareness techniques, mindfulness-based stress reduction (MBSR). Kabat-Zinn has studied the effects of MBSR on various emotional states, immune system function, and cancer, as well on varied populations ranging from prison inmates and staff to employees and managers at the worksite.

Today, MBSR is a well-recognized clinical tool. It is a type of mental training that enables participants to actively notice and experience new things in a non-judgmental, non-reactive manner. Practicing mindfulness enhances clear thinking, equanimity, compassion, and open-heartedness.[112] By being present and observing, one becomes more sensitive to context and gains perspective on the attitudes, thoughts and behaviors that are helpful, and those that are not. Mindfulness can also facilitate creative solutions to problems. We believe mindfulness is critical to the total engagement process.

While there are many meditative and relaxation styles that can help you and your patients 'be here now,' "mindfulness may be the most adaptable and acceptable. It is non-religious, yet addresses meaning and purpose. It has secular and academic appeal and is supported by a solid body of evidence." One of the drawbacks of most relaxation techniques is that they require a significant time commitment. This is always an issue for busy physicians.[112]

Researchers at the Department of Family Medicine, University of Wisconsin-Madison sought to determine whether a more abbreviated MBSR might be helpful in reducing physician burnout. They recruited 30 primary care clinicians who took part in an abbreviated mindfulness course consisting of 18 hours of class training, the use of a practice audio recording, and a specifically designed website with mindfulness techniques for the doctors to use with patients. The physicians were encouraged to practice their mindfulness techniques daily for 10-20 minutes. Participants were evaluated with the Maslach Burnout Inventory and validated research tools to assess quality of life, the DASS-21, PSS, and RS-14.

Physicians participating in this mindfulness course experienced reductions in indicators of job burnout, depression, anxiety, and stress. While the study had a small sample size and lacked a control group, it did indicate that abbreviated mindfulness training could be a time-efficient tool to help support clinician health and well-being, both of which may have implications for patient care.[113]

Don't Forget the Fun

When brought into daily life, the practice of mindfulness begets rather than consumes energy. As David Sobel, MD, MPH, notes, it can also be fun. Sobel is the medical director of regional health education for Kaiser Permanente Northern California. He is also a primary care physician, and author of eight books including *Healthy Pleasures* (Perseus Books) co-authored with Robert Ornstein, PhD.

CHAPTER TWO

Sobel encourages his patients and fellow physicians to focus on healthy pleasures, and on putting the fun back into life. This runs counter to so much of modern day health advice, which typically takes a negative tack and revolves around the all-too-common admonitions to give up pleasurable habits: 'Stop smoking! Stop eating so much! Lose weight!!'

Of course it is important for people to avoid 'pleasures' that have clearly detrimental health effects. But it is equally important to help people identify harmless and healthy sources of pleasure and joy.

Drawing from evolutionary biology, Sobel points out that humans are designed for pleasure and we need daily doses of positive sensory stimulation. The pleasurable stimulation we derive from our five senses has helped humans thrive for centuries. Only in the last fifty years has technology intruded upon the more basic human sensory pleasures.

For example, mindless eating—often in front of a TV or computer screen—is at the core of over-consumption of poor quality food, and is in part responsible for the epidemic of obesity and metabolic syndrome in industrialized nations. The basic pleasures of preparing and sharing healthful meals with family and friends have been replaced by the quick-fix sugar surges of junk food and the disembodied communication we get from the media.

In contrast to mindless eating, nutritional mindfulness involves savoring the taste, smell, and textures of food; chewing completely; breathing; smiling and relaxing the body during the experience.

Even if the food being consumed is less-than-healthy, the odds are good that with mindfulness, someone will eat less of it. Our natural cravings for different taste sensations will steer us to consume a broad range of naturally flavorful and healthful foods. By becoming mindful of what we eat, we start to appreciate herbs and spices, many of which have medicinal qualities.

For example, capsaicin, the active ingredient in chili peppers, has been shown to loosen congestion, decrease cholesterol, enhance metabolic rate, elevate mood and inhibit platelet aggregation.[114] There are many other examples: oregano, rosemary, turmeric (curcumin), garlic, fenugreek, cinnamon, in fact most of the culinary herbs and spices humans have discovered and cherished over the centuries have very definite medicinal properties. There are reasons why we enjoy them.

Our sense of smell is mediated by the olfactory nerve. The first and shortest of the twelve cranial nerves, it connects directly to the limbic system, the part of the brain that deals with emotions. This accounts for the fact that individual reactions to smell are rarely neutral; we have strong olfactory likes and dislikes. Smells also evoke memories. The smell of the fall leaves, for example, might remind us of a long-ago camping trip; cinnamon and nutmeg might evoke Thanksgiving meals with the family. One study indicates that the smell of spiced apple can help reduce stress, pain, insomnia, nausea and depression and reduce food cravings.[115] Eating mindfully includes careful attention to the sense of smell.

The same general principle holds for our sense of hearing. Our ears not only alert us to danger, they allow us to enjoy the sound of leaves rustling through the breeze or the sweet chirping of a bird. Listening to music before surgery has been shown to be as relaxing as a dose of Valium®. People who exercise to music report less pain and more gain from their activity.[116]

Sobel notes that the stimulation we receive via touch is a vital nutrient. Most of us are not getting our daily requirement. Studies on the healing power of touch have shown that in addition to inducing relaxation, touch can help diminish pain, shorten labor, help infants gain more weight, strengthen the immune system, and reduce anxiety prior to surgery.[117]

We were also evolved to look at nature, not at computer screens. Many people who view natural settings recover more quickly from surgery and overcome stress faster. In the work setting, employees who have a view of nature or have plants close at hand tend to work more effectively and have greater work satisfaction. Watching fish swimming in a tank can lower blood pressure and reduce pain sensation.

Your personal search for health and happiness revolves around answering just a few simple questions in an honest way:

- Where do you find your pleasures?
- What gives you joy?
- When was the last time you did something that makes you happy?
- What is keeping you from these experiences?
- Why?
- If not now, when?

CHAPTER TWO

The Power of the Pause

"I'm too busy. I have too much to do. The demands are so great. I have no time." The excuses are many. In the moment, they seem true. Yet all of them are pale overlays on a life that could be more enriching, self-nurturing and vibrant.

In the course of your day you have multiple opportunities to get off autopilot and be present by noticing your surroundings, thoughts and emotions, and doing so without judgment. You have the power to control your physiology through breathing and the practice of gratitude. You just have to be willing.

Given our cultural addictions to the Internet, social media, and multi-tasking, the thought of taking time for stillness seems counterproductive. Yann Martel, author of *The Life of Pi*, puts quietude into the larger perspective.

> "I got to thinking about stillness. To read a book one must be still. To watch a concert, a play, a movie, to look at a painting, one must be still....Life, it seems, favours moments of stillness to appear on the edges of our perception and whisper to us, 'here I am. What do you think? Then we become busy and the stillness vanishes, yet we hardly notice, because we fall so easily for the delusion, whereby what keeps us busy must be important, the busier we are with it, the more important it must be. And so we work, work, work and rush, rush, rush. On occasion, we say to ourselves panting, 'Gosh, life is racing by.' but that's not it at all, it's the contrary: Life is still. It is we who are racing by.'"[118]

You always have the choice to practice stillness—even if it is just for a few minutes. Sometimes those few minutes can make all the difference in the world. The mental and physiological pause that you can gain from meditation, coherence or mindfulness resets your perspective; it also opens up choices. Austrian psychologist and Holocaust survivor Viktor Frankl, MD, PhD recognized the importance of this mini-moment:

> *"Between stimulus and response, there is a space. In that space lies our freedom and power to choose our response. In our response lies our growth and freedom."*[119]

The incredible power of the pause may well rest in its ability to allow us to refocus and obtain moments of greater clarity. In the low-control medical world where events and situations are constantly being thrust upon you, this simple technique may be able to move you toward greater self-efficacy. Rather than always being 'at cause,' you move to being 'at effect' and in this transformation come the powerful benefits that together can be summed up as happiness.

Diet and Exercise: We Know You Know but Sometimes Forget

Coherence, meditation, and mindfulness techniques address the inner game of health and happiness. Total engagement and well-being also require attention to the physical aspects of health, namely diet and exercise.

There is so much nutrition and fitness advice available to both clinicians and consumers these days that there is little point in trying to reiterate it all in a book like this. Our view on nutrition is quiet simple, and best summed up by Mark Hyman, MD, leading functional medicine expert, contributing editor of *Alternative Therapies in Health and Medicine*, and author of the *New York Times* bestsellers, *The Blood Sugar Solution* (Hodder & Stoughton), *Ultraprevention* (Atria Books), and several other popular books.

Hyman started The Functional Medicine Foundation, based out of New York, with the intention of promoting awareness, funding research, and educating the public about this growing area in medicine. Hyman is collaborating with The Cleveland Clinic to open a new Center for Functional Medicine. He incorporates the most current research in nutritional science into his Nutrigenomic Index shown below.

The Nutrigenomic Index[120]

A whole, unprocessed predominantly plant-based diet provides the highest nutrigenomic index based on the following properties:

- Low glycemic load—the overall balance of the meal
- Proper fatty acid composition with a high level of healthy omega-3 fats vs omega-6 fats, low in saturated fats and no trans fats
- High phytonutrient density—high level of phytonutrients and antioxidants
- Healthy protein—lean, healthful, predominantly plant-based

proteins or pasture-raised animal products
- High micronutrient density—high amounts of vitamins and minerals
- Low allergenic burden—low in foods that are highly allergenic (gluten, dairy and others based on personalized prescription)
- Low toxic burden—no/few added hormones, pesticides, antibiotics, or other artificial additives
- Healthy pH balance—provides proper balance between acidity and alkalinity
- Healthy sodium: potassium ratio—low in salt and high in potassium
- High fiber content—high in fiber to help slow the insulin response and optimize digestive health.

A complementary, but abbreviated nutritional philosophy is offered by real-food advocate and author Michael Pollan, in his book *In Defense of Food: An Eater's Manifesto* (Penguin Press). His recommendation: "Eat food. Not too much. Mostly plants."

The Inner Game of Exercise

When it comes to fitness, we will assume that you already know that a sedentary lifestyle is a greater risk factor for CVD that being overweight.[88] You are also aware of the benefits of fitness, as noted by the Centers for Disease Control and Prevention,[121] namely that regular exercise can help:

- Control weight
- Reduce risk of CVD
- Reduce risk of type 2 diabetes and metabolic syndrome
- Reduce risk of some cancers
- Strengthen bones and muscles
- Improve mental health and mood
- Improve ability to do daily activities and prevent falls, if you're an older adult
- Increase longevity.

The CDC's fitness recommendations are clear-cut: 150 minutes a week (2.5 hours) of moderate-intensity aerobic activity. Add some resistance training 2-3 days a week to help sustain muscle and bone mass, as well as exercises for the core, and some regular stretching and flexibility exercises, and you have an algorithm for a great deal of disease prevention and health promotion.

For healthcare professionals who have not yet acted on what they know about exercise, or who have fallen off the fitness wagon, we offer these thoughts in the hope that one or more of them will resonate:

1. Exercise, best done outdoors, provides you the opportunity to get out of your head and into your body. It is a grounding phenomenon. One can find a voluntary simplicity in just placing one foot in front of the other. In our world of complexity, this is a very good thing.

2. Aerobic activity allows you to synch your breath with your movement. This gets you into the rhythmicity of life, and helps with your practice of coherence.

3. Protect your morning. Even thought studies show that strength and endurance are greater in the afternoon, and the likelihood of injury is decreased, most consistent exercisers guard their early morning as if were Fort Knox. Resist the temptation to check email or texts until you have put in 30 minutes of activity.

4. Sneak movement into daily life. Take the stairs whenever you can. Park farther away in the parking lot. Get a digital tracking device and put in 10,000 steps a day. Have to discuss an important issue with a staff member? How about a walk and talk?

5. Use exercise to tap into creative solutions. Good ideas come to people in four settings: in the bathroom; while commuting; just before bedtime or when arising; and, in the course of doing non-work related physical activities. Exercise fits into the last category. Got a problem or issue for which a solution doesn't seem evident? You could sleep on it, or you could literally run it by your mind. The grounding and rhythmicity of exercise clears the mind and allows new ideas and solutions to rise to the forefront of your consciousness.

6. Catch yourself sooner. Never allow more than three days to elapse between active workouts. Research has shown that as few as two days of inactivity can decrease insulin sensitivity;[122] with 3 weeks of

CHAPTER TWO

deconditioning the body loses 5-10% of its aerobic power.[123]

7. Remember that as you age you just can't eat as much. According to the American College of Sports Medicine, "a gradual loss in muscle cross-sectional area is consistently found with advancing age; by age 50, about ten percent of muscle area is gone. After 50 years of age, the rate accelerates significantly. Muscle strength declines by approximately 115 percent per decade in the sixties and seventies and by about 30 percent therafter."[123] While regular exercise and strength training can slow the decline, you need to get used to the idea of consuming less fuel.

Lone Wolf or Member of the Pack?

As a generalization, physicians are not very social. We often lack the time and energy for social activities. Many of us also lack the natural inclination toward extroversion. Yet, the social environment and social connections can have a buffering effect on physiological stress. The same stressor that increases plasma cortisol by 50% in an animal left alone does not increase cortisol at all when the animal is surrounded by familiar companions.[124]

Like optimism, gratitude and joy, more social connection is better than less. In one study of social support, 276 healthy volunteers were given nasal drops containing rhinovirus; all were shown to shed virus. The researchers looked at 12 different types of social relationships such as parental, childhood, informal groups, etc., among the volunteers. Those who had the least number of positive social relationships developed cold symptoms four times more frequently than those with the highest number of positive relationships.[125]

In additional to illness prevention, the support of family and friends exerts a positive effect on longevity.[126] In a meta-analysis of 148 studies that followed more than 300,000 people for an average of 7.5 years, researchers showed that more socially connected people lived an average of 3.7 years longer than those with fewer social connections. They concluded that "the influence of social relationships on the risk of death are comparable with well-established risk factors for mortality such as smoking and alcohol consumption and exceed the influence of other risk factors such as physical inactivity and obesity."[127]

Most doctors find their social support systems are centered around family and most closely aligned with their significant other. The illness-preventing benefits of marriage have been backed by numerous studies. Happily married individuals are less likely to get pneumonia, have surgery, develop dementia, or cancer.[128]

It is no surprise that marriage affects the heart. One study examined 1,400 men and women post cardiac catheterization and asked two questions of the participants. "Are you married?" and "Do you have someone you can confide in?" Those people who were not married and had no close confidant had over three times the death rate of the other groups over 5 years (15% vs. 50%).[129]

It's not marriage status itself that confers health benefits; it is the level of happiness in the marriage. It is the union of two happy people who enjoy being together that provides the attendant mental, physical and spiritual benefits. Optimistic couples enjoy happier and more satisfying romantic relationships, a consequence that may be linked to better cooperative problem solving abilities.[130] In optimistic couples, the partners tend to view each other as supportive. They are able to resolve conflict faster, and are more likely to live up to the other's ideals.

In happily married couples, partners often motivate each other to engage in healthier lifestyles. This may, in part, explain the findings of a retrospective study of 3.5 million people between the ages of 21 and 102 who were evaluated for peripheral artery disease, cerebrovascular disease, abdominal aorta aneurysm and coronary artery disease. Carlos L. Alviar, MD, of New York University Langone Medical Center, the principal investigator, found an independent association between marital status and CVD after adjusting for age, sex, race and disease risk factors. Compared with single people, married participants had lower odds of any vascular disease, regardless of gender or condition.[131]

A study of unhappy marriages, on the other hand, showed 34% more coronary events independent of gender and social status.[132]

Regardless of your relationship status, or whether you consider yourself a 'social person or not' keep in mind that you don't exist in a vacuum.

If you are currently practicing medicine, the truth is that more than 40 % of your waking time is spent in a healthcare environment, which is a social environment. Variables such as the quantity and quality of relationships with your colleagues, staff and patients, the norms of the groups in which you participate, the pace of your workplace, and the intrinsic and extrinsic rewards you derive from your practice are all important social determinants of your happiness.

Have a Nice Day

Whenever groups come together they form cultures. And these cultures have norms: unwritten, but powerful determinants that shape group member behaviors.

Starla Fitch, MD, relates how she helped transform a negative operating room culture into a positive one. Seeking greater cost efficiencies, her hospital had recently brought in a consulting team whose recommendations resulted in many of the more senior personnel taking early retirement. This transformed the operating room experience into one large complaint session. The staff were scared and angry; they allowed these emotions to spill over into the surgical procedure. Fitch explains:

> "I realized that I was having a hard time dealing with all this negative energy while I was trying to repair an eyelid damaged from cancer, or perform a perfect blepharoplasty. So I announced at the beginning of each surgical day that we would go around the room and everyone would name three things they were grateful for. I let them know I was serious and that we would not proceed until everyone participated. I thought they would throw wet gauze at me, but to my surprise, the team went along with it. After a while, the word got out, 'Oh, you're scrubbing with Fitch, today. Better have three things you are grateful for.'"

Fitch then began to modify her technique. Influenced by the work of one of the earliest integrative medicine pioneers, Rachel Naomi Remen, MD, author of *My Grandfather's Blessings: Stories of Strength, Refuge and Belonging* (Riverhead Books, 2000), she began asking her team other insightful and positive questions: What surprised you? What warmed your heart? What inspired you today?

Fitch also remained sensitive to the needs of her team. One of the nurse's husbands died of an MI and rather than further inflame the nurse's emotional wound, whenever they worked together, Fitch would introduce a more light-hearted query such as identifying three songs that have the word 'happy' in them.

The power in Fitch's approach lies in her ability to use her influence as a physician to recast the norms of her immediate environment away from the negative, energy-draining complaining and toward health-enhancing, positive behaviors.

Happiness and Resilience Go Hand in Hand

Established in 1986, the *American Journal of Health Promotion* (AJHP) was the first peer-reviewed publication devoted exclusively to the proactive enhancement of health. Founded by its Editor in Chief, Michael P. O'Donnell, PhD, MBA, MPH, it has helped close the gap between health promotion research and practice. It has also served as a forum for many diverse disciplines. In this chapter we've introduced a handful of the newer techniques such as MBSR, nutrigenomics, coherence, and culture change, subjects that are comprehensively discussed in issues of AJHP.

One of the latest paradigms to emerge in the field of health promotion is known as *resilience*. Similar to coherence, the definition of resilience has its roots in the physics, in this case in elasticity and the ability of a substance to spring back into shape after deformation. As used in health care, resilience is that ability to regain health and strength while bouncing back from life's obstacles.

The internal, psychological nature of resilience is best described in a quote by Phillips Brooks, an Episcopal clergyman from Boston, who during the Civil War, vigorously opposed slavery. He is also remembered as the lyricist of the Christmas hymn, "O Little Town of Bethlehem." Brooks remarked:

> *"Make the best use of what is in your power, and take the rest as it happens. Do not pray for easy lives. Pray to be a stronger person. Do not pray for tasks equal to your powers. Pray for powers equal to your teaks. Then the doing of your work shall be no miracle, but you shall be the miracle."*

The ability to become a stronger person involves an inner fortitude, but it also requires that we pay attention to other dimensions of health. Figure 10 below presents an encompassing view of resilience, developed by Rollin McCraty, PhD, director of research at the HeartMath Institute. As you view the diagram, you might ask yourself: In which areas are you doing well? Which could use greater attention?

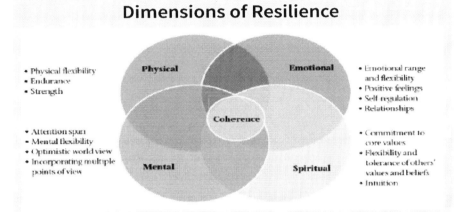

Figure 9: The Dimensions of Resilience. McCraty, R. (2010). Coherence: Bridging personal, social, and global health. Alternative Therapies in Health and Medicine, 16(4), 10-24. Reprinted with permission.

Physicians who pursue the art of medicine with dedication, over time, develop a unique type of happiness: wisdom. McCraty and Maria Zayas, EdD, define wisdom as "an intuitive intelligence that physicians can bring to bear in deepening the important relationships in their lives." They state:

> "The ability to alter one's responses and behaviors in order to build and maintain loving relationships and a supportive social network, as well as to effectively meet the demands of life with composure, consistency, and integrity, arguably becomes central to good health, effective decision-making, and success in lifting consciousness and living a life of greater collaboration, kindness, and compassion. If one's capacity for intelligent, self-directed regulation is powerful enough, then regardless of inclinations, past experiences, or personality traits, people can usually do the adaptive or right thing in most situations they encounter."[133]

To date, we have been discussing situations in which you can either control the stressors you face or modify your reactions to them. No one else has the power to turn on your stomach acidity, give you a headache, or make you eat the entire pizza. You are responsible for your own levels of happiness. There are; however, environments which chronically make it more difficult for you to apply the four dimensions of resilience. The context for this discord is found in the person-environment fit, an explanation of which follows in the next chapter.

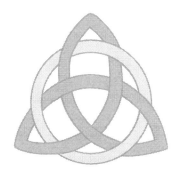

And I realized that there's a big difference between deciding to leave and knowing where to go.

— Robyn Schneider, *The Beginning of Everything*

3
Should I Stay or Should I Go?

In the last chapter, we discussed how you can change your inner dialog, attitudes, emotions and health habits to become more resilient and ultimately happier. While you have the capacity to become the embodiment of the Dara Celtic knot on our cover, the powerful and self-grounded oak, you will need to take the environment into account, as well. If your workplace is constantly subjecting you to harsh storm conditions, these forces can strip your leaves, break your branches and wither your roots.

The Assault on Physician Autonomy

Many physicians believe that the good old days in medicine are gone, lost in the storm that ceded control of care to insurance companies, the federal government and healthcare systems. Medicine has lost some of its luster as a profession; many of us no longer have the same level of autonomy or self-direction that previous generations of physicians enjoyed. We no longer control the content of our work or the organization of our practice, to the same extent we used to. One critical review of the physician's current role even calls into question the entire notion of medicine as a profession: "lacking this authentic autonomy (the physician profession) may alternatively be given designations as quasiprofession, paraprofession, semiprofession, subprofession, or a trade."[133] Designating healthcare professionals as 'providers' further erodes the pivotal and irreplaceable role of the clinician. Along with the death of autonomy has been the traumatization of its sister value: control.

Multiple studies across all workplaces cite a perceived sense of control over the amount and pace of work as being critical for well-being, and its absence as a major contributor to stress-related illness.[135] Control and an abiding commitment to the organization are two of the key factors that go into the definition of hardiness, a psychological state defined by Chicago psychologist Salvatore Maddi, PhD, and colleague Suzanne Kobasa, PhD. Maddi and Kobasa studied the lives of business executives and lawyers—people who dealt with large amounts of stress on a daily basis—and noted that those with a perceived sense of control, a true belief in the mission of the organization, and an ability to define obstacles as challenges, all fared better than those who scored lower in these variables.[136]

By their very nature, some medical specialties are more stressful than others based upon the ability to have a controllable lifestyle with better management of work hours. One study has shown that physicians in specialties defined as 'controllable' (including dermatology; emergency medicine; neurology; ophthalmology; otolaryngology; and child, adolescent, and adult psychiatry) scored higher in career satisfaction than those designated 'uncontrollable' (including family practice, general practice, internal medicine, internal medicine and pediatrics–combined, obstetrics and gynecology, orthopedic surgery, pediatrics, general surgery, and urology).[137]

Loss of control is not unique to physicians: this psychological variable touches all healthcare workers, with nurses perhaps being the most affected group. As Milisa Manojlovich, PhD, RN, of University of Michigan, explains:

> "As long as nurses view power as only having control or dominance, and as long as nursing does not control its own destiny, nurses will continue to struggle with issues of power and empowerment...There are at least three types of power that nurses need to be able to make their optimum contribution. The various types of power can all be categorized as stemming from nurses' control in three domains: control over the content of practice, control over the context of practice, and control over competence. The continued lack of control over both the content and context of nursing work suggests that power remains an elusive attribute for many nurses."[138]

It is not surprising that loss of control is something felt by all segments of the healthcare profession; indeed, it's a human motivation to want to influence our surroundings. If we aren't in control, who is? Often, the answer that question can be found in the physician-administrator relationship.

Can You Bridge the Cultural Gap?

Similar to the ever morphing power relationships between allied nations, the status of the physician-administrator relationship has seen an ebb and flow in both direction and influence succinctly summed up in the historical description below:

> "In the United States, managers gained more control over the allocation of resources and started to play a more central role in the hospital starting in 1974 with the passage of the Health Planning and Development Act. However, the implementation of the Medicare Prospective Payment System in 1983 created competing incentives for managers and physicians, as managers' most important incentive became cost containment, while physicians only concern remained patient care. Consequently, managers realized the importance of obtaining physicians' cooperation, and a new period of physician-manager relationships developed, characterized by shared authority and increased physician involvement in governing and strategic decision-making.
>
> In the 1990s, the relationship became even more complex as factors such as declining reimbursement rates, cost containment pressures, relationship with Health Maintenance Organizations (HMOs), increasing malpractice costs, and regulatory pressures intensified (Kaissi, 2005; Burns, 1993).
>
> That period also witnessed a trend of hospitals' acquisition of physician group practices and employment of physicians. But the trend was reversed by the late1990s and early 2000s as hospital financial losses accumulated (Kaissi and Begun, 2008). The last decade has witnessed two opposing trends in physician-hospital relationships in the US: on the one hand, physicians have separated from hospitals and competed with them by developing their own specialty hospitals, ambulatory surgery centres and ancillary services; on the other, they are working with hospitals in joint ventures and employment agreements (Berenson, Ginsburg, and May, 2006). The passage of healthcare reform in 2010 and its implications for reimbursement has created real incentives for a repeat of the 1990s wave of physician acquisition, and physician

employment by health systems has been on the rise in the last few years."[139]

Throughout these transitions, one thing has remained constant. Physicians and non-physician managers still have different worldviews, training, expectations, and socialization experiences. This gap, and the pressures placed upon healthcare organizations for quality and cost effectiveness, often generates physician distrust, skepticism, and disengagement.

In the opening pages of this book, we defined total engagement as, "A rekindling of the spirit and the inherent joys in the practice of medicine in which passion is in great evidence, time flies, and meaning and purpose prevail." This view of engagement involves looking from the lumen out into the periphery. It begins with you. It is a perspective that is in contrast to the working definition of physician engagement adopted by most healthcare systems in which engagement is "the active and positive contribution of doctors within their normal working roles to maintaining and enhancing the performance of the organization which itself recognizes this commitment in supporting and encouraging high quality care."[140]

The organization-centered definition takes the viewpoint of looking from outside in. It begins with them, the system, the administration, the hospital. Yet, both definitions are both valid and valuable. At issue is whether you can find your total engagement within the construct of theirs. In short, is there a person-environment fit? For this to occur, there must be a match of values, but equally important, a commitment to honesty and openness in communication, the kind of communication that builds trust.

Physicians Need PERKS

In the mid 1980's I (Mark) worked with Marjorie Blanchard, PhD, president of Blanchard Training and Development examining the types of organizational behaviors that contributed to either employee illness or wellness. We trained managers and supervisors in the skills necessary to not just drive productivity, but to also create mental and physical hardiness in subordinates. In today's world, an increasing number of physicians are employees, and the principles of the health-promoting organizational behaviors that were valid three decades ago still ring true today. Blanchard and I summarized these principles with the acronym PERKS. For a healthcare organization to engage physicians and successfully navigate in the white waters of change, doctors, nurses and all other employees must be provided with PERKS. These include:

- **P**articipation in decisions that affect them. Physicians, nurses, and in fact any and everyone who is close to the patient, must have a voice in the patient experience. Those closest to the patient, the caregivers, have the most accurate and actionable information. Those closest to a problem also have the best chance of solving it. In contrast, administrators who are steps removed from direct patient care receive a watered down and incomplete view of reality. Those managers who exhibit an authoritarian style with little listening ability rarely get the buy-in that is necessary for organizational improvement. For an organization to be successful in any of its quality, safety, or revenue-generating mandates, physicians and nurses in particular must be able to state their viewpoints, have them respected, and know that they will be heard. A participative environment also allows the enablement of physician champions who are critical for any organizational change effort.

- An **E**nvironment that embodies a healthy culture. Fred Kofman and Peter Senge, noted author of the classic book, *The Fifth Discipline: The Art and Science of the Learning Organization* (Doubleday), cite three key examples of cultural dysfunction: fragmentation, competition, and reactiveness.[141] Healthy organizational cultures are ones that address complex problems through the application of systems thinking, that focus their energy on bettering themselves, and that provide a space for imagination and experimentation. In contrast, an unhealthy organizational culture glosses over serious issues, focuses on 'beating the competition' rather than bettering the organization, and has cultural norms that discourage innovation and growth. And of course, you can tell how healthy an organizational culture is in medicine by judging its ultimate effect on the patients.

- **R**ecognition for hard work and compassionate care. The most common feedback most employees receive is no feedback at all. The next most common type is negative. Those organizations that actively focus on recognizing and rewarding effort, as well as on doling out-task specific feedback and praise, become magnets, thereby attracting the best clinicians and the most grateful patients. This makes everyone's job easier. When was the last time you were acknowledged by your organization's leadership? And, because we believe in the saying that, 'what goes around comes around,' when was the last time you praised one of your co-workers for a job well done?

- **Knowledge** of the importance of the work and how it contributes to the organization's success. Believing in the mission is one thing, observing that the system makes its decisions based upon its mission, is another. For a position in healthcare to be more than a job, the individual must feel that it is part of their calling with an overarching meaning and purpose. Good leadership continually lets people know they are making a difference. This creates confidence in the organization's success.

- A **Style** that is open, honest and encompassing. Communicating any organizational imperative or change requires both clarity and context. None of us like the feeling that we are being sold a bill of goods. Yet all too often, organizations leap to selling the benefits of a new program, system, or initiative only to find resistance from the physician, nursing or staff groups. It is human nature to first want to understand the 'why,' before the 'what' and 'how.' Context is a prerequisite for understanding. How good is your organization at setting the stage for change? For providing the critical rationale that allows for buy in? Open and honest communication is essential. Clarity of communication needs to follow context. Physicians will attend to and believe in the message of leaders if they believe that doing so will benefit them in meaningful ways. The benefits may be more money, better time utilization, process improvement, or fewer errors and distractions.

Are you getting your PERKS? How healthy is your person-environment fit? How many of the five ingredients are you receiving and to what degree? If many of these nurturing factors are in place, you will have a better chance of implementing a set of evolutionary changes (if you so desire): working within the system to modify it. When all of these factors are absent, however, the best course of action may be revolutionary change; finding meaning and purpose within a different practice structure.

Stick it Out? Or Venture Out?

Considering that 50% of the marriages in the United States end in divorce, many healthcare providers have more than a passing acquaintance with the stages, pains, and sometimes, the benefits of the process. One of the most commonly searched Internet questions, and the one promoted by divorce attorneys, is "Should I stay or should I go?" For those disengaged physicians who are contemplating changing the nature and scope of their practice, these questions may provide some guidance:

- Can I make my current situation better? If so, how?
- Is it possible to improve interpersonal communication with administration, staff, and patients?
- Are there processes and procedures that could be streamlined to improve workflow, or better serve patients?
- What do I really want out of my practice? And, can I acquire it in my current arrangement?
- If I can't get my PERKs at work, are there ways I can find enough joy and satisfaction outside of medicine to keep me fulfilled?
- Can I reframe and adjust my perspective or appeal to a higher power to get by?
- If I improve my personal health and wellness skills, will this provide me with the stamina I need to handle the stress?
- Can I obtain support from friends, family, and members of my communities to buffer my negative feelings?
- Should I seek professional psychological help?
- Is this situation not going to get any better no matter what I do?
- Should I stay...or should I go?

Finding Your Calling Right Where You Are

Staying or going, in part, depends on how you view your work. One way to address this pivotal question is to ask yourself the type of questions routinely posed to workers by Yale psychologist Amy Wrzesniewski, PhD. Wrzesniewski categorizes one's relationship to work in three different ways: either as a calling, a career, or a job. The strongest alignment for professionals in healthcare is to view their work as a calling, and the majority start from this viewpoint. Wrzesniewski notes that there is often a precipitous slide away from viewing work as a calling, and instead seeing it either as a career or a job. The passion shown by idealistic young doctors, nurses, and therapists is eroded by the system. At worst, the profession becomes just another job, a way to make enough money to maintain a life that may provide joy outside the workplace.

For those who have identified their calling and are content to remain in their current practice situation but want improvement, it usually takes a healthy dose of vision and an even healthier dose of persuasion and persistence to effect positive organizational change.

This combination of attributes, along with a palpable passion for fitness, was the motivation for Robert Sallis, MD, a family medicine physician, to create a thriving culture for patient exercise within the Kaiser Permanente system. Sallis is the chairman of Exercise is Medicine®, a multi-organizational initiative coordinated by the American College of Sports Medicine and the American Medical Association, which was started in 2007 to encourage primary-care physicians and other health care providers to include exercise when designing treatment plans for patients. The result of his activity within Kaiser Permanente is the Exercise Vital Sign initiative. Sallis speaks to the need for a universal prescription and how he was able to champion its use throughout the Kaiser Permanente system.

> "In the same way that we routinely ask a patient if they smoke, we check their blood pressure, heart rate, and respiratory rate, and height and weight so we can calculate their BMI, so too must we ask about their exercise habits. No patient should leave the doctor's office without knowing they need to do 150 minutes of moderate exercise a week if they are an adult and 60 minutes a day if they are a kid. The message has to be the same from every provider. This isn't just a primary care problem. All specialists need to get behind this message. The goal of Exercise is Medicine is to make physical activity assessment and exercise prescription a standard part of the disease prevention and treatment paradigm around the world. It needs to be a part of routine medical practice and integrated into electronic medical records."

To back up his contention that the lack of fitness has reached epidemic proportions, Sallis notes that an entire recent edition of the medical journal *Lancet* was devoted to the global problem of physical inactivity and its adverse health effects. The concluding statement of this series of articles was that "in view of the prevalence, global reach, and health effect of physical inactivity, the issue should be appropriately described as pandemic, with far-reaching health, economic, environmental, and social consequences."[142]

The challenge with any good idea in medicine is to scale from the one-to-one assessment and individual intervention to the larger community care system. Sallis notes that this was not an easy task:

"My practices have been at Kaiser Permanente my entire career, and it was a big fight, but I was able to get this done and now every single one of our over 9 million patients gets asked how much they exercise at every visit whether they are going to the cardiologist, the gynecologist, or the allergist.

After they have taken the patient's blood pressure the medical assistant simply asks the patient two questions that they enter into the electronic medical record. 'On average how many days a week are you doing moderate exercise like a brisk walk?' They click 0-7 based on the patient's response. The following question is 'on those days how many minutes do you exercise at that level?' They click 10, 20, 30, 40, 50, so on. The computer then multiplies those responses together to give us a minutes per week of self-reported exercise. Those adults who are doing at least 150 minutes per week are labeled with a best practice alert encouraging the provider to mention to the patient, 'Good job I see you are doing 150 minutes a week.' For patients doing less than 150 minutes per week the alert encourages the physician to say something like, 'I notice today you are not doing any exercise and your blood pressure is high. Before we start you on a medication for high blood pressure, why don't we get you on a walking program? I want you to go down to the health store and buy a 5-dollar pedometer, give me 8-10 thousand steps a day, cut back on your salt. Before we go to medication, let's start that first."

CHAPTER THREE

The results of Sallis' initiative were explored in a published study that examined the electronic health records of 1,793,385 Kaiser Permanente Southern California patients ages 18 and older. It revealed that, "86 percent of all eligible patients had an exercise vital sign in their record. Of those patients who had an exercise record, one-third were meeting national guidelines for physical activity, and two-thirds were not meeting guidelines. Of those not meeting guidelines, one-third were not exercising at all."[143]

Having made a measureable improvement in the outpatient setting, Sallis set his sights on the inpatient experience.

> "Not surprisingly I noticed that when I round in the hospital my patients who just lie in bed don't do as well; when my patients get up and start walking they get discharged sooner. They also have fewer complications. In fact, study after study has backed up what I see everyday when I go on hospital rounds. That patients who get up and walk have shorter length of stay and fewer hospital related complications.
>
> I began looking for a monitor because we have no accurate way of measuring how often and for what distance patient ambulate. The standard process in most hospitals is an inquiry by the nurses: 'How many times did you get up? How many times did you walk around the ward?' And, since we know that it's 200 feet around the nurse's station, the nurses actually write that in the chart. 'The patient walked 5 times 200 feet, so he walked 1000 feet.' When we were able to actually monitor the patient's walking we found it wasn't even close; the nurse's estimates were completely wrong. So I started experimenting with monitors. First, I used a $30 Omron pedometer, but it wouldn't pick up very slow gate. Then I found an accelerometer by a company called Tractivity. It's a very simple device and inexpensive device, and it's reusable. We put it around a patient's ankle with a soft Velcro band. The activity sensor works via USB stick to the in-room hospital computer. It will automatically upload how many minutes and steps the patient took, so when I come in to round in the morning the first thing I do is take a look at the result."

Clearly, Sallis is in the "contented-staying" category. He has had success on a national and international level and been able to lead change efforts that are totally aligned with Kaiser Permanente's mission, vision, and image as the place where its members can *thrive*. For many physicians, however, the struggle for alignment of beliefs, values, strategy and culture with administration is a chronic wound with potential for either cure or sepsis.

Quantum Leaps in Systems Change

Is it possible for the culture of an entire healthcare system to change so it is more supportive of quality and well-being for all constituents? Stephen Beeson, MD, a board certified family medicine physician who began his career practicing with Sharp Rees-Stealy Medical group in San Diego, personalizes this question for physicians asking, "How can we create a physician experience that allows us to not only be successful as measured in traditional terms such as quality, cost, the patient experience and revenue, but also allows us to personally thrive?" Beeson shares many of our concerns about the pervasive cynicism in medicine eroding the common ground of a noble calling, and laments the fact that many physicians no longer get a chance to either be part of something great or do something great.

Beeson's road toward creating a model that integrated healthy organizational change and physician engagement began in 2002, when he was selected by Sharp HealthCare leadership to serve as a "physician champion for the Sharp Experience," a sweeping performance improvement initiative to improve care for patients, as well as the work environment for staff and physicians. The Sharp Experience has touched all facets of this not-for-profit integrated regional health care delivery system.

This initiative is notable both for its scope and its size. Sharp includes four acute-care hospitals, three specialty hospitals, two affiliated medical groups and a health plan, plus a full spectrum of other facilities and services in San Diego, California. Sharp has over 2,600 affiliated physicians and more than 16,000 employees. The Sharp Experience has resulted in numerous advances in clinical outcomes, patient safety, and organizational and service improvements. In 2007 Sharp was named a recipient of the Malcolm Baldrige National Quality Award.

In 2001, Sharp was a notably different organization than it is today. Bottom line, the Sharp Experience delivered results.

CHAPTER THREE

"We went from struggling financially to a healthy operating margin. We went from physicians leaving the organization to our highest physician satisfaction levels in the history of our group. We went from the 6th percentile in patient satisfaction to one of the highest in the state. We rebuilt the leadership by creating a high degree of accountability. We went from physician as passive observer and often victim, to team leader of the clinical microsystem.

Now at Sharp we have a code of conduct. Physicians are paid based on contributions to the group in quality, patient satisfaction and peer review metrics that supplement a productivity model. We have three visit types, down from over 50—new patients, established patients and physicals—to improve flow and improve access. We huddle with our teams in the morning to focus on efforts for the day. We are working as multi-disciplinary teams taking care of both individuals and populations of patients."

In his role as a physician champion, a leader who serves as both role model and change agent, and later as an author of two best-selling books, *Practicing Excellence* (Fire Starter Publishing) and *Engaging Physicians* (Fire Starter Publishing), Beeson's goal was clear.

"As the doctors go, so goes the healthcare organization. We are 80 cents of every dollar, 90% of clinical activity and a key influencer in the patient experience effort. If physicians aren't supporting, leading and contributing, an organization's capacity to do the work of today can be lost. Physician participation is vital for healthcare performance and culture, not only for the patients we serve, but for us and what it feels like to serve a common purpose, to make an impact, to work in high performing teams and to become the sort of physicians we thought we were going to be when we joined this profession in the first place. Our efforts are as much about revitalizing physicians as it is about improving health care delivery."

One technique to implement this movement involves the skill of coaching physicians to build skills in patient engagement, team leadership and high reliability/safety principles. In coaching thousands of doctors,

Beeson had the opportunity to streamline and scale the process. One of the techniques of coaching physicians included a method to assess physician coachability.

"What is their level of self awareness and insight? We have found self-awareness to be a key predictor to response to skill-building efforts and have designed approaches to optimize this. Sometimes the skill is how they include patients in decision-making, how to manage the narcotic seeking patient, how to manage a tough colleague or how to run a meeting. There are virtually hundreds of these skills we need to know. We have found over time that physicians' coachability has really improved and they are hungry to get better. Many have realized blaming others doesn't get the work done and want to get better for both their patients and teams."

Beeson is clear that coaching cannot be a standalone effort. It must be part of an active, comprehensive, organizational strategy to engage and enroll the care team around common ground efforts. To effect organizational change, the necessary skills must reach a critical mass of physicians as leaders of a shared effort built on what's best for patients, delivered on high performing team principles.

Knowing physicians were such a vital part of organizational change capacity, and that physicians were now responsible for skills most had never learned, Beeson founded, along with co-founder Larry McEvoy, MD, an emergency physician and healthcare executive, The Physician Effectiveness Project at PracticingExcellence.com (www.practicingexcellence.com). The Project is a CME certified web-based, interactive skill-building platform designed to advance physician effectiveness in patient centeredness, high performing teams, quality and safety, building collaborative group culture and building physician leadership and influence.

The Sharp Experience shows that meaningful organizational change is possible given the right players, process, persistence and a healthy dose of patience. The ever-changing nature of the healthcare environment, however, continually creates different pain points for systems and practitioners. Organizations change in response to new demands. Some of the changes are positive, others put practitioners at odds with the new reality. When clinicians interpret changes as a shift in the organization's

CHAPTER THREE

values, this can encourage them to take the leap and strike out on their own. Mimi likens this process to that of the trapeze artist who travels through the air with faith and courage as the only safety nets.

Mimi's Story: The Art of the Trapeze

Throughout the 90s I was involved in a great deal of research, however most of it was involved in testing the efficacy of novel cardiovascular devices. My days were spent jumping from cath lab to cath lab placing over 700 stents per year. On one of those days, I opened the cath lab door and was greeted by Dean Ornish, MD. Dean introduced himself and asked if I would be interested in a different type of research study.

Dean asked me to conduct a new study on the effects of an exercise regimen coupled with yoga, group support and a vegetarian diet for patients with significant cardiovascular disease. I listened to the research proposal and thought it was crazy. It wasn't my paradigm; as an interventional cardiologist I had a 'toolbox' of mechanical procedures, and prevention was not in that toolbox. And my education hadn't helped: medical school did not focus on prevention, it focused on diagnosis and treatment.

There is a saying that "When the student is ready the teacher appears." So I was talked into doing this research study—or so I felt at the time—and suddenly I was thrust into this vulnerable position of studying something I knew nothing about. How could I have made it through Internal Medicine at Cornell and two Cardiovascular fellowships and know nothing about nutrition, exercise or mind-body medicine? I did what any physician would do; I found an incredibly smart ICU nurse who was also a Transcendental Meditator of 20 plus years to do the research with me. But I knew that if I didn't personally and actively participate, I would be stuck in the position of studying something I didn't understand. So I became a vegetarian, and started to do yoga and meditation. Basically, I needed to walk the talk if I was going to teach patients about the same practices we were telling them to adopt.

We spent a lot of time with patients and families for this study, and we began to hear their stories. Thoroughly listening to a patient's story is something you rarely do in medicine. We met with families and observed the family dynamics; we got to understand our patients. For the first time I understood what Osler meant when he said, "It is more important to know the patient that has a disease than what disease the patient has." Through a regimen of yoga, meditation, group support, diet and exercise, I saw the magic begin to occur.

What we saw in these patients, and their families was nothing short of transformative. In many ways it was a down right miracle. We observed the things that I expected to see: people lost weight, their blood pressure dropped, and so on. But what I didn't expect was how people began viewing their lives through a different lens. At the beginning of the program our conversations were centered around losing weight and cutting out refined carbohydrates. By the end of the year, participants made the deeper connections between behaviors and the practices that were making them sick. They began talking about how they really wanted to live their lives, what truly mattered and what was their purpose in life.

We witnessed families and relationships being healed. As doctors, we sometimes forget that when someone is sick, it affects the entire family, because everyone is so deeply involved. So we observed this healing take place at a family level. We also learned the power of love and support. Our groups were called cohorts; they were bands of warriors. People made friends for life. They laughed, cried, prayed and meditated together.

As the patients healed so did I. My total cholesterol level dropped from 320 to 100 as a result of the lifestyle changes I had made. I was doing yoga and meditating on a routine basis. Not only was I seeing a transformation in my patients, I was also seeing a transformation in myself.

I started comparing these experiences to what I would see in my role as an interventional cardiologist: the hospital serving roast beef sandwiches to patients recovering from high-tech interventions, serving mashed potatoes to diabetics. I thought to myself, "What are we doing? We are intervening, but we're not preventing disease." More importantly, why hadn't I made this connection earlier?

In medicine, we don't take on medical studies in a vacuum: the purpose is for us to improve the medical care that we offer, to learn how to become better healers. So what did I learn from this study, and from my transformation and that of my patients? I learned that our model of medicine is very good at acute care, but what we're bad at is preventing disease in the first place. The way I was trained was a "pill for the ill;" our emphasis was surgery and drugs. We were waiting for people to

CHAPTER THREE

break down before we treated them. We were treating bodies, not people.

At one point I sat down and made a list of all the ways I was trained versus what a more holistic integrative approach would offer: a reactive approach versus a proactive approach; addressing symptoms versus finding the underlying cause of an ailment; having power and control as a physician versus empowering others; treating bodies versus healing body, mind and spirit. I began exploring ways to heal my patients, drawing lessons not only from Western medicine but also from all Global Healing traditions.

This exploration lead to my being asked to give a lecture at Scripps called "East Meets West." I was asked to talk about some of the integrative medicine techniques I had been learning. This was the first time any such lecture had been given at Scripps, and I fully expected that it would not be well received. But I felt guided to take on this challenge. And so I gave the lecture, all the while expecting a tepid response. Not only did I receive a standing ovation but a gentleman stood up and said: "I will give you $500,000 to start this type of program at Scripps because I have just been waiting for a physician to talk about healing the whole person, body, mind and spirit."

Rauni Prittinen King, RN, and I founded the Scripps Center for Integrative Medicine in 1997 and l served as medical director for 15 years. The center grew, but I was still working as an interventionist cardiologist, putting in my 700 stents a year. I began to ask myself the question: do I stay or do I go? The Center needed my energy, but if I gave up stenting I gave up my livelihood. I was trying to do it all, but I couldn't.

I felt like I was a trapeze artist, swinging back and forth, unsure whether to reach out and grasp that next trapeze bar. I knew I needed to move forward, but I dreaded the moment of free-fall.

I couldn't make the decision to go, so my body decided for me. As a result of the hours upon hours of wearing lead aprons during stent procedures, my back was deteriorating. I went in for a CT scan, and was told to have three bulging discs. Surgery was recommended; I said no! I'm putting down the lead apron and hanging up my balloons. I went to our yoga teacher and talked with her about how to strengthen my core. I never had the surgery. My back healed; and I reached out and grabbed the next trapeze bar.

I began putting my full energy into the Center and lecturing all over the country to raise the level of awareness of holistic integrative medicine. I lectured to physicians, nurses, patients and anyone that would listen.

While I took joy in spreading this message around the country, I confronted some challenges on the home front. I realized it's one thing to have a beautiful building, and calling it an IM Center, and another to having a center that fulfills a mission of healing and functions smoothly as a business. Early on, we struggled financially due to the lack of insurance reimbursement and the need to meet our $1 million annual rent. Administration encouraged us to raise donor money and that we did; millions of dollars. Grateful patients began to provide grants for everything from exercise equipment to CT scanners. We created a truly unique integrative program and even coined the term 'Integrative Cardiology.' Our patients had the best of high tech and high touch. What a journey!

It wasn't long before we realized we needed the help of more health professionals trained in Holistic Integrative Medicine. We initiated programs for training and education both physicians and patients. Through my mentor, Lee Lipsenthal, MD, I joined the American Board of Integrative Holistic Medicine. Here I found my tribe—physicians and health practitioners dedicated to healing, filled with compassion and not afraid to love.

We built out the Scripps IM Center and it became a beacon of light; a model for the world. But with this success came pressures from the administration to transform the Center into a profit-making enterprise. I increasingly began to notice that the administration was pursuing a very different agenda from my own, and their vision was not attractive to me: physicians seeing 20 people a day, administrators measuring our yoga room to convert it into offices, a practice model that eschewed the inter-disciplinary approach that is so essential to the IM model. Their philosophy was not my philosophy. I increasingly felt that the system didn't value or understand what we were doing. So despite our success at Scripps I knew it was time to leave.

Again I felt myself swinging on a trapeze. I began to wonder, do I stay or do I go? And to help answer this question, I asked myself what I was trying to do. What was my mission in life? My vision is "healing people and changing lives through science and compassion." I couldn't do that in a fifteen-minute appointment. Institutionalized medicine felt toxic to me. As one physician said "I am fast or fired; we eat what we kill." And since that was the model that Scripps was embracing, I decided to move on.

Fortunately, my path has always been guided. As I made the decision to leave Scripps, the Atlantic Health System in New Jersey called and invited me to help create a visionary 20,000 sq. foot center for Well Being. At the same time, the Taylor Family Foundation offered me an endowment to form the Academy of Integrative Health and Medicine. The universe opened the doors to my next adventure.

But I love my patients. I was not ready to just be a consultant. I still needed a home for my own IM practice. Again the universe intervened and the perfect building appeared on the market. Pacific Pearl La Jolla is my new home. With the unfailing help and support of Rauni Prittinen King, we were able to create a new model of Integrative Health and Medicine combining the best of naturopathic and conventional medicine with complementary and alternative health practices. At the Pearl, I am free to build the type of innovative practice model that focuses on education and empowerment, not just for our patients, but for the community and our medical colleagues.

The Drivers of Discontent vs. Desire

Mimi's story provides a glimpse into the process by which we choose to initiate major changes in our lives. This is a process that has been subjected to much study within the profession of psychology. Roy Baumeister, PhD, a professor of psychology at Florida State University in Tallahassee, Florida proposed that, as part of the change process, individuals undergo a process of realization called the crystallization of discontent. Crystallization of discontent occurs when our normal coping mechanisms cease being capable of maintaining the perspective that the 'pros' of a situation outweigh the 'cons'. Much of this crystallization revolves around the realization that the future is not going to improve if a person continues down the same path; in fact, it may even become worse.

This moment of realization is both painful and insightful. It can also become the catalyst to initiate positive life change, as the following story indicates.

Steven Bengelsdorf, MD, FACS, is a board certified general surgeon with a thriving cosmetic surgery practice in Franklin, Tennessee, a suburb of Nashville. But this was not always the case. For part of his career, he was a locum tenens surgeon who traveled to rural parts of the country to aid smaller communities struggling with a lack of general surgery coverage.

Like many physicians, Bengelsdorf takes great pleasure in forging positive patient relationships. His reward for hours of grueling general surgery was simple: reasonable compensation for his services, and occasionally, a "thank you" from a grateful patient or family.

As hospital politics increased and remuneration and autonomy decreased, he was still able to find motivation in his noble work, but even that began to erode as patient expectations and behaviors soured and physicians were cast as impersonal providers.

He recounts a moment when these new realities became painfully evident.

> "I had performed a long and complicated surgery on an elderly lady who was critically ill. She survived the procedure and made steady improvement. A week later, I mentioned to her nurse that I believed she was almost ready to be discharged.
>
> I had never been able to get in contact with anyone from her family. Later that afternoon, I received a call from the patient's daughter, who was quite irate. She began yelling at me that her mother was not ready to come home, and that there will be 'hell to pay' if she were discharged. I continued to listen, allowing her to unload on me, for what felt like a very long time.
>
> When I finally had the opportunity to speak, I replied, 'Ma'am, I'm the surgeon who went to the Emergency Department at 2 AM, saw your mother, took her for emergency surgery, and saved her life. I am the one who rounded on her every day in the Intensive Care Unit. I am the one who transferred her to the floor when she was well enough, and saw her every single day since then. I am the one who is involved in planning for her release. Do you honestly think that I would allow her to be discharged prematurely from the

hospital if I didn't think she was well enough to leave?' I then took the opportunity to simply express how hurt I was by her comments. Her tantrum ended and she seemed somewhat apologetic for her remarks. The next day I was approached by a hospital administrator and asked about the interaction. The daughter had called and made a complaint."

Bengelsdorf notes that in the past, physicians had an unwritten contract with society. He states:

"We gave up some of the best years our lives and underwent grueling training to learn to take care of people. We put our patients' health and needs before our own. We often did not charge people who could not afford to pay us for our services. In return, we were supposed to be treated with a modicum of respect and some gratitude. That contract has been violated."

As time went on, Bengelsdorf adapted his skills and knowledge of surgery to elective cosmetic procedures. He opened a small office specializing in aesthetic medicine and laser surgery. Now, Bengelsdorf is able to perform procedures for patients who appreciate his attention to detail and artistry. He is compensated for his time and expertise, as is any professional, and is able to do what is best for his patients without worrying about insurance companies and hospital drama. And he takes the time to volunteer every other week at a local clinic where he performs surgery for the indigent, pro bono.

Bengelsdorf's story illuminates a bit more of the process by which a physician's discontent can crystalize, indicating the necessity for change. Discontent can only show us that change is necessary. But there is still a question unanswered: change to what? Answering that question requires a crystallization of desire, a realization of what you want. This realization will make much clearer the path you need to take.

A Different Approach

Psychologist Jack Bauer, PhD, of the University of Dayton has explored the concept of 'approach orientation' versus 'avoidance orientation.' An individual who uses avoidance orientation focuses on the movement away from an undesired outcome, while one who uses an approach orientation focuses on the movement toward a desired outcome. His studies demonstrated that those whose decision narrative—their stories about a life-changing decision they made—emphasized a crystallization of desire were more likely to have higher levels of life satisfaction than those whose stories emphasized their crystallization of discontent. Different studies of Bauer's also indicated better decision outcomes and lower levels of neuroticism for those with aspirational stories.[144]

Such studies are useful, but not entirely unexpected: it is intuitive that human beings prefer to define our own lives as a process of following our own desires, rather than simply responding to the atmosphere around us.

As chief justice Oliver Wendell Holmes, Jr. once noted, "The great thing in this world is not so much where you stand, as in what direction you are moving." It does not serve you to dwell on what you are trying to give up; the real benefit comes from creating a picture of what could be ahead.

So what do you want to be ahead for you? If your path lies within the clinical practice of medicine, you may wish to cast your mind back to previous times in your life when the way became suddenly clear, when you had a vision for your own future. For many of us, this moment may have come at, or right before, the beginning of medical school. We all had to write a personal statement, a personal narrative about who we were and why we wanted to be a doctor. We had a vision that carried us, that illuminated our path forward and that brought us to medical school.

Or your vision may have crystalized as you chose your specialty. You decided on a course of action, on a specialty, a focus. Now all of a sudden your professional life had direction and purpose. Ambiguity and uncertainty were gone. Something attracted you, fascinated you, or made complete sense to you. You were being pulled by your vision of who and what you would become in medicine. For a growing number of physicians, this vision is intimately tied to an integrative medicine focus for their practice.

Moving to IM

Making the move to integrative medicine is one of the many ways to restructure your practice to be more in synch with a wellness philosophy. One must not assume that creating an IM practice is a panacea for

CHAPTER THREE

all that ails you, nor that simply advertising your integrative services will have patients flocking to your door. There are both market and personal forces at work. Several of the ABIHM/AHMA survey respondents wrote in about their frustrations both within and outside the system.

> I am initiating, as one person, changes in an academic medical center that has been very resistant to change. But over time I have increased student education and see very complicated challenging patients (at virtually no insurance reimbursement--hence the switch to cash-based for my practice within an otherwise contract-based insurance driven practice). I am not allowed to sell products, bill for phone consultations, Skype, etc. and not allowed to email, text, or otherwise use social media (all based on HIPAA fears). When I do group meetings or courses, I am not allowed to charge patients. So making ends meet financially is impossible. So I feel my institution (and perhaps all of medicine) has a ways to go to understand how people get work done and communicate nowadays.

> I left private IM practice because I just could not do everything required in a fee for service practice, even though a large % was cash based. This is a lower income area and paying cash for medical practice just does not compute. In addition, there is a lot of competition from chiropractors; massage therapists and self described health coaches. I was making enough money but working very long hours. Now I'm in a community health clinic. I still do acupuncture and I still do recommendations for supplements and health coaching but I no longer have to worry about the overhead and administrative hassles.

The overwhelming number of participants, however described the joy they obtain from their practice as exemplified by this survey response.

> I began integrating complementary therapies into my practice from the beginning. I knew there was more that I could be doing for patients. I love to connect with patients- partner with them for their health but I too gain from that relationship. It is better than a paycheck to receive confirmation from patients that they are more empowered and healthier because they came to see me. I couldn't just practice without that component of relationship and caring in healing. When I was in a traditional setting, I would try to fit in my integrative therapies, now I get to start there. I can never go back even if I had to go back to a traditional setting, I wouldn't change how I work. They would need to change to fit

me in, not the other way around. I feel more energy, wiser (that sounds egotistical but not meant to be), happier, more helpful to patients and my colleagues. It's the proverbial "sweet spot."

These types of stories were supported by the survey results. For the 150 physicians who changed from a conventional practice to an IM practice, their self-reported levels of happiness doubled, going from 4.4 on a ten point scale to 8.8. They rated their levels of engagement higher as well, going from 6.5 to close to 9.

The ABIHM/AHMA survey also showed that it may be possible to 'stay' and 'go' at the same time. Only 36% of the respondents reported they were in an Integrative Medicine/Holistic practice; an equal number said they were in a conventional practice, but using integrative medicine techniques. Another 10% were in a conventional practice but interested in incorporating IM.

Choosing the Path

Just as we followed our vision into the practice of medicine, so too must we follow our vision if it leads us either to a new professional synthesis or outside of clinical practice altogether. What would you do with your life if you knew you could not fail? If any and all barriers were removed? How would you spend your time? And with whom would you spend it? There is a way to begin removing these barriers and clearing the way toward meaningful change. It is the path of courage.

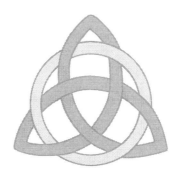

Sign seen at the counter of our favorite coffee shop reads, "Afraid of change? Leave it here."

4
The Courage to Change

A simple ritual occurs at the beginning of many yoga classes across the country. The instructor encourages participants to set an 'intention' for their practice, something to focus on or reinforce during the ensuing hour. A similar type of activity occurs in houses of worship as individuals pray for guidance and direction from a higher power. We'd like to suggest that physicians contemplating change consider courage as their intention or that which they think about, meditate on or pray for. Courage is central to empowerment and accomplishment; it is also critical for happiness. If you have courage in life and work, you will be better prepared for the changes thrust upon you and those you initiate.

We are not talking about the heroic, adrenaline fueled physical type of courage of a Medal of Honor winner, or that exhibited by the fireman who rushes into a burning building to save a child. There is another type of courage, one that is aligned with the inner work of personal understanding and growth. This inner courage exists in five forms, exemplified by the physician-told stories that follow.

1. The Courage to Look Inward

The unexamined life is not worth living.

—Socrates

We live in a society that places greater emphasis on action than introspection. This is especially true for the busy physician who rarely works only forty hours a week. Each day we are subject to the multiple demands of our patients, each of whom commands attention and a care plan. Healthcare decision-making takes place within the compressed time window of the office visit or hospital round; we rely on protocols and algorithms for efficiency. Patients expect us to do something. This penchant for action is often at the expense of stepping back and looking at the big picture. The most common lament we hear from physicians

CHAPTER FOUR

is that they are so immersed in the day to day running of their practice and caring for patients that they have little time for anything else, little time to look inward.

Every major change process begins with honesty and introspection. We all know happiness comes from within, but you have to find your passion. You have to have a reason to get up in the morning. You have to really be honest about whether or not you still have that passion. Are you thriving or just surviving? We see a lot of physicians who are overeating, over-smoking, over doing everything. We encourage you to examine your life with the same analytical, detached skillset you use to diagnose your patients.

Start by taking inventory and ask yourself the tough questions:
- Where am I at? Physically? Mentally? Emotionally? Spiritually?
- What are my core values?
- What is my personal mission statement? Do I even have one?
- What is important to me?
- Whom do I serve?

Draw a Venn diagram of how you are spending your time. Is this time allocation in synch with your core values? Are you spending too much time in front of screens? Are you saying yes when you should be saying no? Are your financial affairs in order?

This taking inventory step is a great time to remember, reaffirm and reset your priorities. Physicians often put the urgent in the way of the important. The important elements of life are health, family, and relationships, yet managing life is an exercise in juggling balls. You can juggle a lot of balls. You drop the ball labeled work, and it bounces back. You drop the ball labeled family or health and it may crack never to be repaired.

With your values and mission clarified, you can begin to identify your passion and purpose. Begin by asking yourself two questions: What am I really good at? And what will people pay me for? Mimi asked herself these questions when she stopped putting in stents and identified that she was a great teacher and a great communicator. She found her overwhelming passion for holism and Integrative Medicine and realized that she had the power to craft a successful practice and lifestyle outside of

Scripps. She also realized she had the skills to aggregate and inspire her healthcare colleagues. Mark identified that he wanted his life work to revolve around synergy, the convergence, expression, and communication of ideas that yield more than additive results. His personal passion for the last 30 years has centered on understanding the factors that keep people mentally strong and resilient. With the passing of each decade, he has deepened and evolved his message to be more inclusive.

This process of introspection or finding one's true purpose in life is summarized in the Venn diagram below.

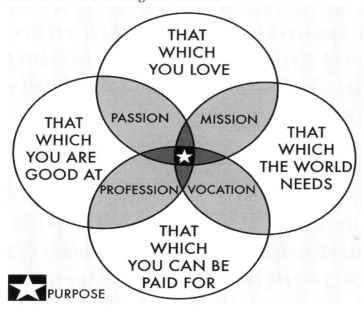

Figure 10: Finding Your Purpose

The circle labeled "that which the world needs" holds particular significance for physicians. It encompasses the altruistic nature inherent in the medical profession. The desire to help and heal others drives physicians toward noble deeds: performing cleft palette surgery in developing countries, volunteering in clinics for underserved populations, fighting for women's health or clean water issues, or providing medical services to those in crisis. Physicians gain as much, perhaps even more from the richness of these experiences than do the recipients of their efforts.

Such was the case for Dore Gilbert, MD, a board certified dermatologist, who left his successful Newport Beach dermatology practice to

CHAPTER FOUR

serve for one year on the front lines in Afghanistan.

Gilbert traces his passion for military service back to 1984 when he first realized he had a deep desire to serve his country because "so much has been given to me." At this stage in Gilbert's life, military service was not a reality, "I would have lost my home, my practice, plus my wife didn't sign up for this," he states. Gilbert channeled his interest in service into other community related areas serving on the school board of education for 29 years, coaching little league and junior hockey. Still, every time he read a book about war or conflict, he felt that stab of guilt that he should serve. When his fifth child joined the Marine Corps, he inquired about enlisting as well.

Gilbert learned he was qualified to join the armed forces until the age of 60. One month short of the qualifying age, he completed all the necessary paperwork just under the deadline. It took 14 months for him to receive his commission, as it required Senate approval, background checks and ample paperwork.

Although he was not required to do so, Gilbert decided he would participate in basic training at Fort Sam Houston. To ready himself, he started doing hundreds of push-ups and sit-ups each morning, working out at the gym and going on timed runs. Looking back, he recognizes that basic training was one of the best experiences of his life.

In 2011 Gilbert volunteered for deployment in Afghanistan where he served along with his son. Functioning as a brigade surgeon, he was thrown into an environment 180 degrees removed from his highly controllable and predictable dermatology practice. Arriving in the war zone, he was immediately in charge of health care for 10,000 soldiers. The experience varied from day to day. It could be mundane, or intense and terrifying.

One thing that Gilbert points to with pride is a "walking blood bank" program he initiated after learning that the base did not store blood. In the event of large-scale casualties from a rocket attack, for example, blood transfusion would only be available to the wounded after evacuation to the regional trauma center. Recognizing the need for a better system, Gilbert asked the commanding general to volunteer to have his blood typed and cross-matched. Every other soldier did the same. Keeping the program really simple, Gilbert elected to use a numbering system for the different blood types. For example, those with blood type

O positive were given numbers 1-40, type A positive 41-50. The numbers were inscribed on a second set of dog tags worn by the soldiers. In this way, fresh blood was always available in the event of a disaster, to be obtained from the appropriately numbered donor.

Gilbert is modest about his accomplishments, and when asked about the benefits he reaped from his service, he notes that, "It relieved me of that feeling of guilt that I never served. In fact, this was the only thing in my life that had really bothered me." But his eyes really begin to light up when he talks about his ability to work with "very committed young men and women who are performing at their best in very difficult situations."

2. The Courage to Be Uncertain

For the great enemy of truth is very often not the lie—deliberate, contrived and dishonest—but the myth—persistent, persuasive and unrealistic. Too often we hold fast to the clichés of our forebears. We subject all facts to a prefabricated set of interpretations. We enjoy the comfort of opinion without the discomfort of thought.

—John F. Kennedy, Yale Commencement, 1962

At the recent annual meeting of the Institute for Functional Medicine (IFM), we overheard the following conversation between two primary care physician attendees. When one asked the other, "How are you doing?" the response was, "Just trying to figure out what I'm going to do when I grow up," to which the other shook his head in agreement and added "me too."

Once you venture outside the rigid boundaries of conventional medicine, you enter into the zone of uncertainty. The psychological safety of evidenced based medicine, while emerging for alternative treatments, is not yet well established. There is more grey and less black or white. Most people, physicians included, don't do well with uncertainty and its attendant stress. Part of the courage to change comes with the ability to handle uncertainty as depicted in Mark's story below.

I remember the moment when my (Mark) dissatisfaction with traditional medicine crystallized. I was in my first year of a family practice residency at the University of Oregon Health Sciences Center in

CHAPTER FOUR

Portland, Oregon. Graduating from Duke University School of Medicine in 1974, I was one of only two physicians in our class who chose the nascent specialty of Family Medicine. I was enthralled by the concept of treating the whole family across the spectrum of illness and wellness.

I was taking care of an elderly woman with disseminated ovarian cancer. She was on a morphine drip and only had a few hours or days to live. When she stopped her output of urine, my resident instructed me to get an IVP to see if the tumors had invaded her GU system. I looked at him incredulously, and remarked, "Do you really want to have this elderly woman spend some of her last hours on a cold gurney, waiting in the hallway, going through the rigors of an IVP just to satisfy your curiosity?" I refused to do it. He took over the case. The patient died shortly after having her IVP. My idealistic balloon of whole person care was quickly deflated.

At this point I already had preventive/wellness leanings. I had become ill with hepatitis A in medical school and housed in the infirmary. I reflected on the fact that between the cigarettes, the fast food, the stress and the lack of exercise, the practice of medicine was likely to lead to my early demise. I took up yoga, adopted a vegetarian diet, worked with a Duke biochemistry professor to create an elective program for medical students in nutrition, trained barefoot doctors in Guatemala, and started keeping a journal.

By the time I had reached the point of the contentious IVP, (and had experienced a number of other similar events), I realized what I didn't want to do. I didn't want to practice conventional medicine. When I left my residency I had no clue what path to take. I was certainly uncertain.

In the late 1970s there were very few role models to which I could turn. Fortunately, a budding movement built around a concept of "wellness" articulated by San Francisco area physician John Travis, MD, and promoted by a handful of other doctors, was just starting to take hold.

As I tried to envision a way to integrate wellness in my work, I asked myself, "If I had a significant health related issue, what type of care would I want? I realized I'd want significant time to be evaluated by and discuss the problem with a physician, and then I'd want to learn what I could do to stay well. Along with another physician, two psychologists, and a massage therapist, in 1977, I founded The Institute of Preventive Medicine in Portland, Oregon. I saw patients for an hour at a time helping them make connections between their lifestyle, emotions and health. I referred them to my colleagues. Together we taught classes in nutrition, movement therapy, yoga, emotional health, fitness, and stress management. Around that time I co-authored my first book, *Whole Person Health Care* with Charles Jennings, a gifted writer. The book advocated a holistic approach and also included a list of holistic practitioners in the Pacific Northwest.

Several years later, my work came to the attention of Marvin Goldberg, MD, then CEO of the Permanente Medical Group in Portland, Oregon. Goldberg challenged me to take the wellness concept to the next level. His goal was simple, when any consumer/member in the Oregon region mentioned the word "wellness," the immediate response should be, "Oh, you mean Kaiser Permanente." It is heartening to see this philosophy embedded in Kaiser's creative and engaging THRIVE campaign today. Goldberg's plan was to have me serve as a health promotion consultant across the region.

Going from a small holistic medical practice to an organization of several thousand healthcare professionals, I was thrust into the realm of uncertainty again. I knew nothing of organizational behavior, professional training and development, occupational health, or managed care. The expectation was that I had to leverage whatever raw talents I had and try to make them scale. I worked on acquiring greater communication skills and started producing videos and programming for a local radio station. Conducting presentations and trainings I realized that I could easily bore people by lecturing at them; instead, I started crafting exercises and activities that fostered introspection and created the 'AHAs' that moved attendees toward greater understanding and personal transformation. I realized that I needed to develop better team-building skills, so I reached out to several trusted colleagues and asked them to help improve my group facilitation techniques.

Toward the end of my career at Kaiser I started looking at the critical role that leaders play in health and wellness and how bad bosses can make people sick and good ones keep people engaged, mentally and physically well. I worked with Marjorie Blanchard, PhD, to develop the first book and training program on how leadership affects the health/productivity connection. I went on to found a consumer/provider wellness publishing company that I ran for ten years and grew to 60 employees before its acquisition by Mosby Yearbook, at that time, the largest medical publishing company in the United States.

Since then, I've invested time and energy consulting, writing and teaching in areas of regenerative medicine, resilience, aesthetics, nutraceuticals, cosmeceuticals, and clinical laboratory services. I have leveraged a passion for Asia into a handful of speaking and training projects.

After conducting more than 700 seminars, workshops and corporate retreats in my 40 years of wellness exploration, I still find that I am enthralled by the power of transformation that occurs in the group setting. This is the work that energizes me. It also humbles me. I know I am not changing people, they change when they are ready. Some part of my message resonates with them. Something we have said or done in the training program sparks them to take action. I am honored to play a minor role in this process.

About every three years, I find an interesting colleague to collaborate with and together we create a book on a subject of mutual interest. Mimi defines the 'interesting colleague' category. I find great joy in the process of identifying synergies, creating new models, and then communicating that synthesis to health care professionals and consumers.

To this day, I am still uncertain as to my future. The joke is that most people—my family included—don't really know what I do. I frequently introduce myself as an MDADHD. But I know what I am capable of doing because of the transferable skills I have gained and this provides me the courage to venture into realms of uncertainty.

3. The Courage to Admit You Don't Have All the Answers

It ain't what
you don't know
that gets you
into trouble.
It's what you know for sure
that just ain't so.

—Mark Twain

All of us like to be right. Whether inside or outside of medicine, the higher up you are in the chain of command, the more you are in a position of knowledge and power, the more likely your identity is invested in always having the right answer. We see this hierarchy physically depicted in the rigidity of the staff meeting where each physician team member has a pre-designated seat around the table. We observe the exaggerated need to have all the answers exhibited when conventionally oriented physicians are asked questions by patients that are outside their knowledge base. "What about nutritional supplements, herbs, acupuncture, or chiropractic?" Historically, medical physicians in large part have dismissed these types of questions because they themselves have not investigated these complementary areas. Some may hold views that are stridently against such practices.

I know for me (Mimi) this was true for many years. I truly believed I was curing cardiovascular disease with my stents and statins. It never occurred to me that I was never getting to the underlying problem, but just "mopping up the mess."

The Science Based Medicine organization (SBM) is a group of physicians that focus on evidence based medicine, and as such, takes a dim view of many CAM practices. For example, with regard to acupuncture, they classify it a pre-scientific superstition that lacks a plausible mechanism of action. Furthermore, they believe that acupuncture claims for efficacy are based upon a bait and switch deception. SBM also points to the acupuncture trials that show acupuncture does not work.[145]

Noting the poor design and over promotion of acupuncture studies, and the fact that many studies have been done by "enthusiastic practitioners rather than trained researchers," the National Institutes of Health (NIH) convened a consensus panel to review the available literature about acupuncture. The NIH Consensus Panel concluded that acupuncture was proven to be evidence-based for two indications: dental pain and nausea (postsurgical, chemotherapy induced, or nausea related to pregnancy). Their panel concluded that "it was time to take acupuncture seriously and that their systematic review of the literature indicated that it might also be useful for a longer list of indications but that better-designed studies were needed to confirm its utility in these areas."[146]

The need for better-designed studies, better data, and, most importantly, better clinical practice patterns is not unique to CAM. A report in the *British Medical Journal: Clinical Evidence* examined approximately

2,500 conventional medical treatments covered by national health insurance. The survey rated 13% of the treatments as beneficial, 23% likely to be beneficial, 8% as trade off between benefits and harms, 6% unlikely to be beneficial, 4% likely to be ineffective or harmful, and 46%, the largest proportion, as unknown effectiveness.[147]

The most blatant disregard of evidence can be found in the continued off-label use of pharmaceutical drugs. Off-label use of pharmaceutical agents is practiced by physicians around the globe, and involves all categories of medication. In cancer treatment in the United States, 45% of cancer patients receive at least one unapproved drug.[148] In a Canadian study that examined more than 250,000 prescriptions over four years, the prevalence of off-label use was 11.0% with 79.0% lacking strong scientific evidence. Most revealing was the prevalence of off-label use for CNS drugs with the following percentages lacking an approved indication: anticonvulsants (66.6%), antipsychotics (43.8%), and antidepressants (33.4%).[149]

Perhaps the largest gap between clinical practice and evidence is revealed in antibiotic prescribing practices. In a recently released study reported in *JAMA*, Jeffrey Linder, MD, and his team at Brigham and Women's Hospital examined the data for an estimated 39 million acute bronchitis and 92 million sore throat visits by adults to primary care clinics or emergency departments from 1996 through 2010. According to Linder, "Our research shows that while only 10 percent of adults with sore throat have strep, the only common cause of sore throat requiring antibiotics, the national antibiotic prescribing rate for adults with sore throat has remained at 60 percent. For acute bronchitis, the right antibiotic prescribing rate should be near zero percent and the national antibiotic prescribing rate was 73 percent."[150] Inappropriate antibiotic use is fueling the growth of bacterial strains resistant to multiple antibiotics.

With regard to the mechanism of action of both alternative and conventional remedies, treatments that show some clinical efficacy are often in widespread use before science and technology can elucidate how they work. Rheumatism has been treated for hundreds of years with decoctions or extracts of willow bark or leaves that contain salicylates. In 1893, following the creation of synthetic salicylate by Felix Hoffman, of the Bayer company in Germany, Aspirin was born. Yet, the mechanism of action of this wonder drug was not determined till 1971, when British pharmacologist John Robert Vane showed how NSAIDs inhibit the activity of cyclooxygenase thereby blocking the formation of prostaglandins that cause inflammation, swelling, pain and fever.[151] Only recently has science uncovered that statins may also exert their benefits by decreasing inflammation.[152] Until the fMRI was developed, scientists were at a loss for explaining how mood changes and mental perception could be affected by changes in heart rate variability.[153]

Respecting the Voice of the Patient

The debate about the efficacy and the evidence of any and all treatment modalities will continue to rage. What is important is that the voice of the patient does not get lost in the debate. When physicians discount or dismiss the possibility of alternative paths, they erode the faith that patients have for self-healing, a health determinant known as self-efficacy.

There is extensive literature to support how the patient- as opposed to the physician-centered model improves healthcare outcomes.[154] The Institute of Medicine has included patient-centered care as 1 of the 6 aims of quality. This shift in empowerment is behind The Patient Centered Medical Home, a primary care initiative that emphasizes coordination of care and teamwork in treatment. Multiple studies have shown that higher patient self-efficacy leads to better outcomes.[155] For example, it has been shown that patients undergoing coronary artery bypass surgery recover better if they have higher self-efficacy.[156] Patient-physician partnership is one of the keys to improving patients' sense of self-efficacy and ultimately their health outcomes.

Patients with high self-efficacy tend to gravitate toward and fare best when they are matched with physicians who view healthcare as a partnership. Both patient and physician enjoy a more satisfying encounter. On the other had "If these patients encounter clinicians who behave in an authoritative, non-collaborative way, they will feel thwarted and diminished."[157] Psychologists Diana Dill, PhD, and Peter Gumpert, PhD, note "Clinicians who do not succeed in partnering with their patients to take control of their health lose a therapeutic opportunity."[158]

We believe that an essential component of this partnering involves taking into account and respecting the patient's belief systems for healing even if they differ from the clinician's. It takes courage to admit you don't have all the answers, and it takes a healthy dose of listening to

CHAPTER FOUR

patients to find meaning in their narrative. Sometimes patients must awaken their physicians and get them off cruise control.

Craig Brandman, MD, an interventional cardiologist in San Francisco and now founder of StepOne Health (www.steponehealth.com) discusses the moment when "a door opened to the path that I am now moving down in terms of understanding how it is that we most effectively interact with our patients." Brandman had agreed to see the wife of one of his cardiology patients for a non-cardiac problem, and according to Brandman:

> "I was beginning to go down my traditional top down, paternalistic 'I'm the Doctor, do what I say' mode of interacting with her, and she stopped me. She said, 'I've already got some ideas about what I want to do about this problem. I think I want to pursue an Eastern medical solution to my problem.' I must have reflexively rolled my eyes and she stopped me and said 'Craig, you western allopathic doctors have been doing this for what, 50 years? And they've been doing it in China successfully for larger groups of people than you guys do for two or three thousand years. And of course you western guys think you know more than they do in China and have no respect for some of the Eastern solutions to problems that trouble everybody.' I realized at that moment that she was completely right. If I was going to be successfully interacting with my patients going forward, I had to open my mind about how I was going to look at what they were telling me and provide them the opportunity to understand what choices were available to address their health and wellness issues."

Confronting the limitations of conventional medicine, and driven by genuine caring, an increasing number of physicians are beginning to look for alternative complementary approaches for conditions that do not respond well to conventional approaches. Writing in his blog, David Katz, MD, MPH, Director, Yale University Prevention Research Center, noted,

> "Clinical decisions are easy if a treatment is known to be dangerous and ineffective, or known to be safe and uniquely effective. But what if a given patient has tried all the remedies best supported by randomized clinical trials, but has

'stubbornly' refused to behave as the textbooks advise and failed to get better? Or what if a patient just can't tolerate the treatments with the most underlying evidence? One option is to tell such a patient: See ya! But I think that is an abdication of the oaths we physicians took. When the going gets tough, we are most obligated to take our patients by the hand, not wave goodbye."[159]

Confronting Limitations in Standard Care

Ahvie Herskowitz, MD, accepted the hand holding challenge. At first it would seem that Herskowitz, a rigorously trained academic physician who underwent residencies in pathology and internal medicine, and fellowship in cardiology at The Johns Hopkins Medical Center would be among those physicians most skeptical of CAM. During his 12 years at Johns Hopkins, he directed a multidisciplinary research team in the study of molecular and immunological mechanisms of heart ischemia, heart transplantation and heart failure. Herskowitz served as Director at the Ischemia Research and Education Foundation, working with over 100 leading heart surgery hospitals around the world, dedicated to reducing adverse outcomes during and after heart surgery. His interest in CAM was born out of finding tools to fulfill the obligation that Katz describes. Herskowitz explains

> "When I was involved as part of the transplant team, there were always a cluster of patients who were not going to get on the list, and yet I felt compelled to offer them something. I thought that if we could help them learn to optimize their nutrition, or acquire some mind-body techniques; this might possibly be of help. I sent a few patients to the acupuncture school to be treated and they had a level of improvement that I could not explain. For example, patients with ejection fractions in the low teens had improvement. In 1995 I spent time in Europe examining ways to improve outcomes in patients undergoing high-risk cardiac surgery. As I traveled all over Europe, I realized how differently patients were treated. There was much lower antibiotic use. Many patients were being treated with homeopathy or botanicals."

As Herskowitz traveled internationally for his work with the Gates

Foundation, he was exposed to other systems of healthcare and healing. Some of the developing countries such as India had global stand-alone systems. Herskowitz's travels sparked the realization that we needed convergent systems with shared language and principles that could provide a better solution than a single form of medical tradition. This belief led him to establish Anatara Medicine (www.anataramedicine.com), a holistic center in San Francisco that specializes in treating patients who are dealing with difficult, chronic diseases. Anatara Medicine includes the services of an osteopath, a naturopath, a chiropractor, a nutritionist, massage therapist, meditation teacher, massage therapist, and oriental medicine specialists.

Herskowitz speaks to the importance of always having an open mind, an inquisitive nature and a keen sense of observation. He will ask himself questions such as, "Why did five children in middle school have asthma? Or, why did two children develop lymphoma?"

Herskowitz also believes in the concept of a larger basket of tools. "We have steroids that can modulate biology, but if we also add botanicals, these two can work in harmony, or for those patients who can't tolerate steroids, we have other methods of modulating the immune and circulatory systems. After personally being treated and healed from five element acupuncture, Herskowitz studied this deeper form of acupuncture and now employs it with his patients.

In examining tools to help his patients, he looks, "for things that are safe, relatively inexpensive and that have a scientific basis. For example, there is extensive science to nutritive medicine. Once you move over to the evaluation of energy you have to go to a different system. This is where the thousands of years old pulse system can be helpful. It is a difficult system to learn and teach, and does not lend itself to scaling."

4. The Courage to be Authentic

This above all: to your own self, be true, and it follows as the night follows the day that thou canst be untrue to any man.

—William Shakespeare

There is no one universal definition of authenticity. However, at its core lies self-acceptance free of envy, an awareness of limiting beliefs, and the richness that comes from embracing both logic and emotions.

For those physicians who are, by nature, highly logical and often introverted, getting in touch with feelings and expressing them is akin to trying to learn Mandarin. It is a foreign language and has its own rules. One of the basics in any type of therapy is the requirement that the subject get in touch with his or her feelings. *How did ____ make you feel? What are you feeling now?* This is the starting point for developing the emotional intelligence that can help you become whole. In the course of caring for others, the logical side of our brain dominates as we seek to rule out, diagnose and prescribe. Our feelings get pushed to the side. Many physicians supress emotions, but the healthier alternative is to have the courage to let them emerge at the appropriate time and place.

Len Wisneski, MD, a renowned integrative medicine physician, expresses how the emotional part of our brain—the limbic system—must often take a back seat to pure logic. Wisneski states,

> "My grandson was born three months premature in 2007. Being just over one pound at birth, he could fit into the palm of my hand. He first visited my home at the age of three months. The visit was wonderful until the night before his return home. I was in my office thanking God for guiding him through the UCLA NICU with no sequelae of retrolental fibroplasia or cognitive complications when my wife and daughter screamed out to me for help. I literally ran upstairs to find him cyanotic with labored respirations. He progressed to stridor within seconds and I shouted to call 911 and began CPR. The ambulance arrived and I led the paramedic team for 90 minutes until he was stabilized. He was then transported to Denver Children's Hospital and recovered fully from what was thought to have been an acute volvulus.
>
> This story is an extreme example of a technique that I taught myself over the years. When I was working on my grandson Kai, he was not a cherished family member to my mind, but a small human and my brain operated on pure logic, similar to Mr. Spock in Star Trek. I remained in that logical, emotionally detached state until his care was turned over to the physicians at the hospital. After the transfer, I allowed myself to cry a river of tears and as I relate this story, I do so this with tears in my eyes. I have taught this technique to residents over the years and call it 'dancing on the corpus callosum.'"

CHAPTER FOUR

Overcoming Self Doubt

In the last chapter, we introduced the work of psychologist Dan Baker, PhD, co-author with Cameron Stauth of the classic book, *What Happy People Know* (St. Martin's Griffith), and the concept that two driving forces are at the root of much anxiety. These two forces are: one, not having enough and two, not being enough. As we work with physicians on their process of transformation, these two fears are among the first things to surface. Their limiting beliefs begin with self-doubt, and are exemplified by remarks such as:

- *I am only good at one thing: surgery, orthopedics, cardiology, etc.*
- *It's all I know how to do well.*
- *I've spent my entire career in academic medicine, I don't know anything about…*
- *The only thing I can be is a conventional doctor.*
- *I'm too old, or it's too late to change.*

Nonsense! Every physician carries an enormous, and well-tested black bag of transferrable skills that he or she has learned in practicing medicine. These tools include the ability to investigate, communicate, plan, analyze, research, coordinate, follow-through…and the list goes on. These are skills that are valuable to success in any number of activities. When you focus on your attributes, the self-doubts pale in comparison. Stephen Beeson, MD, in his book, *Engaging Physicians: A Manual to Physician Partnership* (Firestarter Publishing) affirms doctors' positive abilities as follows, "Physicians are the smartest and best students in the world, and can turn quickly when they decide to do so and are given training on how to do it correctly."

The second of the two anxiety drivers can best be described as the 'golden cage.' This is where we develop a lifestyle we feel we can't live without. We get trapped by our trappings. It becomes very hard to undo and unplug from this lifestyle. For Mimi, the process was relatively easy. She looked at her life and saw, "I don't have kids. I don't need to live an extravagant life, so I could be more true to simplifying my life financially. I could live life differently, and not have the fear of not having this huge paycheck. I realize that this is more difficult for many other physicians."

Financial concerns arise when contemplating any practice transition.

For example, physicians who move from a conventional payment model to a membership model worry that they will be able to retain and recruit enough patients. On one hand, they see the potential and promise, on the other, they logically understand that it will take sacrifice.

When we advise sick and stressed out doctors to unplug and take a break for a period of time to regain their health, many say they can't afford to.

You have to not be afraid to put the brakes on and say 'this isn't working for me.' Also, you have to talk to your partner. A lot of doctors are afraid to talk to their partner, afraid to get in touch with their feelings, to open up emotionally, and admit that, for the survival of their health and spirit, they need a change.

Daniel Friedland, MD, speaks to how his personal experience anchored his purpose and was fundamental to the work he is now doing. The Founding Chairman of the Academy of Integrative Health and Medicine, Friedland's focus is on leadership and resilience training. Through his company, SuperSmartHealth, he delivers a 4-Step Program (The 4 in 4 Framework™) that enables leaders and healthcare providers to leverage brain science to effectively navigate stress and shift from a reactive mindset to a creative mindset. This process allows individuals to lead more consciously and to thrive in their health, relationships and work.

Friedland's passion for this work can be traced to the emotional experiences he went through in medical school, a time of great stress and self-doubt. Originally from South Africa, he arrived in the United States in the 80s and found the transition very difficult. Accepted into the University of California San Francisco (UCSF) School of Medicine, he was hopeful that he could reconnect with a sense of community. This didn't happen. Friedland found himself studying alone. When he broke up with his one anchor, a supportive girlfriend, Friedland describes how he fell apart. He says,

> "Without my familiar surroundings and the validation I'd received from friends and doing well at school before I immigrated, I became overwhelmed and I spiraled into a depression. I reached out for counseling, something I had never done before. In this process I realized how I had run my life around achievement striving to overcome self-doubt. In doing so I understood how self-doubt had run my life. In retrospect

CHAPTER FOUR

this insight was a tremendous blessing. Instead of continuing my futile pursuit to overcome self-doubt, I became determined to learn how to embrace it.

It was also a life changing experience to realize I was not alone. When I asked my counselor if I was the only person going through this he responded that many people struggle with these feelings and that in fact more than 50% of my class was is in counseling too! I was suffering in silence and so too were my fellow medical students. Further, our attendings were suffering in silence, too. The result of this silent suffering is that it frequently strains the compassion out of caring for patients who are suffering too."

Friedland went on to establish a program at UCSF to facilitate student resiliency and well-being, and to promote the compassionate delivery of health care.

Following his residency in internal medicine he wanted to continue his work in healthcare leadership and resiliency, but was advised "to do something more academic." As a second choice at the time he decided to teach on a subject he felt he personally needed to learn something about. Inspired by a *JAMA* article in 1992 on Evidence-Based Medicine (EBM), he went on to author one of the first textbooks on EBM (*Evidence-Based Medicine: A Framework for Clinical Practice* (McGraw-Hill Medical)) and become one of the preeminent thought leaders and program creators in EBM for the next decade.

One of our sayings derives from the Far East: "Don't make friends with an elephant trainer if you don't have room in your house for an elephant." After teaching and training EBM for nearly a decade, Friedland met his elephant trainer in the person of Lee Lipsenthal, MD. Just as Lipsenthal transformed Mimi and countless other physicians with his message of gratitude, love and wellness, so too did he "rock my world," notes Friedland. The depth of Lipsenthal as a man, a teacher, and a physician can be found in his book, *Enjoy Every Sandwich: Living Each Day as If It Were your Last* (Random House), a poignant narrative that chronicles Lipsenthal's relationship to both life and the esophageal cancer that took it, robbing the world of one of its most gifted teachers of holism and physician healing.

Lipsenthal sparked Friedland's introspection and growing sense of self-doubt on his career path. After a decade of teaching EBM, Friedland realized he was immersed in the "mind of medicine" and that he was sorely missing the "heart of healthcare," his early work on healthcare provider leadership and resiliency. Friedland decided to return to his roots as a healer, first by healing himself and then by pursuing his passion for teaching resilience to others.

In undertaking this transformation into the heart of healthcare, Friedland also discovered the value in taking with him the experience he had gained from his ten years of work on EBM. In fact, he states, "It not only became a deep part of the architectural framework of the 4-Step Program I use to build resiliency, it also provided a meaningful way for me to relate to the medical audiences that I work with." He goes on to provide advice for physicians who are considering a career switch, and lamenting that they may have spent too long going down their current path. Friedland encourages them to face their self-doubt, choose the path that feels most meaningful as well as trust that nothing has been wasted. Even in the dark, there is much to be learned in one's struggles. As Friedland says, "This is the gold you can take with you as you move forward."

5. The Courage to Commit/Be Passionate

By natural ability, I mean those qualities of intellect and disposition, which urge and qualify a man to perform acts that lead to reputation. I do not mean capacity without zeal, nor zeal without capacity, nor even a combination of both of them, without an adequate power of doing a great deal of very laborious work. (p. 37) If a man is gifted with vast intellectual ability, eagerness to work, and power of working, I cannot comprehend how such a man should be repressed.

—Francis Galton[160]

In our interviews with dozens of accomplished healthcare practitioners, many shared a trait we call "transferable mastery." Prior to, during, or after medical training, they embarked on a course of mastering skills in fields outside of medicine. Prior to enrolling in medical school some of our interviewees had previous careers in engineering or even art. Others were accomplished musicians, engineers, wilderness guides, or, in the case, below, successful athletes. Mastering the necessary skills

CHAPTER FOUR

for their avocation or previous vocation allowed these doctors to identify and exercise their passion, as well as to test the power of their commitment, two ingredients essential for personal accomplishment. The needs for passion and commitment are directly proportional to the magnitude of the challenges we take on.

Scott Shreeve, MD, CEO of Crossover Health traces his success to a father who instilled in him a sense of creativity and imagination that ultimately created a sense of confidence and belief that he could do and be whatever he wanted, provided he worked hard enough. This viewpoint was reinforced by Shreeve's success in organized sports, where he led his central California high school football team as a star quarterback and captain of his basketball team. He would later play as a quarterback at Brigham Young University behind Heisman winner Ty Detmer. Exposed early and often to team physicians, he naturally gravitated toward a career in medicine. What he found, however, upon entering the clinical rotations of medical school was a shock.

> "I was appalled at the way we practiced medicine. Every morning beginning at 4:30 AM was a ritualistic paper chase gathering labs, xrays, and other reports before morning rounds. Despite best efforts, the educational instructional method was a withering, daily beat down in front of overworked interns, numb residents, and unhappy attendings who took a perverse pleasure from the trembling medical students. No one seemed to be happy. From one specialty to another, it didn't seem to get any better. The obgyns were miserable. So were the surgeons. I kept thinking there must be a medical specialty that would provide for my vision of a creative, fulfilling, and meaningful practice. While I had set on orthopedics entering medical school, I strongly considered anesthesia and ultimately settled on a residency program in emergency medicine,"

It was during his third year of residency that Shreeve got the business bug. During one of his electives, Shreeve determined to do something different and talked his way into spending his only six-week elective as a research analyst with Delphi Ventures. The idea was to see medical innovation at its inception, the tools and technology that would eventually work its way into day-to-day clinical practice.

"My first day I showed up in some guy's garage where he was pipetted DNA fragments using Xerox print technology. At the end of a month, I got to see the entire lifecycle of the deal, and he received a $7.5 million investment to start his company. My mind was on fire. For the first time, I saw a glimpse of how my medical training and background could serve as a platform to engage in the creative freedom and innovation I personally found missing from clinical practice. I though if I could get some experience running a company, maybe I'd be able to do the same."

In 2002, Shreeve and his medical student brother co-founded a company called Medsphere Systems. The Shreeve brothers' vision was to create an open source electronic health record that could be adopted by health systems that could not afford the much more expensive options from Epic, Cerner, and McKesson. Addressing his start up challenges, Shreeve notes:

"It was absolute insanity. We were just two kids, a couple of laptops, no money, and no investors but one really powerful idea that we were absolutely passionate about. But we knew we were smart enough and willing to work hard enough to figure it out. We learned quickly, literally having hundreds of meetings with family, friends, investors, partners, hospital CEOs, and others. We got a lot of good feedback, including that many of the people we really respected thought we were onto something. We ultimately raised $500,000 from friends and family. We spent this money as carefully as we could. It was a really lean time when we had to stare into the void and keep walking. I distinctly remember being down to our last $19 before an investor came in with a $100,000 check. Little entrepreneurial miracles like that fed and watered our dream. We ultimately closed our first contracts, implemented our first systems, and enjoyed several years of unabated growth and opportunity."

Later, the Shreeve brothers would close in on almost $15M through various rounds of venture funding.

In mid-2006, Scott and his brother were unceremoniously escorted out of the company they had built in a painful separation that included them

CHAPTER FOUR

being served with an eight figure lawsuit. While the lawsuit was eventually dropped, Shreeve had already moved beyond the vision of changing medicine with technology and began to examine fundamental reformation of the entire system. Retreating in order to figure out his next step, Shreeve was enthralled by Michael Porter and Elizabeth Teisberg's book *Redefining Health Care* (Harvard Business Review Press). He notes, "It was like a light shining on the crisis in the U.S. healthcare system, a totally new way to redefine the competitive landscape From that moment, I knew I wanted to be on the forefront of the movement to transform healthcare and take it to the next generation of care."

It was at this point that Shreeve realized that if he wanted to change healthcare, he would need to get firsthand experience in new healthcare delivery models. A six-month stint as an entrepreneur in residence with Lemhi Ventures provided the accelerated crash course in health care finance, care delivery, incentive management, and the emerging field of advisory services. Later, he worked with the X Prize to create a nationwide competition where cities would compete to raise the health, wellness, and vitality of their defined populations. His final preparatory consulting opportunity was working with a large San Francisco based practice to convert to a membership concept. With these combined experiences, Shreeve was prepared to jump back into business.

In 2010 he took the plunge. He signed a $1 million lease and obtained enough tenant improvement funds from the building owner to open a clinic in some prime retail space in Aliso Viejo, CA.

> "We hung out our shingle as the first membership based primary care practice in Southern California. While there were plenty of high dollar concierge practices in our area, it was our intent to democratize the experience and service level with our $75 per month membership fee. In addition to care, we provided a health advisory service to guide people through the maze of insurance, billing, specialist network, and the other challenging aspects of navigating a totally disorganized health care system," he notes. Nearly one hundred patients signed up at the grand opening. The patients absolutely "loved the service," but it soon became apparent to Shreeve that for the economics to work, the population base needed to scale. "While we were thrilled with our membership growth, I could see that it was going to take years to sell

our service one by one to people who were having a hard time understanding our value proposition particularly when there were no insurance products that would complimentarily wrap around our primary care service. We realized we would have to find large populations that have already been organized by some aggregator."

Shreeve identified that large, self-insured companies were the best aggregators. Because they pay directly for their own healthcare, these self-insured companies immediately and directly benefit from any health care cost and quality improvements.

Given the increasing prevalence of chronic diseases in the working-age population, employers are concerned about the toll that these conditions take on both the cost of employer-sponsored health coverage and productivity. A recent survey by benefits consultant Towers Watson and the National Business Group on Health reported that 67% of employers identified "employees' poor health habits" as one of their top three challenges to maintaining affordable health coverage.[160] Corporate wellness programs are on the rise. A 2010 Kaiser/HRET survey indicated that 74 percent of all employers who offered health benefits also offered at least one wellness program. This percentage jumped to 92 percent among larger employers defined as those with 200 or more employees.[160] These employers commonly offer both health screenings and interventions. The Affordable Care Act has included incentives for worksite screenings and health promotion incentives.

Taking the wellness program concept a step further, several years ago Shreeve started Crossover Health, a company built upon a next-generation health management model. He believed that by combining onsite clinics with screening, health promotion and proprietary patient management technology, Crossover Health could change the cost, quality and experience of care.

Crossover Health's first pitch to one of the largest, most valuable self-insured companies in the United States was "surreal." Going up against larger and more established competitors, the Crossover Health team challenged the employer to think different and select them. Shreeve vividly recalls taking the phone call notifying him that they were selected.

"It was an incredible rush, several years in the making, when all the blood, sweat, and tears of birthing your vision become tangible. Only mothers and entrepreneurs truly understand the feeling."

This first meaningful corporate success helped Crossover Health obtain other large clients including Facebook, Applied Material and Cummins. Today, Crossover has over 100 employees, services nearly 75,000 employees, and is looking forward to extending their model to even more companies with nearsite, retail, and virtual health services under development.

Through all the ups and downs of healthcare entrepreneurship, Shreeve is clear on one thing.

> "You have got to find your passion. You will never have the courage that you need unless you are passionate enough and believe enough to literally will your dream into reality. The bigger your vision, the deeper you will have to go inside yourself. It is hard to overcome the natural inertia that we all have. Don't keep your head down and settle, fight for what you believe in," says Shreeve. Finally, he notes that, "Crossover Health has become a magnet for awesome physicians who share this same passion, who want to spend their time, energy, and creative best selves building the future of health."

How Clear and Strong is Your Vision?

> *Until one is committed, there is hesitancy, the chance to draw back, always ineffectiveness concerning all acts of initiative (and creation). There is one elementary truth the ignorance of which kills countless ideas and splendid plans; that the moment one definitely commits oneself, then Providence moves too. All sorts of things occur to help one that would never otherwise have occurred. A whole stream of events issues from the decision, raising in one's favor all manner of unforeseen incidents and meetings and material assistance which no man could have dreamed would have come his way. Whatever you can do or dream you can, begin it. Boldness has genius, power and magic in it. Begin it now.*
>
> —Johann Wolfgang Von Goethe

We often ask physicians in our workshops to think about a time when they were totally committed to something or someone and to express that feeling in one word. The responses include terms like, "vital, alive, great, loved, empowered, focused, accomplished…" These are not bad ways to lead a life.

Research in a process called Appreciative Inquiry[161] has led us to understand that the best path to creating transformational change is to focus on what works, to cultivate a process of inquiry, and to focus on potential, all the while keeping in mind ingredients that promote vitality and excellence in living systems. Appreciative inquiry also places high value on seeking positive role models, one of the reasons we have included many stories about physicians who have made the choice to transform their lives and careers for the better. While inquiry is a prerequisite for change; passion and commitment are the drivers for success. And, as we've discussed in this chapter, the major barrier to commitment is fear.

When it comes to change and transformation, each of us deals with this strong sensation. We're all afraid. It's part of the human condition. This fear is well expressed by Lev Linkner, MD, who shares his perspective on change.

> "Most docs are afraid. They are afraid of not getting what they want or afraid of losing what they have. When you have fear you can't be in the now. Visualize what you want and attract it to yourself and then make the necessary changes. Follow your heart and dreams, live with grace, and continually reinvent yourself, have fun and go for it."

As you move forward, there's one important thing to remember. Courage is not the lack of fear but the ability to take action in spite of it.

PART TWO
HEAL YOUR PATIENTS

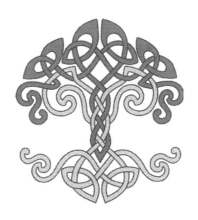

It's supposed to be a professional secret, but I'll tell you anyway. We only help and encourage the doctor within.

— Albert Schweitzer, MD

5
The Art and Science of Patient Healing

Building Healing Relationships

What are the ingredients of a healing relationship with patients? And how can this occur in the course of a clinical consult, defined as the interaction between clinician and patient (and family) in the privacy of the exam or consultation?

Fortunately, medicine has made great strides in identifying these ingredients. With the advent of the patient-centered care model (PCC) we are rapidly moving, in many sectors of healthcare, away from a physician-dominant approach to one that revolves around the patient's needs and interests. Canadian Moira Stewart, PhD, at the Shulich School of Medicine & Dentistry, Western University, proposed a definition of PCC in the late 1990s. She set forth the original six principles that are guiding this transformation in clinical relationships. Stewart defined PCC as that which "(a) explores the patients' main reason for the visit, concerns, and need for information; (b) seeks an integrated understanding of the patients' world—that is, their whole person, emotional needs, and life issues; (c) finds common ground on what the problem is and mutually agrees on management; (d) enhances prevention and health promotion; and (e) enhances the continuing relationship between the patient and the doctor."[162,163]

PCC was catapulted into the national spotlight in the United States when it was included as one of the six aims for high-quality health care in the Institute of Medicine's landmark report *Crossing the Quality Chasm*[164] in 2001. The patient-centered approach has gained increasing prominence as the bedrock of the Primary Care Medical Home.

We now understand that PCC is a relationship and a complex one at that. We have also known that some physicians are better at it than others. Can we use the best practices of these physicians—and the

CHAPTER FIVE

experience of their patients—to help light the way for other clinicians?

John Glenn Scott, MD, PhD, a family practitioner of more than 20 years in Lydonville, VT, and Clinical Assistant Professor at the Robert Wood Johnson Medical School, sought to answer this question.

> "Over the years I began to realize that the quality of the relationships I had with my patients were as important or more so than the pills that I gave them. I wanted to explore this relationship further so I identified a handful of clinicians who demonstrated exemplar patient care. These were physicians who had received special interest awards and were well known for positive engagement with patients. We interviewed each of them with regard to their technique. I had each physician nominate 4-5 patients who could describe the nature of their relationship with the physician. At no time did we attempt to define 'healing' for the patient. We conducted interviews lasting from one to three hours with each patient, transcribed the dialog and subjected the output to both textual and qualitative analysis."

Along with some core competencies, Scott identified three processes that characterized the healing relationship and an additional three outcomes. [165] These are shown in the model depicted below.

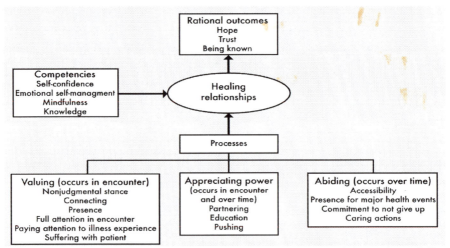

Figure 11: Healing Relationships. Reprinted with permission of the author JG Scott, MD, PhD.

Scott defined the first process as the valuing that must take place in the encounter. He states:

> "Everyone is a person of worth and it is the role of the physician to find some way to commit to the patient as a person, to find something about them that you like and can connect to. This is easier with some patients than others."

Scott points to the importance of being non-judgmental and fully present. Rather than use the term empathy, which we prefer and is described in detail below, Scott emphasizes "suffering with the patient."

Appreciating power is the second of the processes and the one that addresses the inherent asymmetry in the physician patient relationship. Scott points out that much of the physician's language in the encounter has its underpinnings in rigid contract law as opposed to humanism. He emphasizes both partnering and education. Scott also notes that, in the context of a healing relationship, patients were fine with being "pushed," meaning that they could be moved to do some things that they weren't quite ready for if they knew they had the physician's support.

Abiding is the process variable that occurs over time and allows for the creation of a relationship where the patient believes you will neither abandon nor give up on them, even if with pills and technology, you have little left to offer. Abiding is demonstrated by the physician's actions both large and small. Examples included recognizing the major events in the patient's life, doing home visits, telephoning patients after hours, taking time to research answers or doing little things like trimming the patient's toenails or removing wax from their ears when they in for a different problem.

When physicians combine these processes with the appropriate emotional, behavioral and cognitive competencies, both patient and physician are enriched by the experience. Patients achieve the outcomes they desire including a sense of hope, trust in the physician, and the knowledge that their clinician knows them and they are more than just a diagnosis.

Scott points out that the healing relationships seemed to work in both directions. Although the sample was small, the clinicians in his study "have been in practice, some in very difficult environments, for 15 to 30 years and still greatly enjoy what they do." These physician's practices were not unique. They experienced the same financial and time pressures, patient volume requirements and paperwork burdens as their colleagues.[166]

In today's shared risk environment, a supportive and engaged patient-physician relationship can contribute to improved outcomes such as morbidity,[167] mortality'[168] treatment adherence,[169] health status,[170] and improvement in diabetes.[171]

Placebos and Persuasion

Other behaviorally oriented physicians have made great contributions to the field of patient engagement. Jerome Frank, MD, PhD, was an early researcher who combined a passion for folk healing with his psychotherapy research. Frank, an anti-nuclear activist authored *Persuasion and Healing* (JHU Press) in 1961 in which he provided answers to the question, "What heals people?" Frank identified five key factors: a shared belief system; an emotionally charged setting; a confiding relationship; ritual and setting; and hope.

An additional body of research is contributing to our understanding of healing. The placebo effect is derived from the Latin meaning "I shall please." Henry Knowles Beecher, MD, author of the well quoted 1955 article, "The Powerful Placebo," traces its roots back to exorcism trials in the 16th century. Placebos—sham or simulated treatments—have been shown to reverse pharmaceutical effects from drugs such as ipecac, narcotics and stimulants. In the 1960s, patients even reported benefit from the placebo effects of mammary artery ligation, sham surgery that has no effect on coronary circulation.[172]

More recently, Irving Kirsch, PhD, Director of Placebo Studies at Harvard Medical School has clarified how all placebo responses are based on expectancies. Kirsch is author of *The Emperor's New Drugs: Exploding the Antidepressant Myth* (Random House) in which he argues that antidepressants have little or no direct effect on depression but, because of their common and sometimes serious side effects, they are a powerful placebo. Using the Freedom of Information Act, he and his colleagues acquired data from the FDA showing unpublished trial results for six antidepressants. Examining these studies, the researchers determined that the drugs produced a small, clinically meaningless improvement in mood compared with an inert placebo.[173]

Kirsh coined the term "active placebo" to represent a pharmaceutically active agent with no target effectiveness, but with noticeable side effects. The presence of side effects enhances the subject's belief that the drug is working, hence increasing the placebo effect.

The power of the placebo was reinforced by a PET scan study comparing placebo to fluoxetine in 17 unmedicated depressed men. The results showed similar brain scan results in both groups of responders. The researchers concluded "It is therefore emphasized that administration of placebo is not absence of treatment, just an absence of active medication."[174]

Building upon the healing models of Scott and Frank, as well as an understanding of patients' capacity for self-healing, we will now turn to a more in depth discussion of the tools of patient engagement. However, before doing so, we must first address one major objection inherent in the engagement model.

The Constraints of Time

Every time we discuss the concept of healing relationships with our colleagues, the first red flag they raise is the issue of adequate time. An older study that took place before the mandatory introduction of the electronic medical record—which has further compressed interactive dialog—examined 392 physician-patient interactions in primary care that took place between 1998 and 2000. The study revealed that the median visit length was 15.7 minutes and covered a median of six topics. About five minutes was spent by both parties on the major topic; the remaining ones, covering diverse issues, received a little over a minute each. The authors stated, "with only about 2 minutes of talk time on even the major topic from each speaker, we could not help but wonder how much is accomplished during such a brief exchange." They went on to note that when patients initiated the major topic, the physician talked less, perhaps indicating that the physician did not view those topics with the same importance as patients did. When patients displayed mood problems nonverbally, the physician also talked much less, raising the question as to whether physicians "feel disinclined to engage patients who appear depressed or anxious."[175]

Time constraints can be addressed in two ways. The first involves restructuring your practice flow. Increasingly, physicians armed with

CHAPTER FIVE

courage and conviction, are leaving high volume practices and adopting a more scaled down practice model supported by a direct pay component. In these models, physicians usually see between 6-14 patients and have enough time for thorough diagnosis, treatment and behavior change education and support.

Another restructuring approach is built around the team concept and your willingness and ability to utilize other healthcare professionals who can spend more time with the patient and complement and support educational efforts. The ABIHM/AHMA survey revealed the breadth of practitioners that are either part of the IM physician's practice or are available for referral.

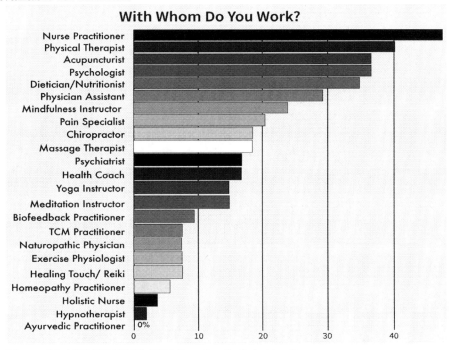

Figure 12: ABIHM/AHMA 2014 Practice Satisfaction Survey

While underrepresented in the ABIHM/AHMA survey—in large part due to the inherent abilities and interests of IM physicians in coaching their patients—the inclusion of an integrative health coach in conventional practices is becoming increasing popular. Integrative health coaching is defined as a *co-creative and dynamic partnership between an individual and professional coach/clinician embedded into a healthcare management system designed to identify, monitor, and motivate behavior in order to maximize physical, mental, social and spiritual health.* Another accepted, well tested, and reimbursable approach to increasing time with patients is the group visit model which is discussed later in this chapter.

Wearable technology, mobile apps, electronic appointment making and patient access to online laboratory results may also improve time management by adding efficiencies to the physician-patient interaction.

These modifications may provide you more time; they don't address the quality of time spent in the clinical encounter. Scott points out that "For patients who feel listened to, cared for, and valued by a physician who is mindful and present, the shorter time seems longer." Expanding quality time begins by better understanding human nature.

The Patient's POV

In 1980 when I (Mark) was working in health promotion with Kaiser Permanente in Portland, Oregon, the head of the health plan received a letter from one of our members that he shared with the medical group. It was entitled, "I am your patient, and I am afraid." In the letter, the female patient went on to share her recent healthcare experience: the fear of words whose meaning she could not fathom, the array of frightening sounds, the cold sensations from her trips on the gurney, the lack of a warm hand and a kind word. While the letter has been lost, the effect it had on me and on many of the other clinicians was profound and remains to this day.

Our patients present to us not just with chief complaints, but also with a coterie of emotions. Anxiety is one. Guilt is another. The first thing we do is put them on a scale and weigh them; if we determine that their BMI is greater than 30, which is the case for more one third of US adults (78.6 million),[176] we now have an ICD-9 code that allows us to label them obese. We've heaped shame on the patient's emotional pile of anxiety and guilt. And while biometrics are important, the first steps we take to assessing our patient's condition colors how we think about them and how they feel about themselves. With this in mind, here are some tips to improve the therapeutic relationship.

CHAPTER FIVE

Put your Patients At Ease

Studies have found that the method of introduction preferred by the patient is the physician's first and last name.[177] When meeting a patient for the first time, you also have the option of setting a warmer tone, should this be conducive to your personal style, by noting that many of your patients call you by your nickname or, if you have a long or difficult-to-pronounce names by your last initial. So Dr. Farhan Taghizedeh, a noted facial plastic surgeon in Albuquerque, NM, lets his patients know that he is often called "Dr T." Many of Mimi's patients refer to her as "Dr. Mimi."

Before entering the exam room, pause and breathe. Clear your mind and appreciate that for the next 15 minutes the most valuable use of your time and attention is to be ==fully present with your patient.== To facilitate engagement, begin each appointment by sitting at the patient's level and making eye contact. Radiate warmth and concern.

When taking your patient's blood pressure, recall that many patients have been conditioned to have 'white coat syndrome' so that their first blood pressure readings are often elevated. You can turn this into a teachable moment by guiding your patient through some deep breathing and relaxation techniques, and then retaking their blood pressure, which is invariably lower. This simple step is empowering and supportive of lifestyle modification and sets them on the road to recognizing the control they have over their autonomic nervous system. The 4-2-7 breath is a perfect exercise for the patient to practice. It is easy and can be used anytime to shift the stress response. Simply instruct the patient to breathe in for four seconds, hold it for two and then breathe out for seven. Breathe with the patient and the blood pressure will definitely go down.

Let Them Tell Their Story

The good news is that physicians seem to be getting better at allowing patients to tell their stories. In the classic 1984 study by Howard Beckman, MD, and Richard Frankel, PhD, on average, patients were interrupted within 18 seconds into explaining their problems. Less than 2 percent were even able to finish their narrative.[178]

A more recent study of 264 audiotaped visits to family physicians showed that the patients were interrupted after an average of 23 seconds. This shows how easy it is to get a 28% improvement when you are starting from such a low base! [179]

Kristi Hughes, ND, founder of the Dynamic Healing Center in Alexandria, Minnesota and Associate Director of Medical Education for the Institute for Functional Medicine, talks about the importance of allowing the patient to tell his or her story and what it may reveal about critical moments. She says, "We have to remember that the patient knows more about their body than you do and that stories make sense out of healthcare." She offers this advice for clinicians:

> "The first leg of the process is to focus on the patient's story. Work with them to develop a storyline: how did they arrive at the disease? Not just their signs and symptoms, but the story of the patient behind the disease. How did the disease manifest over time? Look for what might make their case different from other cases with the same disease. All the answers to these questions come from an ongoing dialogue with the patient.
>
> Be alert for the patient's triggers, the moments in time where the patient expresses that they have 'never been well since.' These are profound moments for the patient, and so they should be profound for the doctor. When a patient says to you 'I have never been well since that accident' or that 'death', or that 'moment', that information is a gift to you as a clinician. It's a critical data point around which you need to orient your response."

And, she points out, patients will often offer this information unsolicited if the clinician allows them to tell their story without trying to control or shorten it.

As for triggers, Hughes summarizes these triggers as "either a person, a place, or a thing. It's somewhere, someone, or something. And it sets things into motion that affect the patient's life and the patient's health."

Healing Through Feelings

This idea, that providing space for patients to tell their story can be a healing technique in and of itself, deserves further exploration. For example, there is an increasing body of literature asserting that having people write about previous emotional upheavals in their life "can result in healthy improvements in social, psychological, behavioral, and biological functioning."[180] Channeling this concept, there has been the development of expressive writing as a form of writing therapy, whereby patients struggling with traumatic events write down their thoughts and emotions regarding the event.

A seminal study by social psychologist James Pennebaker, PhD, on "Writing about Emotional Experiences as a Therapeutic Process" showed that patients who write and talk about emotional experiences utilize fewer physician visits. This emotional expression is also associated with positive benefits on the immune system including t-helper cell growth, antibody response to Epstein-Barr virus, and antibody response to hepatitis B vaccinations;[181] as well as on short-term changes in autonomic activity. Patients who practiced emotionally focused writing experienced lowered heart rate and electrodermal activity as well as decreased facial muscular activity (i.e. wrinkle-associated corrugator activity) as compared to controls. A body of research has also developed linking expressive writing to enhanced memory and cognition; reduction in pain, tension and fatigue; enhanced mood, and sleep quality.[182]

One take-away from this is the idea that giving voice to one's feelings is therapeutic, in the sense that it can bring increased healing. So just having your patient write or otherwise tell their story may provide significant benefit for the patient, besides providing you with additional diagnostic tools to greater understanding. But, to achieve these benefits, more is needed than just letting the patient talk; the physician also needs to listen.

Again, respectful and empathetic listening is a technique that sounds intuitive, but in reality, goes against much of our training as physicians. We have been trained to quickly get to the chief complaint, to judge our patients' behaviors as either healthy or unhealthy, and then to tell the patient what they 'should' do.

Emphasize Empathy

The work of Mohammadreza Hojat, PhD, a research professor at Thomas Jefferson University reveals a rather disturbing phenomenon: the erosion of empathy in physicians during the course of their training.

Hojat is the developer of the Jefferson Scale of Physician Empathy (JSPE) and author of *Empathy in Patient Care: Antecedents, Development and Outcomes* (Springer).

In his study of 456 medical students entitled "The Devil is in the Third Year: A Longitudinal Study of Erosion of Empathy in Medical School,"[183] he concluded that a significant decline in empathy occurs concurrent with the students' shift to patient-care activities. Ironically, it is at this time that empathy is most essential for establishing a therapeutic relationship. Hojat notes that further erosion in empathy occurs throughout internship and residency.

As empathy declines throughout medical school and later residency, it is replaced by the progressive spread of cynicism, a mental state affecting three quarters of medical students and more than 60% of medical residents.[184, 185] The root cause of this cynical transformation can be found in the harsh treatment of medical students, a condition which has been likened to the "battered child syndrome."[186]

Hojat points to the ambiguous and sometimes poorly defined nature of empathy. He defines it in the context of patient care as "as a predominantly *cognitive* (as opposed to affective or emotional) attribute that involves an *understanding* (as opposed to feeling) of patients' experiences, concerns, and perspectives combined with a capacity to *communicate* this understanding." He adds that the physician must also have an "intention to help through the prevention and alleviation of pain and suffering."[187]

One of the key determinants of 'clinical cognition' is detached cognition. Hojat warns against misplaced emotional involvement as a result of being too caught up in a patient's pain and feelings.

Jodi Halpern, MD, PhD, an associate professor of Bioethics and Medical Humanities at the University of California, Berkeley makes the argument for bringing more emotional resonance into the patient-physician encounter, encouraging the clinician to be moved, to some extent, by the patient's experience. When the physician allows emotional attunement to guide the timing and the tone of the encounter, and displays appropriate non-verbal body language, this facilities trust and disclosure. In these quiet, non-judgmental, supportive moments, the patient may share vulnerable information that is critical for her care.

Halpern points to the larger context of clinical empathy, in which emotions help us to focus on that which is significant for the patient. She also notes that deeper connections with patients can make the practice of medicine more meaningful. In order to do this, clinicians must maintain an inherent curiosity about patients' lives. They should also recognize that emotional needs are part of and not separate from the patient's illness. At the same time, it is important to remove your own feelings of anger or disappointment with the patient from the equation as these only get in the way of the patient's healing.

Outcomes of Empathy

For David Rakel, MD, of the Department of Family Medicine at the University of Wisconsin, empathy seems to come naturally. Quick to laugh, and possessed of a youthful chuckle, he seems by nature, the epitome of the kind, caring family physician. Rakel participated in an innovative study to determine whether patients with colds recovered more quickly if the physician provided empathy. The randomized encounters were of two types. In the 'enhanced' version, Rakel and his colleagues were encouraged to make a connection with the patient, relate to them, make eye contact, use supportive body language and get to know more about them. For the 'standard' visit, he was instructed to "just do the job" and get out of the room as quickly as possible. The encounters were videotaped and monitored with a stopwatch.

The normally affable Rakel was not prepared for the emotional upheaval that came not from the provision of empathy, but from withholding it.

Before entering the treatment room, he observed on videotape a happy 12-year-old girl, sitting quietly with her hands placed calmly in her lap as if she were saying a short prayer. Rakel cringed when he drew the 'standard card.' Following the protocol he avoided eye contact, kept his answers curt and to the point. All the while he avoided any bonding. During the exam, the young girl asked the question that made Rakel's heart sink. Attempting to reach out to him, she asked, "Do you have a family?" To which he responded in a sterile voice that he had a wife and three children. Rakel then quickly dismissed any possibility of her asking more questions and ended the encounter. The elapsed time on the stopwatch read 3 minutes and 11 seconds.

For Rakel it was three minutes that ruined his day. With his stomach turning, and a sense of nausea pervading his abdomen, he realized he missed an opportunity for a meaningful moment in medicine. He also began to wonder about the consequences of his actions on the young girl. Was she disappointed? Had he negatively impacted her attitude, beliefs, and feelings about physicians? And, to the point of the study, could his behavior have worsened her cold?[188]

The common cold study evaluated a total of 350 subjects. Physician empathy was measured with the patient-scored Consultation and Relational Empathy (CARE) survey that allocates 50 points to the encounter. A score of 50 indicates "perfect care." Patients reported their cold severity and duration twice daily. Measurements of the immune cytokine interleukin-8 (IL-8) and nasal neutrophils were obtained by nasal wash.

Eighty-four of the subjects gave perfect scores of 50 to the physicians. After accounting for possible confounding variables, cold duration was shorter in this perfect care group as compared to the group with lower scores (mean 7.10 days versus 8.01 days) and there was a trend toward reduced severity. Those patients with perfect scores also had the largest increase in IL-8 levels and nasal neutrophils. The authors concluded, "Clinical empathy as perceived by patients with the common cold, significantly predicts subsequent duration and severity of illness and is associated with immune system changes."[189]

It is normal human behavior to miss something most when it is taken away from you; in this case, for Rakel it occurred when his natural empathetic behaviors had to be removed from the patient encounter. His understanding is summed up by his belief in bonding with patients: "I realized that through crafting a relationship, we allow unknown mysteries to unfold, giving meaning and joy to this work."[190]

Help Patients Move Past Their Ambiguity

"Every therapist knows that motivation is a vital element of change," explained William R. Miller, PhD, psychotherapist and co-founder of the counseling approach known as motivational interviewing. Miller, along with Stephen Rollnick, PhD, developed the concept of motivational interviewing based on the hypothesis that the way clients were spoken to by their counselor would either enhance their motivation to change, or minimize it. Motivational interviewing began in the field of substance addiction, but is increasingly being used in other areas, such as controlling diabetes, eating disorders, obesity and heart disease.[191]

At the heart of this theory is the insight that the client or patient both wants to change and doesn't want to change, at the same time. The goal for any counselor, of course, is to shift her client or patient's ambivalence towards the stance that leads to the patient changing his habits. But given that the patient himself feels conflicted, resistance can emerge when the counselor pushes the patient. Rollnick explains, from the perspective of the client, resistance makes a lot of sense:

> "Resistance might be viewed as we might view resistance movements in war: as an heroic defense and counteraction to a perceived or quite palpable threat. What might the client be defending and maintaining? His/her self-esteem, personal values or the articulating of a particularly important opinion—one, perhaps, that expresses a core belief held dear by the client. Most commonly, the threat is an injunction, not always expressly stated but felt nonetheless, 'think differently, act differently!' Such injunctions rarely elicit the response, 'Of course, whatever you say, You're absolutely right!'"[191]

The technique of motivational interviewing aims at avoiding confrontations and battle-of wills with the patient in favor of empathy, open ended questions, reflective listening and affirmations all of which support self-efficacy. Examples of motivation questions for a condition such as obesity include the following:

"How has your life been affected by your weight?" (Open-ended question)

How would your life be different if you got down to the weight you want? (Open-ended question)

"Sounds like you were really frustrated when you regained the weight you lost." (Reflective listening)

"So, you want to eat more whole grains, but you think that your family may protest" (Reflective listening)

"I know you've got what it takes to get control of your weight." (Affirmation)

Embracing motivational interviewing means being willing to give up a top-down approach and instead provide space for the patient. While this is best done in a visit that allocates enough time to do so, it is possible for clinicians to implement some elements of motivational interviewing into briefer consults. The key is to catch yourself at the moment when you typically provide a directive-type solution to the patient, pause, and then place the burden of solution-finding back on the patient, as shown in the following examples.

Patient: I need to come up with some sort of plan to help me lose this extra weight. The stress at work has thrown me for a loop. I just can't stop thinking about it. What do you think I should do?

Practitioner: Well, I have some ideas about what might help, but first let me hear what you have already considered.

Patient: I am not going to keep that journal tracking my moods and what I eat. How does it help me to monitor how I feel? I'm coming here to lose weight and paying attention to this emotional stuff doesn't seem to help.

Practitioner: OK, you might be right. This works for many folks, but not everyone. Maybe we need to try a different way to approach this. We've talked about other ways to address this issue. What makes sense to you to practice instead?

These are only examples of how conversations could go. But the overall concept is that of an exchange led by the patient; the physician or health coach must step back. Through the dialog, you can gain a sense for how the patient analyzes and processes information. In your interactions, you may wish to mirror this process. Overall, your interactions should enable the patient to become a partner in his or her own journey to better health. Much of this enabling starts with acknowledging the patient's motivation to change

Provide Support for Behavior Change

James Belasco, PhD, and Ralph Stayer the authors and organizational change consultants, note in their book *Flight of the Buffalo* (Little, Brown) that "Change is hard because people overestimate the value of what they have—and underestimate the value of what they may gain by giving that up." It's a reminder that change is often not easy, and that patients who struggle with shedding unhealthy habits have several things stacked against them.

Patients can have a variety of motivations and obstacles keeping them from change: Lack of information or well-defined goals, a lack of motivation to change, lack of confidence in themselves or other psychological or medical issues with which they are struggling, lack of external resources or support, or a conflict between the proposed change and their current lifestyle. To help patients overcome these barriers and build a positive foundation for health behavior change, the physician can do several things:

1. Demonstrate loving-acceptance of the patient.

This approach can be accomplished through questions and statements designed to motivate the patient. The simple inclusion of questions such as: "What's going well in your life? What are you enjoying most?" can provide a platform to validate the patient and provide them with the strength and the confidence to take on lifestyle changes. Integrative physician Lev Linkner, MD, expressed his simple approach to behavior change, "I have a belief that unconditional love is the biggest healer. I love my patients even if they are fat and haven't made any progress. I don't do a guilt trip, I do a support trip."

2. Present options and choices.

Today, patients receive many mandates from us. "Quit smoking. Cut out carbs." This isn't advice; these are orders. Instead, physicians can start by sharing their interpretation of the issues the patient is facing, ending not with a commandment but instead the idea that "These are the issues I think are the most important for you to work on." Then, shift back to the patient, with questions like: "What's most important to you? Which issues are you most ready to work on? How can I help you with that? What other support do you have to help you?" Close by summarizing the specific actions that you and the patient have jointly agreed upon, a plan for accountability, and a commitment to support the patient in this plan.

3. Help the patient establish realistic goals.

Jeff Kaplan, PhD, CEO of the Habit Change Company, encourages patients to only commit to the steps they are confident of taking, and to the goals they are confident in making. Founded in 2005, The Habit Change Company employs psychological assessments, structured educational processes and life coaching to help individuals and organizations enhance vitality and longevity. The company offers a Certified Habit Change Coach program conducted live and online that fulfills some or all of the necessary hours to meet International Coaching Federation requirements (www.habitchangecoach.com).

Kaplan notes that ill-defined goals are one of the major barriers to adopting healthy behaviors. Helping patients set and reach bite-sized, concrete goals allows them to experience a series of wins that can build confidence. Encourage them to establish some mini-rewards for reaching milestones. You can provide information and guidance along their journey, for example, by noting that it takes a 3,500 caloric deficit, from decreased food consumption and increased exercise, to lose a pound. Hence, a reasonable target for weight loss is in the 1-2 pound range per week. One of the easiest formats to remember is the SMART goal: Specific, Measureable, Agreed Upon, Rewarding, and Trackable.

One technique for determining whether a goal is achievable is to get the patient to rate his or her commitment to its success. This can easily be done by asking the patient to rate the likelihood of success, on a scale from one (low) to ten (high). If they score themselves lower than a nine, you can inquire about the barriers that are getting in their way and either have a short discussion about them, or encourage the patient to rework his or her goal.

4. Realize the power of your last words.

The physician's last words are often what patients remember. So end your time with the patient by validating their concerns, letting them know that you have understood them, and closing on a hopeful and optimistic note: "Together, I know we can work to solve this problem."

5. Commit your entire practice to reinforcing the positive.

An encouraging word from a healthcare professional can work wonders for patients. Try to 'catch' patients doing things right, complimenting them on their hard work and progress even before they offer this information up to you. And inculcate this message amongst your staff: for example, when a patient walks into the office, the first person in a position to notice their weight loss is hardly ever the doctor, but the medical assistant or even the receptionist.

One important aspect of strengthening the therapeutic relationship, the "T" in a SMART plan, is to involve the patient in tracking his or her progress in making lifestyle changes. The tracking process provides the vital benefit of holding the patient accountable for their progress.

CHAPTER FIVE

Make Tracking an Active Process

According to a national telephone survey conducted by the Pew Research Center's Internet & American Life Project, US adults like to monitor their health. The study finds that 69% of US adults keep track of at least one health indicator such as weight, diet, exercise routine, or symptom. They may track their status on paper, spreadsheet, with a mobile or wearable device or in their heads.

Among the highlights of the report were the following:

- 46% of trackers say that this activity has changed their overall approach to maintaining their health or the health of someone for whom they provide care.
- 40% of trackers say it has led them to ask a doctor new questions or to get a second opinion from another doctor.
- 34% of trackers say it has affected a decision about how to treat an illness or condition.[192]

The report also noted that as people become more comfortable with mobile devices, tracking is moving from just being done in one's head to relying on the digital device. This movement is fueled by more than 13,000 health related apps available on mobile devices, as well as the explosion in wearable technology that allows for the tracking of biometrics such as heart rate rhythm and variability, blood pressure, oxygen saturation, galvanic skin response, steps taken, calories consumed, and quantity and the quality of sleep.

"Today, there is a lot of excitement about active and passive data gathering and devices that will simply measure things and produce insight or changes for you," mentions Paul Abramson, MD, founder of My Doctor Medical Group, an integrative medical practice in San Francisco (www.mydoctorsf.com).

> "We have experimented with almost all the devices that are out there and have a different perspective when it comes to people with real health problems that want to solve them quickly—whether it's discovering what is going on with their body or making changes to their lifestyle.
>
> We've found that with passively gathered data—where the patient just has to wear something or be around a device—that data is not nearly as useful. The process of change is not

triggered by data; data is not the most actionable part. The patient has to be aware of the process."

To heighten patient awareness Abramson introduced the digital app Mymee (www.mymee.com) into his medical practice last year, as part of his *Quant Coach* program of medically supervised health coaching.

After a conventional medical visit and lab testing, either Abramson or one of the coaches in the practice work with the patient to jointly set goals and then identify the best data to monitor. They then configure the Mymee's app buttons to allow the patient to record things such as symptoms, mood, weight, blood pressure, stress, or even pictures of food. To gather this data, the patient must maintain some amount of mindfulness and awareness of their activities and surroundings. Abramson, who besides being a physician has a masters in Electrical Engineering from Stanford, points out that in control system theory:

> "The tighter the feedback loop, the faster the system can converge on a solution. The typical doctor-patient feedback loop occurs over weeks, months and years. Most physicians don't see patients frequently enough, and when they do, the information they get back is based on very imperfect memory over long periods of time. The feedback is not as accurate and relevant, and there isn't enough quantity of feedback to achieve rapid change in the right direction. So if you have much more active and rapid feedback, then the whole process of practicing medicine becomes more effective and more satisfying for the practitioner. As a physician I don't have the time or the focus to go through lots of raw data. The problem with patients generating large amounts of data is: what do you do with it? How do you make useful?"

The answer is found in Abramson's collaboration with the Quant program coaches. Abramson explains:

> "We have found that gathering smaller quantities of patient-generated data that is meaningful for the patient, and then reviewing it with a coach who can then summarize both the content and the patterns in the data for the physician, has made my job easier. I get a very regular stream of concise information on the patient and I can help guide the process without requiring a large amount of time.

CHAPTER FIVE

Psychologically, it is very hard for a patient to objectively look at his or her own data and then make conclusions about what is happening. The coach is an external force able to impartially interpret the story the data tells. So this is not just data analysis; it's really data-driven coaching.

This is a practice that utilizes self-tracking and self-awareness mechanisms, along with the mindfulness that is generated by that consistent tracking and coaching, integrated into medical care. It's not a different model of care, but it empowers ongoing care to be more responsive and more effective—and more effective, more quickly—because it increases the feedback loop between physician and patient."

Gather the Group

Group visits go by a variety of names: there are Shared Medical Appointments (SMAs), Group Medical Appointments (GMAs), and Group Appointments (GAs). Within this idea of group visits, there are several models: Cooperative Health Care Clinics (CHCCs), Drop-In Group Medical Appointments (DIGMAs), and Physicals Shared Medical Appointments (PSMAs). But the overall concept underlying all these constructs is a simple one: providing a nurturing and supportive environment where patients interact with the healthcare practitioner(s) in small groups, as opposed to exclusively through one-on-one interactions. The group visit model has increasingly been used by major medical institutions such as Harvard, Atrius Health and Cleveland Clinic.

The American Academy of Family Physicians explains that these visits are, "voluntary for patients and provide a secure but interactive setting in which patients have improved access to their physicians, the benefit of counseling with additional members of a health care team (for example a behaviorist, nutritionist, or health educator), and can share experiences and advice with one another."[193]

Edward Noffsinger, PhD, the pioneer developer of group visits, constructed the first model of group visits, the Drop-In Group Medical Appointment (DIGMA), in the early 90s after himself suffering from a serious illness. Noffsinger, who has spent more than a quarter-century at Kaiser Permanente, realized that group visits could offer patients more time, access, and support, both from their doctor and from a network of other patients. Noffsinger has since become a prolific speaker and writer on the subject of group visits, including through his most recent book, *The ABCs of Group Visits: An Implementation Manual for Your Practice* (Springer) and his website www.groupvisits.com.

DIGMAs are follow-up medical visits—usually of between 10 and 16 patients—that are led by the physician and often co-led by a behavioral health professional such as a psychologist. These medical appointments are held for 90-minutes weekly, and patients can drop in or drop out of a specific week, dependent on their medical concerns. Individual vital signs are first taken, and then the session begins, with the physician addressing the medical needs of each patient at a time. The same type and quality of care is delivered: the difference is simply the presence of the group dynamic. Private exams or personal issues are still addressed privately; the goal of group visits being not to overturn the traditional physician-patient relationship, but to supplement it.

The usage of DIGMAs and other models of group visits has been steadily growing; last year, a survey by the American Academy of Family Physicians (AAFP) found that 8.4% of doctors offered shared appointments, up from 5.7% in 2005. The AAFP has concluded that "Research indicates group visits can also provide an improved quality of care and a higher level of patient and physician satisfaction. Group visits have proven to be an effective way to improve patients' dietary compliance and intermediate markers for diabetes and coronary artery disease." The AAFP has also states that "Group visits are one component of the system changes needed for the new model of care."[195]

The primary benefit to such an approach, somewhat counter-intuitively, is time. Instead of the physician's time being divided into regimented fifteen to thirty minute individual interactions with patients, he or she is instead able to interact in depth with small groups. Instead of needing to repeat the same boilerplate points about health practices to each patient—for example, having to provide the "Excess refined carbohydrates are harmful to your health" admonition five times in one day—the physician can more quickly move on to more in-depth discussions about patient preferences, concerns and challenges.

A second benefit is how these group visits help the physician lead a broader conversation about health and wellness, working to prevent further disease and ill health as opposed to just treating existing conditions. Group discussions are transformed into an opportunity for the physician and staff to educate patients in a supportive and interactive environment.

Another benefit of group visits is that the physician and patients, together, are creating social support for health. Patients can encourage each other, commiserate, empathize with and validate each others' progress. Patients struggling with lifestyle change are provided with a powerful tool for accountability: the acknowledgement not only of their physician but also of their peers.

Bring the Coach in From the Sidelines

Karen Lawson, MD, is a family physician and assistant professor in the Department of Family Medicine and Community Health at the University of Minnesota where she directs the integrative coaching program. An early advocate of holistic health, Lawson relates her experience in launching integrative centers in California and Michigan in the 1990s. In working with cross-disciplinary teams of health practitioners she realized that there was a "missing provider." Said Lawson:

> "Everyone had expertise they could share with the patient or client; they would tell them what to do, do something to them, or make recommendations. It didn't matter whether the patient was coming from their internist or acupuncturist, the patient would often stand in the parking lot and go, 'I have no idea how to do this in my life.'"

The missing provider was someone on the team who could sit down with the patient and help them figure out "what they want to do, how they want to do it, what order they want to do things in, what resources—both external and internal— they have, which ones they need and then work side by side going through significant healing work on the patient's beliefs and behaviors." In 1999, Lawson hired a holistic nurse and provided her with extra training in behavior change and advanced communication skills and the position of holistic health coaching was born. The coach soon became the busiest and most sought after provider in the 25-practitioner clinic.

Lawson describes how the philosophy and discipline of coaching fits into a holistic practice.

"Even though, as a holistic physician I worked with people in a different and more collaborative manner than that which I had been trained in during medical school, patients still came to see me for my expertise and knowledge, essentially for wisdom that was outside of themselves. The integrative health coaching model involves believing in and working with clients in a different way, one that nurtures the wisdom inside of them. It involves helping clients recognize their own strengths, desires and passions; and helping them make the choices they want to make and understand the ramifications of their choices. This completely eliminates the concept of the non-compliant patient, who is not doing what I tell them to do. Now, it is their business. They are grown-ups who can make their own decisions."

Lawson started the integrative health coaching program at the University of Minnesota that is now in its tenth year, but is quick to acknowledge that the field, while beyond infancy, is still in a young state. "Most physicians," she notes, "don't even know it exists, despite the fact that health coaching is written into the Affordable Care Act and slated to become a part of all medical homes."

There is a great deal of distortion as to what people think health coaches are and what they do. "We all have our childhood experiences of the gym coach with the whistle, an experience that most of us would not consider nurturing," she relates.

Lawson points out that health coaches are quite different from other supportive health care providers such as case managers, disease managers, or patient navigators who are primarily experts in content areas. Health coaches are experts in a process and work with people in that process. They possess the skills to help patients with discovery and personal change.

"Health coaches trained in integrative techniques do have solid backing in mind-body techniques and can teach relaxation and breathing skills, but their primary mission is to support patients with healthy self-development. In our expert-based medical model, one of the greatest misperceptions is that coaches have greater knowledge about diseases. Their expertise is in the *process* of making change."

CHAPTER FIVE

Coaching is showing up in different mechanisms throughout the healthcare system. Major insurance carriers have some element of health coaching included in their services. Coaching is often provided in the healthcare benefits offered by employers. The quality and methodology of these services varies widely. Coaching may be phone-based, or conducted by a live coach. Some programs are educationally focused; many others are menu driven. The number and length of sessions is often prescribed.

One major distinction between integrative health coaching and that offered by these commercial programs relates to who owns the agenda. In integrative coaching the patient decides what they want to talk about, what they choose to work on, as well as how often they need or want the coach's support. Some patients may choose to be seen only once, some weekly, some monthly, some as needed. The client sets the agenda. In these other models, there is often an externalized agenda in which the coach has been tasked with the assignment to get the patient to do something specific such as lower their cholesterol, or improve their HbA1c. While these are worthy goals, in an integrative holistic model, the patient may decide that she needs to deal with her relationship with her spouse first, before attending to the issue of glycemic control. The following case study, as told by Lawson, shows how an integrative health coach helped a patient both achieve his stated goals as well as improve objective measures of health status.

> "The client, a middle aged engineer, was referred to the health coach by the physician to gain help with a list of seven health problems including obesity, hypercholesterolemia, hypertension, a sedentary lifestyle and a variety of psychosocial issues. The physician's critical goals for the patient were to lose weight and lower blood pressure. When the health coach asked the patient what he would like to get help with, his answer was succinct, focused, and meaningful to him. He wanted to 'gain equanimity.'
>
> Over the ensuing four months the health coach aggressively guided the client through the process of mindfulness and the acquisition of stress management skills, all the while never really focusing on either diet or exercise. Four months into coaching, the quantitative and methodically oriented engineer presented the coach with a flow chart of his markers and

tests indicating a 40-pound weight loss as well as normalization of blood pressure and cholesterol.

You can't put equanimity on the problem list. It is not a problem, nor is it a chief complaint. Lawson believes we may be asking the wrong questions in our health encounters. Perhaps the first questions we ask should revolve around the client's visions, goals and strengths, with the understanding that, "We can help them identify problems and what is broken secondarily."

Given the need for quality control in health coaching, Lawson was one of the co-founders of the National Consortium for Credentialing of Health and Wellness Coaches, an organization that is establishing agreed upon standards and competencies (www.ncchwc.org). NCCWC includes participation from 75 different organizations, professions, and individual leaders.

In her ten years, Lawson can count on one hand the number of physicians who have gone through the intensive integrated coaching program at the University of Minnesota. From a financial standpoint she does not expect a physician to leave practice and become a coach. She does point to the growing interest physicians are displaying in taking a course or workshop on integrative coaching so that they understand its importance and relevance in an interdisciplinary team and look to either hire a health coach or identify coaches to collaborate with in the community.

Partnering for Well-Being

The essence of this transformational path lies in relating to our patients not as passive recipients of our treatments, but as partners in their own health. It requires the uses of patient engagement skills that some of us never mastered, or if we have them, they've rusted from lack of use. Simply put we must listen, instead of speak; teach, instead of command; empathize, instead of insist. Healthcare practitioners carry a heavy burden to help and heal. By engaging with your patients in ways that show you care, and allowing their voice to be equal or stronger than your own, you can gain a valuable partner to take up most of the healing load.

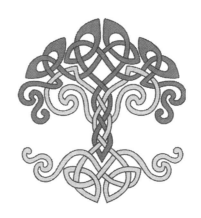

Do you see what you believe, or do you believe what you see?

If the only tool you have is a hammer, everything looks like a nail.

6
The Lifestyle Paradigm

The juxtaposition of these two commonly heard statements frames our discussion of the Integrative Medicine techniques in Part Two: *Heal Your Patients*. The tools you employ with your patients are based both on your belief in their appropriateness and efficacy—supported to some degree by evidence medicine—and your understanding of, training and competence in, and commitment to their use.

In this chapter, we will begin the exploration of three overlapping paradigms—beginning with Lifestyle Medicine (LM) —that *collectively* comprise the tools of Integrative Medicine (IM). They are shown in Figure 13 below, along with short descriptions, and in addition to LM, include Functional Medicine (FM) and Holistic Medicine (HM). For ease of presentation, we have artificially separated our discussion into distinct entities; in reality there is enormous overlap in the three areas.

To help and heal patients the IM practitioner draws liberally upon the modalities that present the best treatment combination for the patient. In part, because of training and belief systems, some clinicians emphasize some of these modalities over others. As we discuss each of these areas in turn, we will also provide examples of practice structures that have incorporated the associated techniques.

Just as the word *wellness* has been broadly adopted and often misapplied in our culture, so too have the terms *integrative* and *holistic*. For many healthcare practitioners holism is the post upon which they hang their shingle, but it has been placed in unsteady ground. Upon closer examination, their "holism" merely involves substituting nutritional supplements, compounded hormones, or homeopathic remedies for prescription medicines. The hammers become vitamins, minerals, and herbs, as opposed to prescription drugs. In the course of diagnosis and treatment, patients are never asked about their relationships, their happiness, spiritual attributes, or their sources of social support. The errors go in the other direction as well. If a practitioner pays too much

CHAPTER SIX

attention to spiritual healing and disregards the best that modern medicine has to offer, an acute disease process may cause lasting damage.

IM embraces a fundamental shift in practitioner mindset from that of being a pharmaceutical prescriber or interventionist to the original meaning of the word doctor from the Latin verb *docére*, which means 'to teach.' Doctors are first and foremost teachers. Your first teaching assignment is lifestyle medicine.

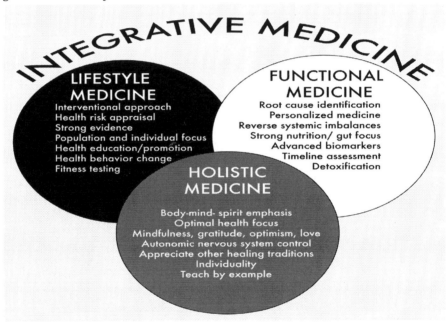

Figure 13: The Three Paradigms of IM

The Lifestyle Medicine Paradigm

Lifestyle Medicine (LM) focuses on an interventional approach to the prevention, treatment and management of disease. The most common interventions are smoking cessation, diet, exercise, and stress management. While LM has a public health orientation that includes both health education and health promotion, it is primarily a clinical discipline administered on an outpatient basis.

The techniques of LM are often used in hypertension, diabetes, osteoporosis and heart disease. For most physicians, LM is intertwined with the guidelines and practices of preventive medicine.

Despite the relentless public health and medical focus on mitigating the major cardiovascular risk factors such as hypertension, hyperlipidemia and diabetes, many Americans still struggle with these issues.[194]

- The JNC-7 reported that only 34% of hypertensives have their blood pressure under control.[195]
- Nearly half of all patients failed to meet the targets for low-density lipoprotein cholesterol.[196]
- Diabetes is at epidemic proportions. Estimates are that if the current rate continues, 1 in 3 people will have diabetes in 2050, up from 1 in ten now.[197]
- Only 37% people with diabetes have HbA1c levels at or below recommendations.[198]
- Chronic diseases such as obesity, hypertension, cancer, depression are draining $153 billion per year in lost productivity.[199]

We are losing the war on lifestyle disease. It has been estimated that four health behaviors: sedentary lifestyles, poor eating habits, smoking and alcohol consumption are responsible for approximately 37% of the annual deaths in the United States.[200] Over half of deaths that occur each year are premature and can be prevented through modification of lifestyle and environmental exposures.[201] Yet many of these interventions are not taught in medical school.

There are other gaps in our management of important health-related behaviors, among them the assessment of patient sleep disorders.[202] Estimates are that 50 to 70 million American chronically suffer from a disorder of sleep and wakefulness, impacting daily functioning and negatively affecting their health and longevity.[203] Sleep disorders lead to overproduction of inflammatory cytokines linked to cardiovascular disease and metabolic syndrome.[204] Sleep deprived patients are at higher risk for motor vehicle accidents and problems associated with altered mood and impaired cognition.

The three most common disturbances, insomnia, obstructive sleep apnea (OSA), and restless legs syndrome (RLS) have high prevalence rates in the general population. Insomnia is present in up to 33% of individuals;[205] OSA is documented in 5%;[206] and RLS estimates are between 5% and 15%.[207] Attesting to the magnitude of the problem, one research report estimates that the global market for sleep aids totaled $54.9 billion in 2013 and is growing at a compound annual growth rate of 5.6%.[208]

Testing for sleep disturbances is becoming increasingly easy for physicians to do given the increasing number of digital devices on the market. One such device is WatchPAT from Itamar Medical (www.itamar-medical.com). The WatchPAT is worn on the wrist with a probe and oximetry band on the fingers. There have been more than 675,000 tests performed with the device and it has been the subject of hundreds of peer reviewed articles. It has a failure rate of less than 2%.

Rising Expectations for Lifestyle Guidance

Today, primary care physicians bear the enormous burden to serve patients with multiple co-morbid conditions. They are caught between the rock and the hard place. On one hand patients look to their physicians as credible sources of advice and guidance on getting help with diet, exercise and problems such as substance abuse. A survey of HMO members showed that more than 90% of subscribers expect advice and help with lifestyle issues.[209] Depending upon the patient and the condition, there are multiple opportunities for the physician to intervene with health-promoting guidance.

On the other hand, many physicians lack the training and time to help patients with lifestyle counseling. They are also ill equipped to provide behavioral interventions for the psychosocial factors that, in one study, accounted for 70% of visits.[210]

While physician competence and time are issues, perhaps an even greater impediment is the physician's 'inner game' of patient lifestyle counseling. Physicians bring a mixture of expectations, and emotions—including both confidence and commitment—to the patient encounter around lifestyle issues.

We often tend to focus more on 'our failures' than our contribution to patient success. Our sense of frustration grows when we are confronted, for example, with a cancer patient who, after diagnosis has not ceased tobacco use. Unfortunately, this is all too common as shown in a recent cross sectional analysis of almost 3,000 cancer survivors finding that nine years following diagnosis 9.3 percent were still smoking.[211]

With this example in mind, physicians may also believe that their counseling doesn't work, and that they don't make a difference. They vastly underestimate their power to steer the majority of their patients to higher levels of health. Physician advice has consistently been shown to be one of the major factors to patients' attempting various lifestyle improvements. These interventions include smoking cessation, weight control, lifestyle changes for diabetes and reduction of CVD risk, and physical exercise for hypertension management. Patients who attempt health behavior change are more likely to remember information provided by their physicians.[212-223]

Commonly held, though erroneous perceptions also discourage physicians from discussing lifestyle issues with patients. There is pessimism concerning the effectiveness of weight loss strategies, yet studies have shown that approximately 20% of overweight individuals will maintain a loss of at least 10% of initial body weight for one year.[224] Physicians may also not believe that patients want to give up smoking. Yet 68.8% of US smokers report that they want to quit completely. Depending upon age, anywhere from 35%-45% of adult smokers stopped cigarettes for more than one day in 2010 because of a desire to quit.[225]

Physicians can also respond with anger when patients are not doing what we clearly know is best for them. Tieraona Low Dog, MD, Director of the Fellowship at the Arizona Center for Integrative Medicine (www.integrativemedicine.arizona.edu) works with their 130 fellows each year and advises them accordingly:

> "Sometimes the fact that a patient is not losing weight, or stopping smoking actually generates physician resentment. We must remember that this is the patient's journey, not ours. They may very well have different agendas for their health. This does not make them a bad patient, or you a bad physician. We must continually partner with, listen to, and support our patients with the understanding that they will make changes on their own timeline, not ours."

CHAPTER SIX

Meet Patients Where They Are

Many models have been developed that describe the motivational and psychological stages that patients go through in making lifestyle change. The Stages of Change, or Transtheoretical Model, developed by James Prochaska, PhD, and Carlo DiClemente, PhD, is the most widely used system in use today.[226] It incorporates concepts from earlier constructs such as the Health Belief model.[227]

In the Stages of Change model (shown in Figure 14 below), patients progress through a series of major stages beginning with precontemplation. In this stage they are unaware of the need for change. They may be in denial or feel that an adverse event can't happen to them. Some patients may be discouraged by past failures and have resigned themselves to the status quo. When patients are precontemplative, direct confrontation may generate anger or backlash. Instead, physicians will have more success by using the motivation interviewing techniques discussed in the previous chapter.

In the contemplation stage, patients struggle with ambivalence. They weigh the potential benefits against the more familiar cons and the overriding sense of loss of the familiar. The physician can help tip the balance by focusing the patient's attention on an improved future state, while also offering suggestions about overcoming potential barriers. Frequently patients will start the contemplation stage after a major event such as a heart attack. This is a great time for the physician to engage the patient in thinking about change.

In the preparation stage, patients ready themselves for making a specific change. They may take some baby steps such as cutting back on cigarettes or alcohol, or switching from a high-fat, high-calorie desert to fruit. Physicians can help determine which behaviors they would like to start with, and to which they will be fully committed.

Most physicians are eager to see their patients reach the action stage in which they have a definite goal, a plan in place, and a mechanism to track and monitor progress. Recognizing and praising the patient for success is important at this stage.

The next two steps, maintenance and relapse prevention revolve around how successful the patient is at integrating the new behavior into the fabric of his or her life. This often requires the support of health-promoting cultures. It is normal for a patient to go through the stages of change several times before the new behavior becomes ingrained into their life.

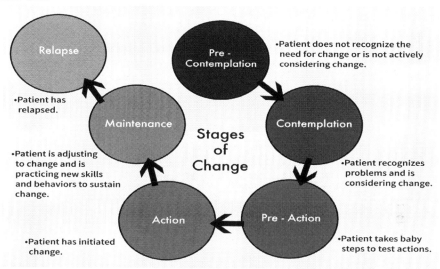

FIGURE 14: Stages of Change Model

The Stages of Change model is often folded into another system of brief patient counseling, the 5 A's model.[228] Originally developed by the National Cancer Institute to help people quit smoking, it is employed for many types of behavior change. The 5 A's stand for:

- Ask about the behavior.
- Advise patients to make changes in a strong, clear and personalized way.
- Assess where they are in terms of readiness with stages of change.
- Assist the patient to create a plan.
- Arrange for the necessary support and follow up.

Closing the Physician Belief-Behavior Gap

Another barrier for lifestyle intervention can be found in the mirror.

In a recent Medscape survey (Figure 15 below), in which physicians self-reported being either overweight (BMI 25-30) or obese (>30), many specialties did not fare well. Seven specialties weighed in at greater than 45%; these included general surgery, family medicine, gastroenterology, critical care, pulmonary medicine, Ob/Gyn and orthopedics. Not surprisingly, the specialties tied most closely to aesthetics—dermatology, ophthalmology and plastic surgery —were the least overweight.

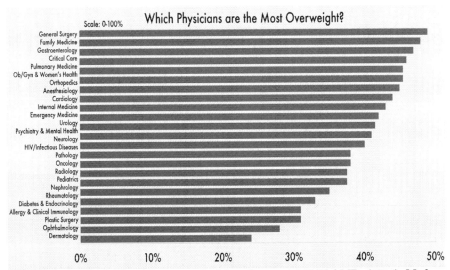

Figure 15: Which Physicians are the Most Overweight? WebMD. (2014). Medscape physician's lifestyle report 2014. New York, NY. Peckman, C. Used with permission from Medscape.

Physicians are contributing to the obesity epidemic of which it has been estimated that almost two-thirds of U.S. adults are overweight and a third obese.[229] Obesity puts individuals at increased risk for CVD, HTN, dyslipidemia, OSA, gallbladder disease, osteoarthritis and several types of cancer.[230]

A sedentary lifestyle is a major contributor to heart disease, as was first documented in 1958 in London bus drivers who were 1.8 times more likely than the more active bus conductors to develop coronary heart disease.[231] A recent study of 7,744 men (age 20-89), initially free of CVD, examined the relationship of time spent riding in cars and watching television and the incidence of CVD mortality. Men who reported riding in a car more than 10 hrs/week or who had more than 23 hrs/week of combined sedentary behavior had 82% and 64% greater risk of dying from CVD than those who reported less than 4 car hours or less than 11 hrs of combined sedentary behavior per week.[232]

Another large scale population study has shown that sitting for more than five hours per day is a risk factor for all-cause mortality, independent of physical activity.[233] The benefits of walking or cycling to work, as opposed to driving, include lowered risk of diabetes and hypertension.[234] Learnable moments for confronting one's own unhealthy lifestyle behaviors abound in practice. One obese physician discussed his moment of enlightenment when he was counseling an overweight teen with acne to engage in more exercise, consume less high fructose foods and eat more vegetables and whole grains. After hearing this advice, the teen innocently (or perhaps passive aggressively) asked the physician, "Is this what you are doing?" The teen's retort was a wake-up call for the physician.

For Owen Meyers, MD, a family physician in Monroe, Louisiana, his moment of enlightenment came when a celebration turned slightly sour.

> "We had our 25th wedding anniversary and went out to eat. While we were there we had a photograph taken of ourselves and the meal was great. At the end of the meal everything was fine until they handed us the photograph, and I looked at it and there I was obese. I couldn't see it in the mirror at home but it was on the photograph. And it really said I need to do something about it. My wife also was obese, and her health issues were worsening because of her obesity. It wasn't just a personal issue but I also had a problem with my own patients. The ones who were diabetic, the ones who were obese wanted extra help and I really couldn't help them. It was a knowledge deficit that when I went through school we really weren't trained about that."

For both himself, and his patients, Meyers turned to the Center for Medical Weight Loss (www.cmwl.com), a structured physician customized weight loss program built around caloric restriction through meal replacement coupled with guided behavioral counseling modules. Tracking and monitoring systems are provided for physicians to use with patients. Meyers learned a tremendous amount about the whole process of bariatrics and has appreciated the company's ongoing support. "The ability to make some quick changes in a patient who has been obese for quite a long period of time and them seeing success and becoming motivated and making the change in themselves has been highly rewarding." Meyers notes that the program has also been very positive from a financial standpoint.

CHAPTER SIX

Physicians' personal struggles with weight, exercise and stress can be a source of reticence to counsel patients, as can their positive health habits be a positive motivator to do so. Studies from the Women's Health Initiative involving a cross-sectional survey of 4,501 female doctors showed a strong correlation between the physician's personal health behaviors and the likelihood of discussing lifestyle changes with patients.[235] Women physicians who exercised themselves were more likely to counsel their patients on the benefits of exercise at least once a year.[236]

Integrating Lifestyle Techniques into Practice

Making a personal commitment to a healthier lifestyle and assessing patient readiness to change are good starting points for addressing unhealthy behaviors. Patients can be moved to greater states of awareness and action through the use of validated assessments, short quizzes and brief interventions related to exercise, nutrition, weight loss and stress. Many of these exist online or on tablets to be used pre- or post-consult, as well as integrated into the EHR. Smart phone apps are increasingly being used for tracking, however there are presently no large randomized, controlled studies providing scientific evidence of the benefits of their use. A large scale clinical trial (Clinical Trials.gov Identifier: NCT02016014) based upon the EVIDENT II study is currently underway.[237]

Among the assessments that can be incorporated into practice are:

Pictorial Models

- These include the Food Pyramid (myfoodpyramid.org) and the Eatwell Plate.[238] A model that we use is the Tree of Health shown in Figure 17 (below). The model depicts a more encompassing view of health that allows for discussion of the root causes of disease and their effects on organs and organ systems. For example, if diabetes is the sick fruit on the tree, we then direct the patient's attention to the soil and the role of a low glycemic Mediterranean diet, an exercise prescription, probiotics to enhance insulin sensitivity, and adequate sleep to regulate cortisol and decrease systemic inflammation. Stress is a major contributor to many of the addictions we see and frequently the solution lies in transforming the stress response. On a daily basis we hear patients state they drink alcohol and eat unhealthy foods as a result of stress. But this is just the tip of the iceberg, since tobacco use, gambling and other addictions are frequently maladaptive responses to stress and tension.

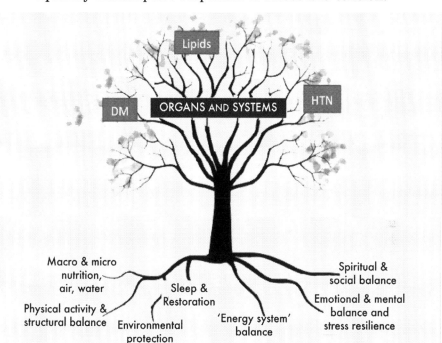

Figure 16: Tree of Health. Reprinted with permission from Atlantic Health

Nutrition, Fitness & Obesity Questionnaires

- The Physical Activity Recall Questionnaire (PAR) is a semi-structured interview process to estimate an individual's time spent in physical activity, strength and flexibility exercises over the past seven days. It can be supplemented with accelerometer data from devices such as Fitbit®, FuelBand, or Atlas along with other self reports.[239]

- The Food Frequency Questionnaire (FFQ) is the most common self-administered dietary assessment tool used in large epidemiologic studies. Participants recall the frequency of consumption and portion size of approximately 125 line items over a defined period of time. An innovative software tool, entitled the VioFFQ (www.viocare.com) is now available both online and in tablet form. The assessment, which takes approximately 20 minutes, collects data on dietary behavior and food use patterns, estimates nutrient intake, and delivers a dietary change report. Representative photographs are used to indicate portion size.

- The Clinical Screening Questionnaire for Eating Behaviors Associated with Overweight and Obesity is available from the American Board of Family Medicine.[240]
- The Weight Loss Questionnaires compiled by the American Medical Association and the Robert Woods Johnson Foundation provide templates for evaluating obesity-related factors.[241]

Stress & Sleep Disorders

- The Beck Depression Inventory for primary care (BDI-PC) is a 21-question multiple-choice self-report inventory, widely used to measure the severity of depression.[242]
- Sleep questionnaires include the Berlin questionnaire (BQ: 10 questions for sleep apnea); Epworth Sleepiness Scale (ESS: 8 questions on inappropriate dozing); STOP (4 questions on snoring, tiredness during daytime, observed apnea and HBP); and the Cleveland Sleep Habits Questionnaire (CSHQ: 2 page combination).[243]
- Stress Assessments: While stress quizzes and tests abound, there are few validated instruments.
- The Perceived Stress Scale (PSS) is the most widely used psychological instrument for measuring the perception of stress and whether situations are predictable and controllable, or overwhelm the respondent.[244, 245]
- Profile of Mood States (POMS) is a psychological test that is often used by sports psychologists. It evaluates one's affective state and provides scores for tension, depression, anger, vigor, fatigue, and confusion.[246]
- The HeartMath Stress and Well Being Survey includes the Holmes Rahe SRE, along with questions related to sources, levels of, and responses to stress; as well as feelings of emotions and quality of life indicators.[247]

The Health Risk Appraisal (HRA)

One tool employed by LM advocates, the Health Risk Appraisal (HRA), is of particular importance, as it will increasingly affect physicians from all primary care disciplines, in large part due to the ACA and the growing corporate wellness movement. Patients who complete HRAs at the worksite are always advised to share the results with their physician. It is becoming increasingly common for patients to have their print out in hand when they come for an appointment. This raises the expectation that the physician will have health behavior change techniques and programs available to utilize with the patient. Hence, some familiarity with this tool is recommended.

HRAs compile self-reported demographic characteristics, lifestyle habits, and personal and family medical history along with basic biometric data including BMI calculation, blood pressure, and lipids. Also included in most HRAs are health behavior change questions related to attitude and willingness to change. This data is electronically compiled and the individual is presented with a printout of their health risks along with suggestions for improvement.

The roots of the HRA come from the Framingham study, an in-depth longitudinal study of 5,000 families in Framingham, Massachusetts. Data on this study are still being compiled by the National Institutes of Health. Using these results, in 1970, Lewis Robbins, MD, MPH, and Jack Hall, MD, of the Methodist Hospital of Indiana, developed hazard tables that were discussed in their publication *How to Practice Prospective Medicine* (Methodist Hospital of Indiana). The guide included the health risk assessment questionnaire as well as the risk computations that went into the results. A decade later in 1980, the Centers for Disease Control and Prevention released a publicly available version that became widely used in early worksite health programs.

Today, there are more than 50 different vendors offering HRAs primarily in the corporate marketplace. Each differs in length, orientation, versions, and customizability. A number of companies have several decades of experience in their use and have compiled an extensive reference database.

In the United States The RAND Employer Survey data suggest that 80 percent of employers with a wellness program are currently screening their employees for health risks. Of worksites offering HRAs, 46% of employees complete them.[248] Benefits to the employer include the ability to better identify high-risk employees, predict health related costs, measure absenteeism and presenteeism and assess return on investment of wellness activities. There is some evidence that, in the absence of other health promotion initiatives, taking a HRA may motivate individuals to engage in positive health behavior change.[249]

HRAs have not found their way into many clinical practices; however, this is set to change with provisions in the Affordable Care Act. The ACA directed the Centers for Medicare & Medicaid Services (CMS) to require that, as part of the Medicare Annual Wellness Visit (AWV), physicians have patients complete a HRA. The HRA requirement became effective Jan. 1, 2012. Similar to its use in the corporate setting, the goals of the HRA are to identify the patient's risk factors as the springboard to discussion and the creation of a personalized prevention plan. Unfortunately, the compensation for additional staff time is paltry. CMS increased the RVUs of the AWV to 4.89 for the initial AWV and 3.26 for the subsequent AWV, thus increasing average reimbursements to $5.39 for the initial and $3.59 for subsequent AWVs.[250]

CMS has required that the HRA must be written at a sixth grade literacy level and be designed so that most patients can complete it in 20 minutes or less. One source, www.HowsYourHealth.org, a not-for-profit service of the Dartmouth Co-Op Project. Dartmouth, provides free interactive assessments that meet the CMS requirements. The HRA is available in both print form and electronically. The commercially available HRAs are ideally suited to the fee-for-service or membership practice model in which they can provide extra value to the encounter. Incorporating a HRA into the initial patient intake can serve as a valuable adjunct to not only determine the patient's risk profile, but also to identify their beliefs around self-efficacy, motivations, and barriers to change.

Integrating Fitness into Your Practice

It has been seven years since ACSM and the AMA jointly launched the Exercise is Medicine initiative, yet exercise counseling has not made great strides in conventional clinical practice. The difficulty, in large part is the lack of payment for fitness evaluation and exercise services within the insured model of care. Ironically, it is possible to get insurance reimbursement for bariatric surgery, but not for exercise counseling. However, a number of physicians have reorganized their practices to include a more comprehensive approach to fitness under a direct-pay model.

Bob Tygenhof, CPT, a ACSM certified personal trainer has been instrumental at incorporating fitness testing and counseling into the Integrative Medical Group of Irvine (CA). Tygenhof's wife, ob-gyn physician Felice Gersh, MD, heads this primarily private pay multi-disciplinary practice. Gersh completed a Fellowship in Integrative Medicine at the University of Arizona's Center for Integrative Medicine and is one of a very select group of gynecologists who have this training. Gersh is nationally known for her unique approach to the treatment of polycystic ovary syndrome.

Getting the fitness model incorporated correctly in the practice took some time. According to Tygenhof,:

> "We initially brought in independent fitness trainers to work with our patients, thinking that this would be a natural and logical extension of our practice. However, we found this did not work well. We would refer the patient and the fitness trainer would see them, but we would have no idea of what was taking place during the visit. These independent agents were also selling their own supplements and weight loss programs. We decided that if we wanted to have a serious fitness program, we would have to tie it into everything else we were doing in the practice. I had always had a personal interest in exercise and fitness so I underwent the certification course offered by the American College of Sports Medicine."

Tygenhof discusses the current process in the practice.

> "The patient will see Dr. Gersh for approximately 30 minutes. During that time she will evaluate the patient and make a variety of recommendations related to nutrition, stress management and fitness. All of these recommendations go into our EMR. Upon checkout, we ask the patient if they have any interest in our fitness services. If so, they see me and I will discuss the benefits in their particular situation. We discuss how fitness can impact their overall health and how it intersects with lifestyle medicine. We try to identify what

will best serve their needs. I present the costs of my services to them.

Many of our patients travel to see us, so while it would be ideal to work with them on a recurrent basis, this is often not possible. So I focus more on a fitness assessment and the creation of an exercise program that will work for them. Some of our patients either belong to or will sign up for a gym, but we also have elderly patients who live in retirement communities that have a small gym and I will go there to find out what equipment they offer. I usually recommend that patients start with a small introductory program consisting of an assessment, an exercise prescription and a small package of one-on-one workouts till they master the exercises. We provide different assessments depending upon age group and physical conditioning."

Since he often deals with older patients in the practice, Tygenhof uses the Senior Fitness Test developed by C. Jessie Jones, PhD, and Roberta E. Rikli, PhD, professors at California State University, Fullerton. The Senior Fitness Test is based on a large database of Medicare aged patients that allow the application of normative criteria to identify thresholds of disability on individuals 60 years of age and above. It focuses on the strength, balance and flexibility needed for everyday activities. "By repeating the assessment over time, we are able to see just when and where disability is occurring," notes Tygenhof. It includes a series of assessments including chair stands, arm curl, 6 minute walk, 2 minute step, chair sit and reach, back scratch and 8-ft Up & Go. The test takes an hour to run, record, and discuss results with the client. Tygenhof uses other standardized fitness tests on younger people.

Tygenhof's balanced philosophy for fitness assessment and counseling mirrors that of the practice. "We walk a thin line sometimes between giving patients what they need and not overwhelming them."

Organizations offering training and certification in fitness include the American College of Sports Medicine (www.acsm.org), and The Medical Fitness Association (www. medicalfitness.org). The American College of Lifestyle Medicine has links to a broader range of wellness and behavior change programs. (www.lifestylemedicine.org/programs)

Taking Clinical Integration to the Next Level

"One of the things that is unique about our health and wellness centers is that we've adopted this clinical integration concept," said Douglas Ribley, MS, Senior Vice President, Health & Wellness at Akron General Health System and a past president and chairman of the Medical Fitness Association.

Akron General Hospital is a national model for health and wellness center development; they have invested more than $100 million in three centers totaling more than 500,000 square feet. The wellness centers cover the spectrum of outpatient care from diagnosis, to treatment to rehabilitation including physical therapy, sports medicine, sport performance, and cardiopulmonary rehabilitation. The fitness centers—open to the community—are located adjacent to 40,000 sq. ft. of physician office space. The mix of primary care physicians and specialists benefit from the powerful sense of community that the centers generate.

Ribley notes that the Medical Fitness and Wellness Centers serve a more mature, deconditioned, higher risk population.

> "The average age is 48-50 years old. Half of our members have never been a member of a commercial health club, rec center, YMCA, or JCC, before. So, 50% are members because they are using physical activity, health education and nutrition to manage or prevent chronic disease.
>
> What that means is when you look at the floor, when you go through the center, there's a blend of patients and community members. So you can walk onto the floor and on one treadmill there could be a physical therapist working with a therapy patient, on the next could be a cardiopulmonary nurse working with a patient that has an oxygen tank, and the third could be an exercise physiologist working with a community member. This complete sharing of space creates a better outcome for the member, for the patient, and for the business.
>
> It is actually a powerful dynamic. The thing you have to understand with this medical fitness and wellness model is this is not a club. It's not a gym. It is a department of the sponsoring healthcare organization just like any other department, with the only difference being the medicine is physical

activity, nutrition, and health education. Every decision is made with physician input. Every center is staffed with qualified personnel who have a minimum 4-year degree in exercise physiology, exercise science, or some related discipline. This clinical integration is what creates the medical fitness difference and attracts people from the community that are not comfortable going anywhere else."

Nutrition

For the practicing physician, there is little disagreement about the role of exercise in health and little confusion over the basics of the fitness prescription. Periodically an interesting article surfaces that sheds additional light on the merits of one type of activity. For example, a study by researchers from Iowa State University, showed that any amount of running—regardless of length, duration, or speed can reduce risk of death.[251]

The issues around meaningful fitness counseling usually boil down to lacking the time and the type of support in the healthcare setting to allow for personalization.

There is also little controversy over stress management techniques. At this point, we know that a handful of techniques such as deep breathing, meditation, gratitude practice, mindfulness and yoga, if pursued with intentionality by the patient, can yield beneficial results. Who can argue with Schneider's Transcendental Meditation study showing a 48% reduction in stroke, heart attack and death?[252] The field of nutrition, however, generates much more controversy, driven to a large degree by three obfuscations that color our interactions and discussion with patients.

The Misplaced Focus

The first is the micro focus on nutrients to the exclusion of the larger focus on food. In his book, *In Defense of Food: An Eater's Manifesto* (Penguin Press), Michael Pollan notes that we have entered an age of *nutritionism*. Our attention is consumed by the ingredients in foods such as polyunsaturated and monounsaturated fats, carbohydrates, fiber, amino acids, vitamins, minerals, polyphenols, antioxidants, probiotics and phytochemicals. In a world of processed and man-made foods, we have had to develop the survival skill of label reading and this has in turn spurred food manufacturers to overhype their products. This absurdity is evident in gluten free claims that appear on vegetables, fruits and fish. The process of acquiring, preparing and eating food has become divorced from the earth from which the foods come. Good nutrition really simple: it is a back to basics approach.

As one of the country's foremost herbalists, Tieraona Low Dog, MD, employs a back to the earth approach in training physicians on herbal medicine. Low Dog takes groups of 24 physicians on retreats to her ranch outside of Santa Fe, New Mexico where they not only learn how to use herbs in healing, but also get hands on appreciation for their origins. Over the three-day retreat, the physicians harvest herbs such as echinacea, marshmallow, sage, skullcap, peppermint, St John's wort, valerian, holy basil, and calendula. Low Dog then instructs the physicians how to dry and store herbs, as well as how to create tinctures, balms, salves, creams, honeys and vinegars.

In the same way that one would attend a wine tasting in Napa Valley, Low Dog holds herb tastings in which the participants use their senses to become more intimately knowledgeable of the herb, along the way, asking them questions such as, "Does it make you salivate? Is it dry, bitter, or sweet? Would a child drink this?"

Low Dog notes that, "One can only learn so much from books. There is no substitute for having a primary experience of being in the field with the plants, and then harvesting, preparing and tasting them."

This same philosophy is the key to nutrition education: help your patients focus on food, whole food that comes from the earth.

The Law of Unintended Consequences

The second confabulation begins with a noble pursuit: eradicating world hunger while also keeping food prices affordable. The American farmer, always among the most productive and efficient in the world, has taken on this challenge. And industry has responded to assist. Genetically modified (GM) crops have allowed farmers to generate higher crop yields by producing plants that have desirable traits such as drought tolerance or the ability to eradicate bacteria such as *Bacillus thuringiensis* (BT).

CHAPTER SIX

Congress has done its share with subsidies that allow for the stabilization of food prices. The end result is the most abundantly produced, most heavily subsidized, and most modified product on the planet: corn.

Corn has turned out to be an amazingly versatile. Not only is it used slightly processed in corn flour, grits, hominy, or sweet corn, it has also found its way into ethanol, animal feed and high-fructose corn syrup (HFCS).

As cheap filler, HFCS contributes to the 156 pounds of sugar the average American consumes each year. This is the equivalent of 31 five-pound bags. Half of this amount comes from the HFCS in processed food such as salad dressings, ketchup and regular soft drinks. In addition to its role in obesity and insulin resistance, the onslaught of this glycemic load facilitates advanced glycation endproducts (AGEs) in which glucose molecules are non-enzymatically bound to proteins. One target of the cross-linked proteins is the structural collagen in the vascular wall where the AGEs contribute to plaque formation, thickened basement membranes and loss of vessel elasticity.[253]

The damage of corn extends beyond the human body. More than 5.6 million tons of nitrogen laden chemical fertilizers, and another million tons of nitrogen from manure are applied to cornfields each year. Much of this fertilizer, along with topsoil, finds its way into our lakes, rivers and coastal oceans where it damages ecosystems.

Pollan points out other unintended consequences of our reliance on corn: the sickness we have induced in cows fed a corn as opposed to grass diet. Approximately 36% of the crop from the 84 million acres of corn [254] produced in the US each year finds its way into animal feed. In order to combat the GI effects of this unnatural food source, the cows are given antibiotics, thus generating resistant strains of E. coli. Unlike meat from grass fed cows, which has a preponderance of healthy omega-3 fatty acids, meat from corn-fed cows are higher in unhealthy omega-6.

Ironically, while most of today's corn crop, about 40%, is destined for biofuels, corn requires just about the highest ratio of petroleum to edible stuff produced. Between fertilizer and transportation, it takes a quarter to a third of a gallon of oil to produce a single bushel of corn.

It will take a concerted effort on the part of all healthcare practitioners to combat the damage that is being done to consumers and to the environment through excessive reliance on corn. You can help your patient reduce their HFCS dependence by first pointing out the relationship to their conditions such as CVD, weight gain, fatigue, dental caries, metabolic syndrome, diabetes, and acne. One of the easiest interventions is to encourage patients to keep a 3-day dietary recall, in which they write down everything they eat and in what quantities. You can then go over this record with them, identify the high glycemic load foods and sources of hidden sugars, and then suggest healthier alternatives.

The Lure of the Diet du Jour

The third confabulation is the diet du jour, or what David Katz, MD, MPH, equates to the latest entry into an unending diet-focused beauty pageant. Katz is the founding director of Yale University's Prevention Research Center and president of the American College of Lifestyle Medicine (www.lifestylemedicine.org), a national professional society that trains physicians how to assess lifestyle 'vital signs' such as tobacco use, alcohol consumption, diet, physical activity, body mass index, stress level, sleep, and emotional well-being.[255] Membership is broadly inclusive and ACLM welcomes all formally trained healthcare professionals both inside and outside the United States. The third edition of Katz's text, *Nutrition in Clinic Practice: A Comprehensive, Evidence-Based Manual for the Practitioner* (Lippincott Williams & Wilkins) has just been released.

Katz points out that in his early years of practice, "Patients didn't know much about nutrition. They came in as empty vessels with the expectation that as physicians we would provide them with information. Given the ease with which patients can Google nutritional information today, our role is to help them go from information alone to knowledge and understanding," said Katz. He acknowledges a dichotomy:

> "Physicians generally don't know much about nutrition, and generally know they don't know much. Some patients also know they don't know much, but more often, patients have surfed the Web, and think they know everything—but much of it is wrong. The way things ought to be are for both parties to be respectful but assertive."

Katz says that physician assertiveness may need to come into play "when patients have allowed the mono-nutrient to be the tail that wags the nutritional dog," and nutrition extremism is causing harm.

CHAPTER SIX

Such was the case for a patient of Mimi's. The 56-year-old woman had interpreted a popular nutrition book as giving her permission to eat all the butter and fat she wanted because it would help to prevent Alzheimer's disease. She also heard that gluten was bad so she switched to tapioca, rice and potato flower. When she was first evaluated, her cholesterol was 320 and she had 'rip-roaring' angina. She was sent her off to the cath lab where it was determined that she had 90% blockage in three arteries.

The preoccupation with healthy eating can also become an obsession, a condition known as orthorexia nervosa, a term first coined in 1997 by Steven Bratman, MD. While it is not officially recognized by the DSM-IV as an eating disorder, it can lead to a fixation on food quality and purity and a preoccupation with what and how much to eat.

Finding the Best in Most

In a paper entitled, "Can We Say What Diet is Best for Health?"[254] Katz and Yale colleague Stephanie Meller compared the major diets in use today: low carb, low fat, low glycemic, Mediterranean, mixed/balanced (DASH), paleolithic, and vegan. They concluded that no diet is clearly best, but there are common beneficial elements across the different eating patterns. They summarize their findings by highlighting the consensus, namely that "A diet of minimally processed foods close to nature, predominantly plants, is decisively associated with health promotion and disease prevention."

Among the specific findings were solid support for:
- Nutritionally-centric plant-based diets and the association with fewer cancers and less heart disease.[256] Ideally, plant-focused eating should be supplemented not only with fruits and vegetables, but also with whole grains, nuts, and seeds.
- The low glycemic Mediterranean diet and its positive effects on cardiovascular disease, cancer risk, obesity, and metabolic syndrome.[254] The authors point to a potential association between the Mediterranean diet and "defense against neurodegenerative disease and preservation of cognitive function, reduced inflammation, and defense against asthma."[254] Features of the diet include a high intake of fiber, moderate alcohol and meat intake, as well as foods

high in antioxidants and polyphenols.
- Carbohydrate-selective diets proving to be better than categorically low-carbohydrate diets. Consuming whole grains lowers the risks for certain cancers and allows for better control of body weight.[257]
- Attention to glycemic load and index is a sensible approach; with high glycemic loads being more tied to negative health outcomes than glycemic index.

There is growing support in the literature for moderating carbohydrate intake. A recent study examined 148 ethnically diverse men and women without clinical cardiovascular disease or diabetes randomized into either a low carbohydrate (<40g/day) or a low fat (<30% cals from total fat, 7% saturated fat) group. Followed for one year, patients in the low carbohydrate group had greater weight loss and cardiovascular risk factor reduction than those in the low fat group.[255]

In an attempt to replace calories lost from carbohydrate consumption, many patients erroneously turn toward over reliance on meat products. Katz and Meller have concerns for how individuals may interpret the Paleo Diet, noting that the composition of animal meats commonly available today is much different from lean grass fed, grazing animals. The Paleo Diet should be mainly plant based with careful consideration of the amount and type of meat consumed.

Katz acknowledges that patients often come in with concerns about a specific ingredient such as fructose, gluten or artificial sweeteners. He advises physicians to acknowledge the concern but also to help the patient distinguish between sensitivity and toxicity. For the patient who may get headaches from aspartame, for example, it becomes sensible to remove it from the diet and to counsel them that aspartame is not toxic; it is something that they just can't tolerate.

In addition to his textbook, Katz points physicians who are interested in learning more about nutrition to his OWCH program, (www.turnthetidefoundation.org), a free 4-hour online training program in weight management. Another resource is Weigh Forward (www.weighforward.info) a third party program that has demonstrated evidence-based standards for weight loss and is certified by the American College of Preventive Medicine. Those physicians who want a more hands-on, and tastier approach to nutrition can take advantage of the "Healthy Kitchens, Healthy Lives" program a joint initiative between Harvard

Medical School and The Culinary Institute of America (CIA). The program, held at the CIA's Greystone campus in Napa Valley—brings together health professionals and world class chefs to explore the delicious possibilities of healthful food and its preparation.

Gaining Content and Credentialing

Mark Houston, MD, MS, MSc, is Director of the Hypertension Institute in Nashville, TN, and author of multiple books on the prevention and treatment of both hypertension and cardiovascular disease. One of the foremost nutrition experts in the country, Houston holds two masters degrees, one in Human Nutrition, another in Metabolic and Nutrition Medical Science, as well as teaches the Advanced Metabolic Cardiovascular Medicine module for the American Academy of Anti-Aging Medicine (A4M), and the Metabolic Medicine Institute (MMI). He is also a Hypertension Specialist (FASH). Houston is a firm believer that any physician who speaks on nutrition should have proper training in nutrition science.

He explains that the most in-depth understanding of nutrition is best gained from acquiring a university degree in nutrition. Houston acknowledges that few physicians will go through the time and expense to go this route. He directs some interested physicians to the University of Bridgeport, which has a 41 credit curriculum program that is exclusively offered online (www.bridgeport.edu).

Houston counsels that the next best step is to acquire one of the certified nutrition degrees offered through the American Nutrition Association (www.americannutritionassociation.org).

The third approach, he advises, "is to pick and choose from symposia offered by associations that offer CME. Some of these organizations now offer Fellowships or Masters of Science degrees from an accredited university such USF or GWU. Others do not grant degrees, but will often offer a certificate from the sponsoring organization."

A unique offering is a program created by A4M in conjunction with the University of South Florida Schools of Medicine. The Master of Science in Medical Sciences with a Concentration in Metabolic and Nutritional Medicine is a 32-credit course covering 480 total contact hours, much of which is delivered as webinars by A4M faculty. A similar program in Integrative Medicine is being developed at George Washington University with MMI.

Houston is often asked his views on supplementation. He counsels that there are only a handful of US based nutritional companies that he believes have both the quality control on all aspects of production and that only sell to physicians. He has personally toured many of the companies and inspected all aspects of manufacturing.

When asked what supplements he feels have the most scientific evidence, Houston, agreed with the American Heart Association on the important role of omega3s and AHA's recommendations to both increase oily fish intake and utilize omega3 fatty acid supplements for the primary and secondary prevention of CVD. The mechanisms underlying omega3's role in the prevention of CVD include anti-inflammatory, antiplatelet, anti-hypertensive, antiarrhythmic, and triglyceride-lowering properties.[258] Then, depending upon how much the patient is willing to spend on nutritional products, he will add a balanced supplement from one of his preferred manufactures that includes vitamins, minerals, Co-Q10, lipoic acid, and many others.

While there is a role for supplementation and for specific recommendations based upon personalized medicine and the patient's history and disease state, Houston agrees that the primary focus should initially be on optimal nutrition with specific supplements depending on the problem or disease that is being treated.

Integrating Lifestyle Medicine into Clinical Practice

When asked how he found his way into medicine, Mark Berman, MD, a physician who practices lifestyle and obesity medicine at One Medical Group in San Francisco, provides an oft-heard answer, namely that he wanted to "help people." Unlike many physicians in previous generations, he states, "Nutrition was the starting point that made me want to be a doctor. My driving passion entering medical school was to prevent chronic disease and co-morbidity. I was always interested in how we could get patients to shift their diets to patterns that were not only healthier but ecologically and humanely oriented, as well." Berman's "winding and non-traditional path" has included studying physical therapy at McGill University, Medicine at Yale University and primary care internal medicine at Harvard's Brigham and Women's Hospital. He was

CHAPTER SIX

a Doris Duke Clinical Research Fellow at UCSF and later served as the Special Assistant to the CEO and President for Childhood Obesity at the Robert Wood Johnson Foundation. Berman is a director of ACLM.

In addition to his lifestyle and obesity medicine practice, Berman serves as medical director for Mark One Lifestyle, a start up company that has produced a computerized drinking cup called Vessyl (www.myvessyl.com). The Vessyl not only tells the user how much they are drinking, it also contains proprietary sensors that identify and break down the liquid's contents to a molecular level. The Vessyl is able to identify fats, calories, sugars, caffeine, alcohol, and other chemical characteristics.

Berman's clinical practice at One Medical involves seeing eight patients a day, each for one hour. His one-on-one work is supported by health coaches and nutritionists, as well as by the use of wearable monitoring tools and home-based devices including remote digital scales. Group visits for stress and anxiety are just starting to be implemented in One Medical's South Bay and Washington, DC locations. Tools and techniques are matched to the patient's motivations for change and state of readiness. Operating in the One Medical environment for the last two years, Berman says, has been "super fun." Noting the increased physician satisfaction with this model of care, One Medical is working to see how other physicians in the group can transition a portion of their practices accordingly.

Berman notes that the structure of the visit follows the hourly time allotment.

> "The goal of the first visit is to provide a comprehensive assessment. We do a deep dive on their weight history and spend time trying to understand it. When did they start putting on excess weight? What was their weight history like as child? What happened over time? Do they binge? What have they tried? Most patients have tried dozens of things, including medication and formal programs. I inquire about patterns such as purging or laxative use. We find out what has worked in the past, what hasn't and why. This process of inquiry, and the sharing that results from it, not only creates an intimacy with the patient, but also provides the understanding that ultimately helps us figure out a starting point. We do a lifestyle history and learn more about their exercise, sleep,

stress and mood patterns. Do they feel supported? Many of the patients who live in the city feel isolated and alone. We inquire as to their work commute, both how long and how they get to work. I examine their chart looking at their medications, co-morbidities and the labs that have been done in the past.

I then conduct a brief physical exam including going over their biometrics to make certain they are stable. I look for rare conditions such as Cushing syndrome or leptin deficiencies. Sometimes an hour is not enough to accomplish this, but usually at about 30-40 minutes into the visit, we have a holistic sense of their readiness to make changes, what's been helpful in the past, and we can begin to formulate the treatment plan.

I try to triage my patients. Do they need a little guidance and some advice or do they need more support? For those that need more support I run through a list of options, including the availability of our coordinated program with coaches and nutritionists, as well as the resources available in the community. If their mental health is not well attended to it will be very difficult to make any lifestyle changes. I will refer them out for mental health counseling. We identify a small number of one to three lifestyle changes to get them started.

Eighty percent of my patients take advantage of our coordinated metabolic program that we began six months ago. It is a highly supportive, highly tracked program conducted by our nutritionist and health coaches. Some people just need a one off consultation with me, however, they are in the minority."

When asked about providing advice to other physicians who may want to establish a holistic lifestyle and obesity management practice, Berman notes that doing so is very difficult if there is little or no support from the healthcare system. He encourages interested physicians to first ask, "How am I going to do something that is economically viable? Even though a physician may see enormous merit in this kind of work, the business side of the equation is the hardest part to figure out."

He outlines several paths. The first is essentially a carve out in which physicians maintain their salary and traditional billing practice but

CHAPTER SIX

allot some time—maybe a day or half-day a week to offer extended time and more in depth visits for patients with metabolic disease. This allows the physician the financial support and freedom to figure out the model that is best for them.

Another excellent starting point involves making use of group models which he believes can be extremely rewarding for both clinician and patient, as well being economically successful. Berman also points to the viability of the concierge model noting that many physicians have made it work, but that it wasn't personally rewarding for him.

Berman is most optimistic about the "box that I fit into," the innovative primary care system as implemented by One Medical Group because of the shared values and their willingness and flexibility to provide a sandbox in which he can play.

Other core services provided by One Medical Group (www.onemedical.com) include same day appointments, on-site lab tests with no appointments required, ease of electronic access to records and providers, 24/7 phone support, and treatment of common medical issues through video visits and mobile apps.

Members of One Medical pay a fee of $150 per year. The company accepts a wide range of insurance plans for the medical services. Berman is able to bill a one-hour consultation that usually involves three to five different comorbidities as a level 5 visit. A modest direct pay fee is charged for coordinated care that involves the services of the health coaches and nutritionists.

Building Upon the Basics

While physicians may find more excitement in technical advances in fields such as genetics, stem cells, robotics, or neuroplasticity, healing patients begins with the back to basics approach. Mitigating health risks, improving diet, adherence to exercise, regular use of stress management techniques—these form the bedrock for helping our patients lead healthier, higher quality lives. In helping patients make these changes, we must first recognize their state of readiness and then meet them where they are in their process. It is important to remember that very often we don't see all of our successes. The patient who takes our advice to heart may not return to see us, not because of dissatisfaction with our services, but rather the opposite: they are too well and don't need further care.

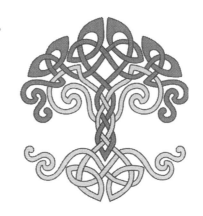

Individuality is the fundamental principle of biology. It is the mechanism for adaptation. Adaptation is what nature gives us to find our solution in the world. The environment is offering us the opportunity to change and we are not keeping up.

— Sidney M. Baker, MD

7

The Functional Medicine Paradigm

FUNCTIONAL MEDICINE
Root cause identification
Personalized medicine
Reverse systemic imbalances
Strong nutrition/ gut focus
Advanced biomarkers
Timeline assessment
Detoxification

A note about the word "functional" is in order. Most conventional physicians were trained that a functional disorder is supratentorial, meaning psychological or psychiatric. In this context, the diagnosis of a functional illness is made after all other physically based causes have been ruled out.

As the term is used today, functional medicine is a multi-factorial approach in search of the root cause of illness. The basic tenets of functional medicine are derived from personalized healthcare and a systems orientation to illness and wellness. The therapeutic approach aims to restore balance in the system; imbalances are regarded as a two-way street. On one hand a condition such as obesity drives inflammation, creates imbalances in hormones, affects mood, creates absorption and digestion disturbances, and ultimately affects epigenetics. On the other hand, one imbalance such as inflammation may lead to many conditions such as heart disease, depression, arthritis, cancer and diabetes.

The functional medicine concept was created by noted nutritional biochemist Jeffrey Bland, PhD, who in 1991 cofounded The Institute for Functional Medicine (IFM) (www.functionalmedicine.org). IFM has been the driving force in teaching this encompassing, personalized, patient centered model of care to thousands of clinicians both domestically and internationally. Bland served as Chief Science Officer for Metagenics and President of MetaProteomics for 12 years. In 2012, he formed a nonprofit organization called the Personalized Lifestyle Medicine Institute

CHAPTER SEVEN

(www.plminstitute.org) based in Seattle, Washington. A prolific author, his latest book, along with Mark Hyman, MD, is *The Disease Delusion: Conquering the Causes of Chronic Illness for a Healthier, Longer, and Happier Life* (HarperWave).

Bland's approach takes into account genetics, biomarkers and lifestyle based therapeutics, a combination he likens to the secret sauce of personalized medicine. "Genomics decode out the hardware, phonemics assess the software through a dizzying array of more affordable biomarkers and deeper diagnostics, and lifestyle medicine provides a smarter therapeutic approach to prevention before the disease even sets in."[259]

FM acknowledges the many factors that impact upon health and affect the human organism. This was well expressed by IFM President David Jones, MD, in an IFM monograph entitled *21st Century Medicine:*

> "Each human emerges from a mold that has but one model. Uniqueness continues to develop throughout life as a result of myriad influences. Family, school, work, community diet, exercise, stress and environmental toxicity all communicate information from outside the organism to the epigenetic translational structures that are married to nuclear DNA and that create powerful downstream effects on the genome, proteome, and metabolome."[260]

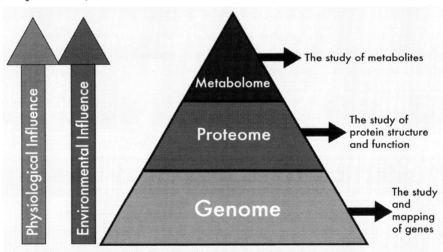

FIGURE 17: A Functional View of Physiology and Environment

In the IFM model, clinical imbalances are organized along seven nodes, examples of which include:

- Assimilation: digestion, absorption, macro- and macrobiotics, and respiration
- Defense and Repair: the state of the immune system, inflammation, infections and microbiome health
- Energy: Cellular energy and mitochondrial function; the relationship of oxidative stress
- Biotransformation & elimination: toxicity and detoxification
- Transport: the movement of fluids, arterial and venous circulation, the state of the lymphatic system
- Communication: the hypothalamic-pituitary-adrenal axis, endocrine function, neurotransmitters and immune messengers
- Structural Integrity: ranging from subcellular membranes to musculoskeletal structures.

The Functional Medicine Perspective

Functional medicine presents a different approach to evaluating and treating patients. As with any emerging paradigm, there are critics who take issue with both the science and approach. For example, functional medicine practitioners place a high priority on assimilation, and defense and repair as it pertains to the GI tract. One of the axioms of functional treatment is "First, repair the gut." This axiom is consistent with every global healing tradition except for western medicine. One of the first principles of Ayurvedic Medicine is "with proper food there is no need for medicine."

Given that 70 million Americans have digestive disorders that prompt nearly 60 million healthcare visits, addressing imbalances in the GI tract is fertile ground for improving health. Many patients are so accustomed to the assorted symptoms of GI distress—bloating, constipation, burping, belching, flatulence, infrequent heartburn—that the subject may not even come up in a routine office visit. Sales of Nexium® alone, reached $7.9 billion, ranking it number six on the top global pharmaceutical products in 2013.[261]

CHAPTER SEVEN

Researchers are increasingly appreciating the complexity of the GI system. Its enteric nervous system has been labeled "the second brain." Similar to the brain, the gastrointestinal nervous system utilizes more than 30 neurotransmitters and is responsible for producing 95% of the serotonin in the body.[262] The gut is also home to an estimated 500-1,000 species of bacteria. While the human genome features 23,000 genes, the genomes of the viruses and bacteria in our intestinal tracts is estimated to encode 3.3 million genes.[263] Microbial balance between 'good' and 'bad' bacterial is essential for health, and imbalances in the microbiome can contribute to generalized inflammation.

One area of research is garnering increasing attention from both the scientific and lay community. Known as 'leaky gut,' this condition is sparking research that substantiates the importance of maintaining the GI tract's barrier function. The gastrointestinal tract is a single contiguous layer of cells separating the inside of the body from the external environment. Along with the neuroendocrine network and the gut's lymphoid tissue, the tight intercellular junctions in the epithelium prevent non-self antigens from entering the circulation. Another way of stating this is good fences make good neighbors.

In genetically susceptible individuals, these non-self antigens can potentially lead to an immune response directed toward extraintestinal organs. Increased intestinal permeability has been observed in several autoimmune diseases as well as a host of others. These include patients with GI diseases such as Crohn's disease, celiac disease, and irritable bowel syndrome, but also patients with multiple sclerosis and diabetes. "In several autoimmune conditions it appears that increased permeability is a constant and early feature of the disease process."[264] New treatment approaches are being directed at counteracting this increased intestinal permeability.

Alessio Fasano, MD, at Massachusetts General Hospital for Children, has shown that zonulin, a protein that modulates the permeability of the tight junction is critical for its integrity. Disturbances in this mechanism may underlie the pathology of food sensitivity.[265] Exposure to antigenic triggers causes zonulin upregulation and an opening in the tight junctions. The dietary peptides stimulate macrophage pro-inflammatory gene expression and the release of inflammatory cytokines. "Pathophysiological regulation of tight junctions is influenced by many factors, including: secretory IgA, enzyme, neuropeptides, neurotransmitters, dietary peptides and lectins, yeast, aerobic bacteria and anaerobic bacteria, parasites, proinflammatory cytokines, free radicals and regulatory T-cell dysfunction."[266]

The Argument for Chronic Exposure

Functional medical providers also place significant emphasis on the concept of toxicity and the tools to detoxify the body. This paradigm has drawn controversy from some conventional physicians who view this treatment approach as nebulous and unproven at best, and as "voodoo" or "woo," at worst. Heated debates and personal attacks, by established physicians on functional medicine practitioners can be easily found on the Internet.

Environmental toxicants include heavy metals such as lead, arsenic, mercury and cadmium, volatile organic pollutants, plastics, pharmaceutical wastes and pesticides. These chemicals enter our systems through the skin, lungs, and gastrointestinal tract. Potential food related toxins include nitrates, hormones, xenoestrogens, colorings, and antibiotics provided in animal feed. In its first ever report, the Food and Drug has estimated that 29 million pounds of antibiotics were sold for use in food animals in the United States in 2009.[267]

Agreeing with their functional counterparts, opposing conventional physicians have no quarrel with the physiological effects of the food-related 'toxins' in a high glycemic index, alcoholic beverages, or hydrogenated, saturated fat laden products. These conditions can be measured with validated clinical laboratory tests such as HbA1c, BACs, LFTs and lipids. In comparison, many of the tests for toxins are less well validated; so too are some of the treatment methods. Physician critics of functional medicine warn that these treatments are not proven and may cause harm. Research demonstrates that toxins such as lead, mercury and cadmium are linked to vascular disease, yet few western physicians are trained to assess for heavy metal body burden.[268] Discussion of the magnitude of harm done by integrative-type treatments including chelation, pales in comparison to the incidence of Adverse Drug Event (ADE) caused by pharmaceutical agents.

More than 8.6 million ADEs are reported in the United States each year, with 2.2 million of them being severe. After heart disease, cancer and stroke, ADEs are the fourth leading cause of death.[269] More than

CHAPTER SEVEN

700,000 patients present to the emergency department annually with ADEs. This accounts for 2.5% of ED visits for unintentional injuries.[270] Dose-related drug problems, a potentially avoidable complication, abound in the elderly. One study examining admissions and in-hospital reactions in an elderly population identified that 80% of ADEs were dose related.[271]

The divergence of belief around environmental toxins begins with concurrence; it has been established that exposure to high levels of certain elements can cause illness. The question is whether repeated sub-clinical exposure to relatively low levels of environmental toxins such as heavy metals, volatile organic chemicals, pesticides, etc. may lead to chronic adverse health effects.

For example, lead poisoning in young children is an established disease that affects the developing nervous system and can cause abdominal pain and cramping, anemia, low appetite and energy, headaches, irritability and difficulty sleeping. At the highest levels of exposure, lead poisoning may also cause muscle cramps, vomiting, staggering walk, seizures, and coma.[272]

The susceptibility of children is driven, in part by their enhanced gastrointestinal absorption (30-50%) as compared to adults (5-10%).[273]

While lead is no longer used in gasoline and house paint in the United States, it continues to be a health issue. In 2012, of the 2.5 million children tested in 39 states in the US, 121,344 had levels between 5-9 ug/dL; approximately 16,000 had levels greater than 10 ug/dL. The CDC notes that these data may be underreported because certain states do not report the higher levels. Could sub-clinical lead exposure be at fault for delayed development in some children?

Acute pesticide poisoning is a well-recognized clinical entity in farmworkers exposed to the estimated 5.1 billion pounds of pesticides applied to crops worldwide each year—with the United States making up about 20% of that amount. Signs and symptoms of acute pesticide poisoning[274] include headaches, nausea, shortness of breath, or seizures. When a farm worker presents with cancer, infertility and other reproductive problems, neurological complaints, or a respiratory condition, how likely is it that the offending agent is pesticide related?

In addition to identifying traumatic brain injury as the signature injury of the Iraq War, the Veterans Administration recognizes other environmental hazards suffered by veterans who served from 2003-2011. These include conditions caused by exposure to dust and particulates; burn pits, sulfur fires, machinery chemicals and paints, chromium, depleted uranium, noise, heat, and Mefloquine used to treat malaria. The VA also notes that a prominent condition affecting the earlier Gulf War veterans is "a cluster of medically unexplained chronic symptoms that can include fatigue, headaches, joint pain, indigestion, insomnia, dizziness, respiratory disorders, and memory problems."[275] Illnesses qualifying for disability include chronic fatigue syndrome, fibromyalgia, functional gastrointestinal disorders and a variety of undiagnosed illnesses. The VA associates presumed toxin exposure with these conditions.

While exposure to toxic chemicals and other environmental irritants can be linked to military service, it is more difficult to establish relationships or causality with the environmental factors that are ubiquitous in everyday life. For example, Americans spend an average of 1.5 hours in their cars every day. According to The Ecology Center, a non-profit environmental organization based in Ann Arbor, Michigan, this is where we are exposed to more than 275 chemicals, "some of which are associated with allergies, birth defects, impaired learning, liver problems, and cancer. They included chromium and lead, as well as volatile organic compounds that come from brominated flame retardants and other additives in some cars' plastic parts."[276] Carpets, dry-cleaned clothing, the flame retardants on our mattresses are all treated with compounds that are potentially hazardous to our health. Does this subacute exposure play a role in disease causation?

Just as chemicals are omnipresent in the air we breathe and the water we drink, additives are also ubiquitous in our foods. Seeking to quantify the level of danger posed by food additives, the FDA has coined the acronym GRAS that stands for Generally Recognized as Safe as defined "under sections 201(s) and 409 of the Federal Food, Drug, and Cosmetic Act (the Act), any substance that is intentionally added to food is a food additive, that is subject to premarket review and approval by FDA, unless the substance is generally recognized, among qualified experts, as having been adequately shown to be safe under the conditions of its intended use, or unless the use of the substance is otherwise excluded from the definition of a food additive."[277]

The study of environmental toxicity has led many researchers to single-mindedly focus on analyzing and quantifying the offending agent.

CHAPTER SEVEN

Little attention has been paid to the individual who is subjected to the insult. Ira Goodman, MD, an IM physician in San Diego, California notes that people react differently to the same stimulus; their reactions reflect genomic variability combined with exposure levels; and one toxin can cause a variety of pathology even in the same person.[278] This focus on the individual was perhaps best expressed by the 19th century French chemist Louis Pasteur who was famous for his insistence that germs were the cause of disease, not the body. Toward the end of his life, however, he modified his position about disease causation, noting, "It is the soil, not the seed." Pasteur recognized that an infecting agent (the seed) causes disease when the host's body (the soil) provides a favorable environment.

Hearing The Voice of the Patient

Every discipline, be it cardiology or orthopedics, has its own unique acronyms, an abbreviation for the diseases and procedures that comprise the specialty and frame the patient-physician relationship. Mastering the language of medicine poses one of the greatest challenges to medical students and residents during their training. We learn shorthand: CVD is cardiovascular disease; THA stands for total hip arthroplasty. During our training, we were also subjected to a longhand version of the medical language, a unique combination of phrasing that, in part, sets the tone for how we view the physician-patient relationship. In his article, "The Military Metaphors of Modern Medicine," Abraham Fuks, MD, Dean of the Faculty of Medicine, McGill, notes that much of our medical language has a violent connotation:

> "Medical discourse is replete with the language of war and such phrases as 'the war on cancer,' 'magic bullets,' 'silver bullets,' 'the therapeutic armamentarium,' 'agents of disease,' 'the body's defenses,' and 'doctor's orders' are deeply engrained in our medical rhetoric. The mindset engendered by this discourse of war renders the patient as a battlefield upon which the doctor-combatant defeats the arch-enemy, disease. The reified disease becomes the object of the physician's attention, displacing the patient as the interlocutor in the doctor-patient relationship. This shift of attention is exacerbated by contemporary imaging methodologies, and patients,

who in Foucault's clinic became open to the medical gaze, are rendered totally transparent, perhaps virtual. Diagnostics becomes centred on the putative agent and therapeutics revolves around extirpation and conquest. Arguably, the most important effect of this framing of medicine is the eradication of the patient's voice from the narrative of illness."[266]

Growing up in the Midwest, Kristi Hughes, ND, Associate Director for IFM was first attracted to chiropractic school and attended Western States Chiropractic in Portland, Oregon for a year, before determining that she wanted to learn more about naturopathic medicine. She enrolled in the National College of Naturopathic medicine so that she could pursue medical training that incorporated a more robust discussion of nutrition and botanical medicine. Her introduction to chiropractic provided her with solid grounding in physical and structural medicine.

Hughes talks about "her moment of enlightenment" that came when she attended her first IFM conference in 2000 and was exposed to one of the key tools, the Functional Matrix. The Matrix helped Hughes, "organize the aspects of systems biology. It provided me with a framework onto which I could hang all the information I had been exposed to. It provided safer ways to integrate nutrition and greater depth to identifying and treating disease."

Hughes describes functional medicine as "a unique blend of science, philosophy and tools that drive patient engagement organized around three steps."

She goes on to explain the steps from the clinician's perspective: "The first is to acknowledge the importance of lifestyle and the key elements such as diet, sleep, stress, movement and relationships and their effect on health. We deal with the lifestyle factors upfront."

The second step marks the departure from history taking as practiced by conventional practicing physicians. "We view the history as the beginning of the therapeutic partnership. This encounter allows us to bring the patient into the storyline and to create a medical history based upon the functional timeline."

Thirdly, patient and physician work to identify the ATMs that are plotted on the timeline. "ATM stands for the antecedents, triggers, and mediators that affect the patient's condition. Working cooperatively, patient and physician seek to identify both key patterns and key times in an attempt to identify critical patterns," said Hughes.

The Timeline, the Functional Matrix, and a treatment algorithm summarized by the acronym GO TO IT are included in the Appendix.

While these tools help clinicians appreciate the art of the patient encounter, physicians who practice functional medicine also strive to balance these data with evidence. Jones notes that, "Appreciating the narrative nature of the illness experience and the intuitive and subjective aspects of clinical presentations does not require us to reject the principles of evidence-based medicine. Nor does such an approach demand an inversion of the hierarchy of evidence so that personal anecdote carries more weight in decision making than the randomized controlled trial."[279]

One Mechanism with Multiple Manifestations

Brad Bale, MD, is co-founder of the Bale/Doneen method, adjunct professor at Texas Tech Health Science Center and Medical Director of the Heart Health program at Grace Clinic in Lubbock, Texas. He started to make changes in the substance and structure of his therapeutic approach after practicing for 25 years as a conventional family practice physician. Bale felt a growing frustration that, despite practicing the standard of care, his patients were continuing to experience strokes and myocardial infarcts. He remembers the moment when one of his patients, whom he had referred to a cardiologist, died several weeks later of a massive MI despite having passed a treadmill test. These types of cases led Bale to have an early interest in coronary artery scans, advanced biomarkers that identify inflammation, and lifestyle and functional medicine approaches to halt and reverse the disease process.

Bale's move to a membership model came at the insistence of his wife, who early on was managing his practice. Early in the formation of his functional/lifestyle approach to managing cardiovascular disease, Bale took pride in the great results he had achieved with a challenging patient who was referred to him by another physician. The patient was a man who had undergone bypass surgery for angina only to have a repeat MI four months later. The patient's disease was so aggressive; the referring physician had told the patient he would be dead in less than a year.

"I spent an hour and a half with this patient going through the testing results, explaining the role of exercise, diet, supplementation—all the key components of the Bale/Doneen Method. We were able to halt the vascular disease. The patient died years later from liver cancer. When the practice received insurance reimbursement for the 90 minutes I had spent with the patient, my wife, who was managing the practice, pointedly asked me 'Do you want to know how much the insurance company paid you for that visit?' The answer to that question sparked our move to a membership type practice," said Bale. Bale's belief in his anti-inflammatory approach is so strong that he provides his patients with a unique guarantee. He returns their annual membership fee back to them if they suffer a cardiovascular event.

Along with nurse practitioner, Amy Doneen, DNP, FNP, who practices in Spokane, WA, Bale is pioneering an expansive view of disease and a methodology of assessment and treatment built around the concept of "arteriology." The two clinicians have recently completed a book entitled *Beat the Heart Attack Gene: A Revolutionary Plan to Prevent Heart Disease, Stroke, and Diabetes* (Turner) and routinely conduct training courses in the Bale/Doneen method to preventing and reversing CVD.

According to Bale, "We have evidence that inflammation is the cause of atherothrombotic disease from inception to progression and to culmination in a cardiovascular event. Our method rests upon maintaining the arteries in a non-inflamed state, so we routinely monitor our at-risk patients every three months."

The role that inflammation plays in cardiovascular disease has been recognized for decades. In 1976, Russell Ross, PhD, at the University of Washington published a sentinel paper entitled "The Pathogenesis of Atherosclerosis."[280] Ross clearly outlined two components of thrombotic disease: an injury and a response. It is inflammation, the response to the insult that is the culprit. Oxidized LDL is but one of many independent factors that can damage the body's 60,000 miles of blood vessels. Others include dental bacteria, smoking, sleep apnea, insulin resistance and stress. The stress-related activation of the sympathetic nervous system, the hypothalamic-pituitary axis, and the renin-angiotensin system increases levels of catecholamines, corticosteroids, glucagon, growth hormone, renin, and homocysteine. It has been estimated that stress-related events may account for the approximately 40% of atherosclerotic patients with no other known risk factors.[281]

Bale relies upon a handful of diagnostic companies to assess, monitor,

CHAPTER SEVEN

and manage inflammation in his patients. Vasolabs Inc (www.vasolabs.com) and CardioRisk Laboratories (www.cardiorisk.us) are two mobile ultrasound testing companies that specialize in abdominal aortic aneurysm testing, echocardiograms, Ankle Brachial Index (ABI) and Carotid Intima Media Thickness (CIMT). Another valuable test of endothelial function is EndoPAT by Itamar Medical (www.itamarmedical.com). Genetic testing can be obtained from labs such as deCODEme, or Quest Diagnostics. For the advanced biomarkers that he uses to diagnose and follow his patients, Bale partners with Cleveland Heart Lab (CHL) (www.clevelandheartlab.com), a full service clinical reference laboratory specializing in next-generation cardiovascular disease prevention, diagnosis and management. CHL has developed a specialized panel of advanced inflammation testing (IT) biomarkers that allow practitioners to assess CVD along a severity and time-phased continuum.

Bale uses these biomarkers to gauge the "heat" of the arteries. He routinely evaluates F2-Isoprostanes (F2-IsoPs) in his patients. This urinary biomarker, formed from arachidonic acid, is considered the 'gold standard' to assess oxidative stress on the body as it relates to lifestyle choices. The more oxidized a patient is, the more likely they are to form clots. Urinary F2-IsoPs levels are increased with a high intake of red meat, lack of exercise, poor sleep and smoking.[282,283] Levels can be lowered through lifestyle improvements.

The F2-IsoP marker is a way to assess compliance with lifestyle adherence. "When asked how they are doing on their program, many patients reflexively answer 'fine.' When their F2-IsoPs come back high and we confront them with this, we get a more accurate history. I've had one patient remark, 'I can't get away with anything with you'" noted Bale.

Bale also gets OxLDL levels on his patients to assess the amount of LDL cholesterol that has been modified due to oxidation. OxLDL is an early warning sign of vessel damage. High OxLDL levels predict the risk of metabolic syndrome and are closely associated with risk of heart disease in healthy individuals with lifestyle risks.[284, 285]

Bale utilizes three additional tests to assess endothelial functioning. These include the well-known tests of hsCRP and fibrinogen, along with the microalbumin/creatinine ratio. Bale cites the Framingham data on this urinary marker. "We know from these data that the microalbumin/creatine ratio was an independent predictor of heart attack. Most conventional labs put the cut off point at a value of 30, which is the point of end stage renal disease. When the ratio was above 4 in men and above 7.5 in women, the risk of a cardiovascular event in the next six years was three times greater."

In his work with at risk patients, Bale uses two tests that specifically assess the inflammation in the walls of the artery. Lipoprotein-associated phospholipase-A2 (Lp-PLA2; The PLAC® Test) is a vascular specific inflammatory enzyme that binds to LDL cholesterol and releases a chemical inside the artery wall. The PLAC® test looks at the level of vessel wall inflammation beneath the collagen cap. Recent data indicate that Lp-PLA2 is not just a marker in the wall but also a factor in the disease process itself.[286]

The second vascular specific test is known as myeloperoxidase or MPO. MPO identifies the body's inflammatory response to vascular damage due to vulnerable plaque, cellular erosions, and cracks in the artery wall. Because it is a marker of plaque instability MPO is an indicator of near-term risk of a cardiac event. MPO is also important for predicting risk in apparently healthy people who may not otherwise have been identified with traditional testing.[287]

Serial management of inflammatory biomarkers is critical for optimal management of the at-risk cardiovascular patient. According to Bale, "Numerous pathologies can cause arterial inflammation and some can be occult in nature. We use these markers to follow the patient with known arterial disease to make sure nothing is rekindling. This happens more frequently than we'd like."

Functional Medicine in Action

A functional medicine approach emphasizes going back to the basics to identify the root cause(s) of illness, employing the timeline and paying close attention to the interaction of pharmaceuticals and adverse reactions. These factors came into play in the evaluation and treatment of a patient that Mimi saw for gastrointestinal and joint complaints.

> The patient, a 54 year old female was referred to Mimi by her husband who called the office and said, "My wife is really, really sick and we heard what you do. Would you please see her?"
>
> During the first visit, I (Mimi) asked the patient "When

CHAPTER SEVEN

were you last well?"

To which she replies, "Three years ago."

I then ask, "What were you doing in your life at that time?"

She went on to note that, "I was doing great, I was exercising, I was doing Pilates, doing everything." At this point she went to see a new family practice physician who reviewed her medications and advised her to stop her thyroid medication. She stops her thyroid medication and gains 30 pounds. Unsettled by the weight gain, she restarts the thyroid medication and goes to a different family practice physician who notes her hyperlipidemia and puts her on a statin. The new primary care physician reviews her medications and says, "Why are you taking hormones? Women shouldn't be on hormones." This physician instructs her to stop her hormone treatment.

This sets off a mélange of symptoms including hot flashes, insomnia, postmenopausal joint pain, and memory loss. A urinary tract infection secondary to serratia was treated with two courses of antibiotics: an aminoglycoside and an antipseudomonal beta-lactam. She consulted a rheumatologist for joint pain and was put on a course of steroids, so by the time she presents to me, her hair is falling out and she is 35 pounds over weight. She complained of frequent bloating, constipation, and mild abdominal discomfort. What actually drove her in is the recommendation that she go on Humira® for a presumed diagnosis of rheumatoid arthritis. In my first meeting I told her "You may have that or you may not, but let's go back to basics."

This involved first focusing on her gut. Given the recent course of antibiotics, we needed to restore proper nutrient absorption, digestion and assimilation. We put her on an elimination diet to identify potential food allergies and intolerances, then orally supplemented her with glutamine, zinc, pre- and probiotics to start the process of healing her GI tract. A closer look at the timeline revealed that her arthritis and joint pain started when she was put on the statin.

While statins offer significant cardiovascular benefits, they also affect

immune regulation and may potentiate autoimmune diseases such as rheumatoid arthritis.[288] They also increase the risk on new-onset diabetes.

Statin adverse events are a common occurrence. A study conducted at the Brigham and Women's Hospital and Massachusetts General Hospital examined records of over 107,835 statin patients. Statin-related events were documented for 17.4% of the patients. More than half of the patients, 57,000 in total, discontinued statins at least temporarily for a variety of reasons; some of which were fatigue, digestive distress, muscle pains, headaches or changes in liver function. While many of the patients were able to restart on a different statin or take a lower lose, there were still patients who were unable to tolerate the statin.

Joint pain is a commonly reported adverse event. In the clinical study for atorvastatin (Lipitor®) arthralgia, arthritis and joint pain were frequently occurring reported adverse events in excess of placebo.[289]

Genetic testing revealed that the patient had C/C genotype SNPs for the SLCO1B1 genotype. These SNPs affect statin metabolism in the liver, an effect that is enhanced depending on whether the patient has the heterozygote (T/C) or homozygote (C/C) genotype. The T/C heterozygote type has a four-fold increased risk for developing statin induced myopathy. With the C/C genotype of SLCO1B1, affecting up to 5% of the population, the risk of statin induced myopathy jumps to seventeen-fold.[290]

> Discontinuation of the statin, coupled with dietary improvements, elimination of potential food allergens, and attention to rebuilding the gastrointestinal tract has led to dramatic improvement in the patient's symptoms.

Healthier Mothers: Healthier Children

Leslie Stone, MD, is a board certified family practitioner with Stone Medical, PC in Ashland, Oregon, who for 30 years has specialized in women's health and healthy childhood development. Stone feels that her primary role in medicine is "to help women enjoy, appreciate, and maximize every passage in life, from infancy through aging." Along with David Jones, MD, and Michael Stone, MD, the group provides comprehensive care to families. The clinicians share a belief in early recognition of health issues and early intervention to correct imbalances that

CHAPTER SEVEN

can lead to chronic disease.

Stone traces her integrative thinking back to her childhood, in part driven by her experiences in a dysfunctional family and her sister's struggle with mental illness. As an undergraduate Stone became intensely interested in the psychological and biochemical underpinnings of behavior. "I was trying to understand my sister's troubles with life and all the while I was wondering about the complexities of these interactions. I later understood from my medical training that a single solutions fits well for an acute problem but does not work for the types of complex problems we see each day in practice. A functional medicine approach allows me to gather information, think about it, and apply it in a very individualized, very fluid and adaptable way to each individual."

Stone rejects the notion of exclusivity and the limitations of scope that a concierge practice can impart.

> "I wanted to take my integrative approach to people who have insurance, who are on the Oregon Health Plan, or who are poor and can only afford to pay every once in a while. We will bill insurance for the maximum allowed. My tools are primarily based on the tests that are readily available at the local clinical lab and imaging center. Because we appreciate that nutrition is the common currency of molecular and sub molecular biology, we have two nutritionists in our practice. While nutrition and lifestyle make up the language of our practice, we also recognize that energy may be a better language for the patient. We practice in a very robust integrated community with Naturopaths, Chinese herbalists, Reiki therapists, so we will refer patients to these resources as well."

Between 25-30% of Stone's practice is related to pregnancy, and it is in this area that much of Stone's integrative approach is focused. She relates the case study of a 36-year-old woman pregnant with pregnancy induced hypertension and a history of difficult pregnancies.

> The patient's story begins with her own birth, as a twin delivered by cesarean section. Raised by a psychotically depressed mother, the patient experienced a non-nurturing and nutritionally depleted upbringing. She recalls struggling with anxiety as a very young child, and by the time she reached

early adulthood she developed reflux esophagitis treated with proton pump inhibitors quickly followed by new allergies and eczema.

Her asthma was treated with a steroid inhaler and her gestational hypertension with induction of labor, producing a small, but otherwise healthy newborn. Post-partum depression plagued the early days of the neonatal time period, requiring an antidepressant starting with and continuing up to her second pregnancy. Her previous physician prescribed a baby aspirin as a preventive measure for preeclampsia, but provided no other advice on how to reduce her now chronic environmental allergies and eczema, inhaled steroid-dependent asthma, gastro-esophageal reflux disease, anxiety and depression.

In the second trimester of her second pregnancy, she experienced asthma exacerbations requiring four courses of oral prednisone. By the third trimester she had developed pregnancy induced hypertension (PIH) again, but this time with proteinurea, a low platelet count, and elevated liver enzymes (PIH/HELLP) with suspected fetal growth restriction. Induction of labor with magnesium prophylaxis for eclampsia produced a stressed, small for gestational age neonate requiring resuscitation and intensive care.

Her provider recommended sterilization because of the near 100% recurrence of PIH/HELLP syndrome with the very real possibility of seizures and disseminated intravascular coagulopathy (DIC).

She arrived on our doorstep thirteen weeks after her tubal blockage failed, paralyzed for fear of the very worst outcome. Recognizing that PIH is a dysfunction of the microvascular system our management of this high-risk pregnancy centered on gut restoration, immune integrity, mitigation of inflammation and fear reduction.

We evaluated her particular genetic vulnerabilities and nutrient insufficiencies, and developed an individualized functional medicine-based dietary and lifestyle plan. This included supplementation of nutrients not adequately addressed by

CHAPTER SEVEN

her diet. We also initiated stress reduction techniques consistent with her belief system.

With this treatment model, we believed we would obtain significant improvement in her symptoms and reduction in her medication use. In her second trimester she eliminated her antihistamine use for allergies, and rarely used her steroid inhaler and proton pump inhibitor. Activated B vitamins intended to help her mood and reduce the risk of PIH proved useful, but did not eliminate her need for a low dose SSRI. By the 3rd trimester she stopped all medications except the SSRI and the very rare PPI (even though she had no reflux symptoms). She developed no signs or symptoms of PIH, and her fetus grew well based on serial ultrasound evaluations. Her fears slowly and steadily abated.

She did experience right flank pain secondary to hydronephrosis, a benign pregnancy related swelling of her right kidney collecting system, and requested induction for maternal discomfort at 38+ weeks gestation. She experienced an uneventful vaginal delivery of a vigorous normal weight neonate, who did not require resuscitation and was able to recover on maternal chest, skin to skin, breast-feeding immediately. Three months later the patient self-elected to eliminate gluten, resulting in the complete resolution of eczema and reflux esophagitis.

One and a half years later this mother remains without allergies, asthma, eczema, and reflux disease, and her mood is very well controlled on a low dose SSRI. She maintains her diet and lifestyle with individualized nutrient supplementation. Her one and a half year old is very healthy.

Case studies can be compelling but provide limited and less valuable data than does a more rigorous clinical study. Stone and her team performed a retrospective observational evaluation of more than one hundred pregnant women treated in their practice over a one year period and compared them to a community treated group of nearly 600 patients. They hypothesized that diabetes, hypertension, large and small for gestational age complications would be reduced. Stone collected detailed diagnostic data including serum zinc, carnitine, iron, 25-hydroxy vitamin D and MTHFR and COMT polymorphisms on her patients. She had used these values to create a customized nutritional program for each patient along with supplemental nutrients adjusted based on genetics, trimester, and previous pregnancy history. The aggregated occurrence rate of the four conditions under study was significantly lower in her study population than in the comparison group of nearly 600 pregnancies.

The challenges of delivering nutritional education lie in making it understandable, actionable and trackable by both patient and physician. Stone has compiled her experience and techniques into a website called growbabyhealth.com. The site features an electronic platform for physicians to monitor their patient's nutritional habits, a mobile app for moms, and four e-learning nutrition modules. To simplify the process of nutritional supplementation, Stone has created a reproductive health dietary supplement called preGenesis that is available on the growbabyhealth website.

Functional Medicine Group Visits

With the modern-day adaptations that are reorienting the field of medicine away from simply reacting to disease, and instead working to prevent disease and promote wellness, group visits offer a new and impactful tool for modeling health behavior change for our patients. With its emphasis on 'teachable moments' for overall wellness, the physician-client relationship, and a supportive environment for patients, the group visit is increasingly utilized by physicians focusing on treating the underlying causes of disease.

Shilpa P. Saxena, MD, IFMCP, is one such physician. Saxena, a board-certified family practice physician founded SevaMed Institute, an integrative and functional medicine practice on the outskirts of Tampa, Florida. "Seva" is an ancient Sanskrit word that translates to "selfless service," one of the driving principles of her practice. Joined by an Integrative Advanced Registered Nurse Practitioner, an AFAA-certified Personal Trainer and certified lifestyle educator, and an Institute of Integrative Nutrition certified health coach, the team emphasizes care based upon a uniting principle: 'Patients Powered by Knowledge.'

In designing her own center, Saxena has been able to create a unique healing environment. Patients enter SevaMed through a large teaching

CHAPTER SEVEN

kitchen with granite tops. The waiting room features butcher block style tables, comfortable armchairs and accent walls with mirrors to invite patients into a true medical home environment. Colorful niches, nice artwork, and exam rooms that feel more like inspiring home offices allow a Sevamed patient to feel like a person, not a number. The center features a 1,000 square foot functionally equipped fitness center featuring bosu balls, light weights, yoga mats, and kettle balls—equipment that easily transfers to the home environment

For years Saxena worked 100% through insurance reimbursement and she continues to accept it for those situations that call for reactive, disease-based care. More recently, she has moved the practice to a membership model that allows patients to establish their truest health goals and to avail themselves of her comprehensive health-focused expertise and services such as advanced cardiovascular technology for earlier detection and prevention, small group personal training, and her unique contribution to field: the lifestyle medicine based group visit.

Saxena's approach to group visits is built around the idea that patient groups can be oriented around the modifiable lifestyle factors that cause conditions, not just how to manage symptoms and diseases with medications and procedures. She explains:

> "In integrative and functional medicine the paradigm is not reactive, but rather it involves looking for the root cause. We can find different patients who manifest different downstream effects of the same root cause. So if I see 14 patients in a day, six of them may have the same root cause manifesting itself in different ways.
>
> Let's take as an example the idea of an allergic or adverse reaction to the consumption of gluten. If we use this root cause as the organizing principle for a group visit, then we can have patients in attendance who have celiac, Irritable Bowel Syndrome, or auto-immune diseases. We gather them not on the principle of disease diagnosis, but because they have the same root cause and the same need for education."

Saxena describes how a typical lifestyle medicine group visit goes:

> "I spend 30 minutes on education, discussing gluten and its effects on the body. Then we move into a 60-minute question-and-answer session, and during that time we are discussing

the patients' various downstream effects resulting from this specific root cause. Patients, as they're listening, can better understand the connection between their own symptoms and the root cause. So understanding increases, their connection with their provider increases, and ultimately their ability to help themselves increases.

Discussing the unique aspect of her group visits, Saxena says, "Instead of the organizing principle where we are putting people who are bitten by the same 'disease bug' into a room, we are creating a situation where the patient becomes part of the solution." Saxena concludes by noting that "So much of functional and integrative medicine is common-core educational topics, so it behooves us to use our time wisely and appropriately."

Speaking about the issue of time, Saxena notes that:

"One benefit of this model is there are many doctors who are popular in their communities, and people want to access them, which leads to the problem of fitting new patients into the practice. Group visits for current patients meet their needs and they increase accessibility for new patients. Wait time for new patients can dramatically drop. So, this model of care is especially useful for specialists."

A gifted and experience educator, Saxena recognized that other physicians might need help organizing the content behind the functional approach to GVs. She developed a series of four training kits, on subjects including: advanced prevention for cardiovascular disease, the connection between blood sugar and blood insulin, gastrointestinal foundations for whole body health, and stress and hormone health. As Saxena explains:

"The whole concept of having time for one's patient, of gathering a group together and educating them on their health, that is something that is universally desired by physicians. These training kits are designed so that physicians don't need to have expertise in how to perform such a task in a group setting. The toolkits focus on four topics, so that they can get the ball rolling, but with the intention that as they learn how to utilize group visits, they can develop their own versions customized to other issues they manage with their unique patients." More information on the kits can be found at www.groupvisittoolkit.com.

Saxena points out that, with group visits, "This is not a support group, because true medical information is transacted. You are giving medical information, medical advice; it's not just a general lecture." Hence, group visits qualify for reimbursement. More information on coding and reimbursement for group visits can be found in a white paper on the groupvisittoolkit.com site.

Back to the Soil

In medicine, we develop a focus on the 'seed' of disease. Functional medicine is an encompassing discipline that has arisen in response to the concern that this focus has become myopic, that we are ignoring the importance of the 'soil' of the individual patient. From toxins to GI health, functional medicine is focusing in on aspects of the patient's wellness that have been under-examined otherwise. And, in various specialties, physicians are utilizing a functional approach to their patient interactions and treatments. The above stories offer examples as to how we can orient our treatment approach and our practices to create 'soil' that is more fertile, not for disease, but for health and wellness.

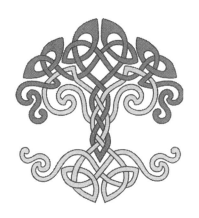

We do not "come into" this world; we come out of it, as leaves from a tree. As the ocean "waves," the universe "peoples." Every individual is an expression of the whole realm of nature, a unique action of the total universe.

— Alan Wilson Watts

8
The Holistic Paradigm

HOLISTIC MEDICINE
- Body-mind- spirit emphasis
- Optimal health focus
- Mindfulness, gratitude, optimism, love
- Autonomic nervous system control
- Appreciate other healing traditions
- Individuality
- Teach by example

The term 'holism' came into the western literature when it was coined in 1926 by South American statesman Jan Smuts. In his book *Holism and Evolution*. Smuts defined holism as the "tendency in nature to form wholes that are greater than the sum of the parts through creative evolution."[291] Holistic health practitioners define this wholeness as the unity of body, mind and spirit. The roots of illness can be found in all three dimensions; conversely, to obtain wellness, a state of optimal health, requires balance in all three dimensions.

In the late 1970s this concept became the dominant view of a small cadre of health care professionals who advocated for a more integrated, as opposed to reductionist approach to medical practice. Formed in 1978 by Norm Shealy, Gladys McGarey, Evart Loomis and Jerry Looney, the American Holistic Medical Association provided a "safe space" for medical doctors to network and collaborate. In 2008, the AHMA opened membership to other licensed holistic practitioners including naturopathic physicians, acupuncturists and massage therapists.

The formation of the AHMA later inspired the creation of the American Board of Integrative Holistic Medicine, which has offered certification to physicians since 2000. More recently ABIHM and AHMA have transformed into the American Academy of Integrative Health & Medicine (AIHM, www.aihm.org) with the inclusion of other healthcare practitioners including advanced nurses, DCs, NDs, LAcs and members of all the global healing traditions.

CHAPTER EIGHT

While the functional perspective focuses on the biochemical and genetic uniqueness of the individual, the holistic perspective takes a more encompassing view of uniqueness. Just as imbalances in hormones, or vitamins and minerals can cause disease, so too can imbalances in emotions, thoughts, and energies. This viewpoint is reflected in all traditional healing arts.

Traditional Chinese Medicine

Traditional Chinese Medicine (TCM) is a system of healing that originates from 200 BCE. As represented by the yin and yang symbol, it is based on the marriage of two opposite principles such as hot and cold, wet and dry, inner and outer, or winter and summer. TCM treatment seeks to balance five elements: fire, earth, metal, water and wood that are responsible for energy flow through the body. This bio-electric energy is known as *chi*. Chi flows through the body along meridians. Blockages in the energy flow result in disease that is diagnosed through questioning, visual assessment, listening, smelling, and palpation. One TCM diagnosis may encompass a variety of biomedical diseases. Alternatively, one energy blockage may be responsible for a variety of symptoms. Techniques used to restore harmony include acupuncture, acupressure, tai chi, qi gong, massage, cupping, and Chinese herbs.

The growing popularity of TCM is reflected in statistics gathered by the 2007 National Health Interview Survey (NHIS), which estimated that 3.1 million U.S. adults had used acupuncture in the previous year. The number of visits to acupuncturists tripled between 1997 and 2007. According to the 2007 NHIS, approximately 2.3 million Americans practiced tai chi and 600,000 practiced qi gong in the previous year.

In addition to growing consumer support for acupuncture, there is deepening appreciation for its use among practitioners, in large part because new techniques are validating its method of action. Acupuncture has shown promise in reducing postoperative dental pain, and chemotherapy induced nausea and vomiting. In addition to pain relief, it appears to be beneficial as an adjunctive, complementary treatment for asthma, drug addiction, stroke rehabilitation, and chronic pain.[292] While its effects are thought to occur by stimulation of multiple regions of the central nervous system, only with the advent of functional magnetic resonance imaging (fMRI) has one of its mechanisms of action been identified, in this case the activation of the limbic system. Researchers at Massachusetts General Hospital and Medical School used fMRI in a study involving needle manipulation at the LI 4 acupuncture point. This point was selected because it is one of the most commonly employed regions used to obtain anesthesia and sedation. For a control group, superficial tactile stimulation was also perform over the LI 4 region.

All subjects who experienced acupuncture sensation evidenced prominent decreases of fMRI signals in multiple areas of the limbic system. In these individuals, signal increases were also observed in the somatosensory cortex. When superficial tactile stimulation alone was used in the same L1 4 area, it elicited signal increases in the somatosensory cortex but no signal decreases were detected in the deeper limbic structures. According to the authors, "these preliminary results suggest that acupuncture needle manipulation modulates the activity of the limbic system and subcortical structures and...may be an important mechanism by which acupuncture exerts its complex multisystem effects."[293] It was not until the invention of the fMRI that we can even begin to understand this ancient healing tradition.

Ayurvedic Medicine

Another ancient healing system is Ayurvedic medicine, originating in India more than 3,000 years ago. Today, the majority of India's population either uses Ayurvedic medicine exclusively or combines it with conventional Western medicine. Ayurveda is derived from two Sanskrit words: *ayur* (life) and *veda* (science or knowledge).

The holistic framework of Ayurveda is reflected in a belief of universal interconnectedness and the importance of balance among three elemental substances known as *doshas*. The unique combination of these three life forces, known as *vata, pitta* and *kapha*, determines a person's unique temperament and characteristics. *Pakriti,* an important concept in Ayurveda, broadly reflects nature and the concept of a primal driving force within human beings. In Ayurveda, balance can be achieved through behavior modifications or changes in the environment including the use of herbal compounds and special diets. Emphasis is often placed on the moderation of food intake. A vegetarian diet supports the belief in *ahimsa,* the principle of non-injury of living things.

The most well recognized Ayurvedic technique is the mind-body

CHAPTER EIGHT

practice of yoga. Yoga combines physical postures known as *asanas* with breathing exercises and meditation or relaxation. The postures emphasize flexibility, strength and balance. While there are many forms of yoga, the most practiced forms in the United States are varieties of *Hatha* yoga. Examples include *Ashtanga, Bikram, Iyengar, Kundalini* and *Vinyasa*, each of which differs in the intensity of practice, the types of positions emphasized and the breathing or meditation techniques. Most yoga classes are led by an experienced teacher and last 60 to 90 minutes. Classes follow a basic format of meditation or relaxation for the first few minutes, followed by a series of postures, and conclude with a period of rest and mental relaxation known as *shavasana*. Throughout the postures participants are encouraged to heighten their body awareness by focusing on their breathing and bringing both their mental attention and their breath to the area of the body that is experiencing tension. Instructors in yoga classes often accompany the practices with positive dialog that includes messages of self-acceptance, gratitude, respect, intention, and unlimited potential.

The growing popularity of yoga is reflected in the 2012 "Yoga in America" study conducted by *Yoga Journal* (www.yogajournal.com). It shows that 8.7 percent of U.S. adults, or 20.4 million people practice yoga, compared to 15.8 million from the previous 2008 study, an increase of 29 percent. The study also highlights the economics of yoga practice, noting that practitioners spend $10.3 billion a year on yoga classes and products, including equipment, clothing, vacations, and media. This was a dramatic jump in spending from estimates in the 2008 study of $5.7 billion.[294]

Yoga participants not only benefit from the stress relief that the discipline provides, they also experience more energy, calmness and focus. Within the context of medical practice, yoga is increasingly showing efficacy in the treatment of chronic low back pain (cLBP). In a systemic review of ten randomized controlled trials meeting the inclusion criteria, yoga was demonstrated to "significantly improve quality of life and reduce disability, stress, depression, and medication usage associated with cLBP in 8 of the 10 analyzed trials when compared with usual care, self-care book, or exercises."[295] Other studies are demonstrating that yoga may be effective in the treatment of hypertension,[296] schizophrenia,[297] and weight loss.[298]

TCM and Ayurveda are two well-established examples of traditional medicine systems of healing. The World Health Organization (WHO) defines traditional medicine as:

> *"the sum total of the knowledge, skills, and practices based on the theories, beliefs, and experiences indigenous to different cultures, whether explicable or not, used in the maintenance of health as well as in the prevention, diagnosis, improvement or treatment of physical and mental illness."*

Often referred to as indigenous or folk medicine these are knowledge systems that have been developed well in advance of modern medicine. The WHO estimates that as much as 80% of the population in Asia and Africa utilize traditional medicine for primary care. WHO also cautions that their inappropriate use can have deleterious health effects.

Examples of traditional healing systems can be found among the Vietnamese, Koreans, Iranians, South American and African tribes; and closer to home, among the Hopi Indians and Mexicans. It is not uncommon for Mexican farm workers in the United States to seek treatment from a traditional Mexican healer, the most holistic of which is the curandero. Curanderos are healers who function at the interface of disease with spirituality. They may also employ traditional treatments such as herbs and manipulation. Curanderos treat ailments related to envy—the evil eye known as *mal de ojo*—or to sudden shock—the fright sickness known as *susto*. Yerberos are specialists in herbs and plants. Among the most commonly used herbs are chamomile to achieve calming, aloe vera for skin irritation and eucalyptus as a tea for colds.[299]

From Either/Or to Both/And

The principles of the Western medical model, based primarily on the germ theory, differ from holistic healing disciplines. Medical training has taught us to identify physiological causes of disease and to create treatment plans based upon the underlying pathology or the symptoms of illness. In essence, we are trained to treat after illness arises with little focus on disease prevention. Systems such as TCM or Ayurveda are based upon observations of natural phenomena and an appreciation for their interrelatedness. These global healing traditions emphasize the prevention of disease. The schism further widens whenever dialog involves less-easily identified and quantified energy concepts such as auras, chakras, or meridians.

CHAPTER EIGHT

The rhetoric tends to become further divided whenever the term spirit is included to expand the body-mind concept. How do we define spirit and the soul and not confabulate it with religion?

Leonard Wisneski, MD, FACP, a thirty-five year proponent of holistic medicine and the CAM practices that are part of it, is often posed this question. Wisneski is a clinical professor of Medicine at George Washington University Medical Center, a past board member of the American Holistic Medical Association and author of *The Scientific Basis of Integrative Medicine* (CRC Press).

He uses an example to explore an interesting distinction:

> "I can be the attending rounding in the hospital with the residents, interns and medical students and come upon two patients side by side in the ICU. They both have pneumonia and their presentation and status are very similar. If I say—in the absence of any objective data—that I have a 'gut feeling' about Mr. Jones doing well, but that I am more worried about Mr. Smith and that I need to keep a closer eye on him, that rhetoric is acceptable. If I take this a step further and discuss this feeling as 'intuition,' then I could be considered a 'flake.' We are inundated with information, but we don't talk about the intuition that we have gathered from our years treating patients. Self-growth is a process of deepening intuition."

Wisneski's own process of self-growth developed through an active questioning of the process of medical education. At an early age, Wisneski became enthralled with what now is described as the science of cultural anthropology. He entered Thomas Jefferson Medical College with the perspective that every civilization holds beliefs around spirituality, religion, compassion, and the importance of family and that these beliefs are central to healing. His medical school experience provided none of the above. The residents displayed gallows humor, had a militaristic style; surgery was the competitive race to tie the fastest and most perfect knots. While Wisneski learned to be an excellent technician, he was also being subjected to "subtle, subliminal messages that I was something special. I was above the nurses, the technicians, the people who drew the blood."

This false sense of modesty was in direct contrast to his humble beginnings. Wisneski's father died when Len was seven years old. In a childhood marked by early suffering, he learned to make his way in the world by engaging with others. He notes that the most compassion and understanding shown to him during medical school came not from the other physicians or staff, but from an older female housekeeper who mopped the entrance way of the hospital and each morning "greeted me with the biggest smile."

Wisneski's sense of wonder of complementary techniques can be traced back to his first week of internship and a grand rounds story of acupuncture treatment by the cardiologist leading the session that "spun my world." The cardiologist recounted Pulitzer Prize winning journalist James Reston's story of experiencing acupuncture. In July 1971, Reston suffered appendicitis while visiting China with his wife. His appendix was removed through conventional surgery conducted at the Anti-Imperialist Hospital in Peking (Beijing). While there, Reston's post-operative pain was successfully treated with acupuncture by Li Chang-yuan a 36-year old practitioner without formal medical training. Reston's report of his treatment, printed in the *New York Times*, fueled public and medical interest in learning more about this ancient Chinese healing art.[300]

This sparked Wisneski to learn traditional Chinese medicine and acupuncture, tools that he continues to use to this day. He believes that the only way for physicians to change their belief systems around complementary techniques such as acupuncture is to experience them. When presenting to conventional medical physicians he will often bring a box of acupuncture needles onto the podium with him and offer to treat those in attendance. It is not uncommon for a half-dozen or more of the house staff or attendings to shed their white coats and get a first hand experience of acupuncture.

Belief in integrative medicine deepens as a result of cumulative experiences. One of these occurred when, as a young endocrinology fellow researching calcitonin, Wisneski had the occasion to lecture at an osteopathic school in Des Moines, Iowa on the subject of osteoporosis. On route to the lecture he twisted his back the wrong way and was in significant pain throughout his discourse. J. Gordon Zink, DO, a leader in osteopathic manipulation and originator of the Common Compensatory Pattern that identifies dysfunction in the neuromyofascial-skeletal unit, saw that "I was in discomfort. He had a table brought out. In front of

CHAPTER EIGHT

about 500 people, he told me to lie on the table and that he would come up and treat me. I had a picture in my mind of anything from going directly to the hospital, to immediate paraplegia. And yet it was hard to say no. It wasn't hard; it was impossible. He manipulated my back, and I sprang off the table, feeling phenomenal, feeling full vitality and no back pain," said Wisneski.[301]

Somewhat later Wisneski became director of medical education within the George Washington University Medical System. There he encouraged the Indian and Chinese medical residents to open up to their healthcare backgrounds. "Some of them felt thrilled to have honor accorded to their cultural roots. We started having group discussions on various CAM techniques, based on the traditions of their homelands. This deepened my love affair with integrative medicine." Wisneski went on to become one of the earliest members of the AHMA in the late 1970s.

In an interview of Wisneski conducted by Molly Roberts, MD, current president of AHMA, she points out that "humility is an attractive quality in a physician," albeit, one that is usually present in either small quantities or often non-existent. When she asked Wisneski how physicians can become more humble, he drew from his teaching experience and how he framed his words of advice for the house staff.

> "I began by acknowledging the difficulty of having to make many decisions about life and death, sometimes 30 or 40 in a day. There is an enormous fear of making mistakes. One of the defense systems we use is arrogance, which has the effect of distancing ourselves from our patients. It can also distance us from our families and family and the compassion and love we need. We can become lost souls.
>
> I remember one time when I was making rounds with the interns and residents. The captain of the code blue team had lost a patient that night, and his response was arrogant laughter. I asked him why he was laughing, what was he truly feeling? At this point he broke down into tears and started to share his feelings of fear and remorse. His colleagues rallied around him and provided emotional support. This episode paved the way for the team to share, on future rounds, not only clinical information but also emotions as well.
>
> It is imperative that we share our vulnerabilities with

colleagues and allow our humanity to always be front and center when dealing with patients, our families, friends, and most importantly, ourselves."

In addition to training and teaching generations of healthcare practitioners Wisneski has tirelessly advocated for a holistic voice in public health policies. He is currently chair of the Integrative Healthcare Policy Consortium (www.ihpc.org), an advocacy group for integrative medicine. Wisneski is finding an enormous sense of optimism in the greater receptivity to holistic health coming from government, the insurance industry, and the military.

Much of the support for IM can be traced back to a groundbreaking 2005 Institute of Medicine report noting that patients seek CAM because:

- Conventional medicine does not work well for the complaint
- Lack of trust in and disenchantment with healthcare system
- Dissatisfaction with previous treatment outcomes
- Looking for a more patient-centered approach
- CAM enables the patient to play a more active and participative role in care
- CAM enables the patient to manage and conserve the use of valued conventional medications
- Desire to prevent future illness or to maintain health and vitality.

Wisneski adds that the strong winds of the Affordable Care Act are propelling plurality in healthcare services. Seven sections of the ACA spell out increased roles for non-physician healthcare practitioners in our system. Section 2706 relates to non-discrimination for reimbursement. All state licensed or certified healthcare practitioner including massage therapists, chiropractors, acupuncturists, naturopathic physicians, and nurse midwives are entitled to benefits by third party carriers. Section 3502 contains provisions that include CAM practitioners in the medical home, important recognition that a pluralistic team working together for thousands of patients in a community setting is the bedrock of healthcare transformation. He notes that we are at the dawn of a revolutionary integrated approach to medical care that will be occurring over the next five to ten years.

CHAPTER EIGHT

The Voice of the CAM Professional

Wisneski's passion and optimism is shared by Pamela Snider, ND, who along with John Weeks are the founding executive director and current executive director, respectively and co-founders for The Academic Consortium for Complementary and Alternative Health Care (ACCAHC). The ACCAHC consists of councils of colleges and schools, accrediting agencies, and certification and testing organizations associated with the five distinctly licensed integrative health and medicine professions recognized by the United States Department (Secretary) of Education. Traditional World Medicines and emerging professions are also represented. These five licensed groups include acupuncture and Oriental medicine, chiropractic, direct entry (home birth) midwifery, massage therapy, and naturopathic medicine. Together, these licensed and accredited disciplines account for more than 375,000 practitioners nationwide, as shown in the chart below.

Development of Standards by the Licensed Complementary and Alternative Healthcare Professions

Profession	Accredited agency established	US Department of Education recognition	Recognized schools or programs	Standardized national exam created	State regulation*	Estimated number of licensed practitioners in the US
Acupuncture and Oriental medicine	1982	1990	61	1985	44 states + DC	28,000
Chiropractic	1971	1974	15	1963	50 states + DC, Puerto Rico, and all other US territories /insular areas	72,000
Massage Therapy	1982	2002	350	1994	44 states + DC	280,00
Direct-entry Midwifery	1991	2001	10	1994	26 states	2,000
Naturopathic medicine	1978	1987	7	1986	16 states, DC, Puerto Rico, Virgin Islands	7,000

*For chiropractors and naturopathic Physicians, this category uniformly represents licensing statutes; for acupuncture, virtually all states use licensure; for massage, there is a mixture of licensing, certification and registation statutes.

Table 3: Development of Standards by the Licensed Complementary and Alternative Healthcare Professions. Reprinted with permission.

Snider received her ND degree from Bastyr University of Natural Health Sciences. She serves as Vice Chair on the board of the Integrative Healthcare Policy Consortium where she takes a macro viewpoint of our country's health status. She has been deeply moved by the Institute of Medicine's 2013 report on the abysmal state of health in the United

States. When compared with 16 peer nations—affluent democracies that include Australia, Canada, Japan, and many western European countries, the United States ranked at or near the bottom in nine key areas of health. These included infant mortality and low birth weight; injuries and homicides; teenage pregnancies and sexually transmitted infections; prevalence of HIV and AIDS; drug-related deaths; obesity and diabetes; heart disease; chronic lung disease; and disability.[302] Snider is a strong voice for a common, perhaps even radical approach to improving our global health standing by actively creating rather than simply promoting, health.

The unifying message of ACCAHC, as created by Snider and Weeks and the ACCAHC board revolves around the concept of *health creation*: the values that society, practitioners and patients need to focus on. According to Snider, "These values must be infused in leadership, teamwork and all aspects of patient care. We need health creation for all people, not just some. To do this, we must make health creation such an ingrained part of our culture that it is talked about in living rooms, on buses and trains, and is totally integrated into our communities."

Snider works to make certain that the silo approach to conventional medicine does not create discord among complementary practitioners. Membership in ACCAHC has always included organizations representing Traditional World Medicines and emerging professions such as homeopathic medicine, Ayurvedic Medicine, Yoga Therapy, and herbalism. Citing the reason for making a seat at the table for these healers, Snider notes:

> "These traditional world medicine practitioners have immense cultural authority. Just because they are not licensed in the USA does not diminish their value. We are also seeing emerging disciplines such as homeopathic medicine—200 years old—and herbalism becoming more 'professionalized' by developing accreditation, regulation etc. This is exactly what professions do when they 'emerge.' Becoming 'professional' does not mean becoming conventional—it does mean that they are becoming more rigorous and publicly accountable in their work."

Snider also reacts strongly to the political discord between certain groups of conventional physicians and professionals of the five disciplines. She equates this schism to the "ghettoization of the complementary practitioner," and remarks:

> "These are federally accredited, licensed health care professionals, not second class citizens. And like our conventionally trained colleagues we have burnout too, although it is more closely related to the stresses of inequity in access and payment systems. For example, In the field of naturopathic medicine we do the same depth of work as conventional physicians, with equivalent responsibilities, but receive less reimbursement."

The newly launched Academy of Integrative Health and Medicine Snider believes, represents the growing convergence between conventional and CAM professionals and a forum for transformative collaboration among diverse practitioners for health creation.

John Weeks, ACCAHC's co-founding executive director is a 30 year veteran in the integrative space and publisher-editor of The Integrator Blog News & Reports (www.theintegratorblog.com).

Over the last two decades, Weeks sees that we have made great strides in eroding polarization between conventional and complementary practitioners. Today, there is significant national dialog taking place on the role of ACCAHC's 375,000 licensed practitioners.

Some of the growing acceptance by conventional physicians is related to a more realistic viewpoint of the practice of evidence based medicine. Weeks remarks:

> "For a single diagnosis like throat cancer, it is highly likely that six different physicians will prescribe six different mixtures of radiation and drugs. We portray we are evidence based when we are not. I recently observed a panel with leading academic physicians discussing this issue. One of the university based chief medical officers noted that '25% of what we do has a strong evidence base and we only do that half the time.' I think there is growing appreciation of the double standard in comparing conventional to complementary medicine."

Weeks is adamant about the avoidance of another generalization:

> "Conventional physicians need to appreciate the difference between working with a therapy, for example, acupuncture,

and working with a skilled practitioner who uses that therapy. It is one thing for a practitioner to know some limited use of acupuncture needles; it is another for them to have 3-4 years of comprehensive training as an oriental medical practitioner. We exist in a fundamentally interpersonal world, and just as conventional physicians want to refer patients to the most skilled medical and surgical specialists, this should hold true for referral to complementary providers as well."

Weeks was recently honored for his 30 years as a leading advocate of integrative medicine with a lifetime achievement living tribute at the 2014 International Research Congress on Integrative Medicine and Health Conference in Miami, Florida. Weeks is looking forward to another decade—or more—as a powerful and proactive force for IM. He states:

"In recent years we are seeing some terrific movement from progressive forces in US medicine to set a course on a values-base rather than a production base. The more we focus on patient experience, on outcomes and on creating health, instead of more procedures, the more openness we see to fashioning the appropriate use of integrative health values, practices and professions."

Gathering Evidence for IM

Margaret Chesney, PhD, is director of the Osher Center for Integrative Medicine at the University of California San Francisco (UCSF). Chesney was the first deputy director of the National Institutes of Health's Center for Complementary and Alternative Medicine (NCCAM). She also served as the director of the Center's Division of Extramural Research and Training, which included responsibility for oversight of the Center's research portfolio examining the efficacy of CAM treatments. Similar to trials for pharmaceutical agents, Chesney learned that, "When the results of randomized clinical trials are reported, the statements often do not sufficiently capture all the clinical and scientific insights the trials provide."

She points to the glucosamine/chondroitin arthritis intervention trail (GAIT), a randomized placebo control study of 1,583 patients at multiple sites within the USA. At the two-year follow-up, when the analyses examined all the patients combined, the outcomes were not statistically significant between those who took celecoxib and those who took the placebo. While the combined data showed no difference, a smaller subgroup of 354 study participants with moderate-to-severe pain did gain significant relief with the glucosamine/chondroitin supplement.[303]

Chesney notes that she prefers the terms complementary and integrative rather than "alternative;" which connotes that people are using approaches in place of conventional medicine. " The survey data indicate that the vast majority of people using complementary approaches for health do so in conjunction with some forms of conventional care." She stresses that we need more research on the optimal timing of integrative and conventional treatments, for a wide range of conditions. "As acupuncture is used more in inpatient settings, patients may be interested in trying to manage post-operative pain with acupuncture first before turning to conventional strategies," said Chesney.

Chesney acquired insights into the potential promise of what is now integrative medicine from her work at NCCAM and the UCSF Osher Center, but more significantly in her earlier work with Ray Rosenman, MD, who along with Meyer Friedman, MD, developed the Type A/TypeB concept in the etiology of CVD. The two physicians put forth their treatise in the popular book, *Type A Behavior and Your Heart* (Alfred A. Knopf). Chesney and Rosenman collaborated on research grants at SRI International in Menlo Park, and she practiced as a clinical psychologist in Rosenman's San Francisco clinical practice, counseling his patients in meditation, stress management, and lifestyle change. Even more enlightening was the work Chesney did at UCSF helping patients cope with HIV/AIDS during the days before effective medicines, when patients knew they were not going to live long.

> "This totally changed my understanding of stress and coping. The people I studied taught me about coping and how, when truly confronted with the universal truth that our time is limited, our views of health take on a larger context. We need to ask 'How do you want to invest your time—the most valuable resource you have? What do you want to do that adds meaning to your life?'"

The path to helping patients find greater meaning—and greater adherence to health promoting treatment—may lie in having more choices.

"Patients come to the Osher Center from all directions. Some are referrals from other physicians in the medical center. Some patients sign up for a class and then migrate to one of our complementary practitioners. We will often help direct patients to the appropriate provider when they phone in. Some want to start by seeing a general physician whose diagnosis and treatment are covered by insurance. Others want to go straight to acupuncture," said Chesney.

The Evidence Based Evolution of the Chiropractic Profession

According to William Meeker, DC, MPH, President of Palmer College of Chiropractic, San Jose campus, the integrative ethos is inherent in chiropractic medicine. Meeker emphasizes that the field, started in 1895, "hasn't lost the values of our profession, one that was founded on a holistic, and sometimes a spiritual focus. What has changed most recently is our embracing evidence based healthcare. We now teach evidence-based decision-making in our school. On a larger, national level, we are working with many of the government agencies and have received significant funding from NIH and others."

The NCCAM summarized the evolution of evidence for chiropractic medicine as follows:

"In 2007 guidelines, the American College of Physicians and the American Pain Society included spinal manipulation as one of several treatment options for practitioners to consider when low-back pain does not improve with self-care. More recently, a 2010 Agency for Healthcare Research and Quality (AHRQ) report noted that complementary health therapies, including spinal manipulation, offer additional options to conventional treatments, which often have limited benefit in managing back and neck pain. The AHRQ analysis also found that spinal manipulation was more effective than placebo and as effective as medication in reducing low-back pain intensity."[304]

Two government organizations that have embraced chiropractic to a large extent are the Veterans Administration and the Department of Defense. According to Meeker, "Chiropractic physicians have been working in these organizations for about the last 15 years." Chiropractic students from Palmer rotate through these organizations. Increasingly the

CHAPTER EIGHT

large Silicon Valley companies are also including chiropractic physicians on their teams. Chiropractic physicians are also successfully joining with their conventionally trained colleagues to produce better outcomes for low back pain and other musculoskeletal conditions.[305-307]

The teachers of chiropractic education are clear about the profession's mission as reflected in their practice paradigm statement:

Chiropractic focuses on neurological and musculoskeletal integrity, and aims to favorably impact health and well-being, relieve pain and infirmity, enhance performance, and improve quality of life without drugs or surgery.

Meeker adds the following, "We are a hands-on profession that stresses alignment, posture and function of the spine and locomotor system. On one hand we do see patients with aches and pains, particularly as a specialty approach to back pain, but our emphasis has always been on the wellness side of the continuum."

Surveys show that most DCs regularly provide instructions to patients regarding health promotion and wellness including health risk reduction, physical fitness, diet, self-care, and stress reduction.[308] "In the same way that dentists are positioned as the primary healthcare professionals for the mouth, we want to be the PCPs for the spine and locomotor system." Meeker also points to the large number of chiropractic physicians involved in sports medicine.

Understanding Naturopathic Medicine

ACCAHC has produced an excellent Clinicians' & Educators' Desk Reference (CEDR) (available at www.accahc.org) that provides complete descriptions of the background, training, and emphasis of the five accredited and licensed CAM professions. While most conventional physicians have familiarity with chiropractic, massage, acupuncture and midwifery, naturopathic physicians are less well understood, in part because only 16 states offer licensure in naturopathic medicine. While still small in number—some 7,000 in North America—naturopathic medicine is growing; there were only 2,000 licensed naturopathic physicians in North America in 2000, and several hundred in 1978.

As defined in the CEDR:

"Naturopathic physicians act to stimulate the inherent

self-healing abilities of the individual through lifestyle change and the application of non-suppressive therapeutic methods and modalities, including clinical nutrition, botanical medicine, homeopathy, physical medicine, and health psychology. Naturopathic physicians are also schooled in and able to apply conventional clinical practices including emergency medicine, minor surgery, pharmacology, and natural childbirth."[309]

The CEDR also notes the rigor of the preclinical training:

"At naturopathic medical school, students take two years of graduate level studies in the biomedical sciences. Although naturopathic medical students receive training in the same biomedical sciences in which allopathic medical students are trained, there are differences in the emphasis in the courses and in the way that knowledge is applied. For example, slightly less emphasis is placed on anatomy, requiring an average of 350 hours in a naturopathic curriculum, compared to 380 hours in an conventional/osteopathic curriculum. However, in naturopathic programs, greater emphasis is placed on physiology. Naturopathic students receive approximately twice as many hours of physiology as conventional medical students (250 hours compared to 125 hours)."

The philosophy and practice of naturopathic medicine is closed aligned with the tenets of an integrative approach to healthcare. Naturopathic medicine was founded in 1902, as an integrative medical discipline based on the concepts of Therapeutic Universalism and the Vis Medicatrix Naturae (the Healing Power of Nature).[310] The field grew into a profession which today continues its integrative approach through which "diagnostic and therapeutic methods are selected from various sources and systems, and will continue to evolve with the progress of knowledge."[311]

It is a profession that stresses a whole person, systems and nature-focused approach, prevention, health promotion and education, and the philosophy of first do no harm; treating causes rather than symptoms. The services of naturopathic physicians are increasingly being called upon in primary care, wellness-oriented care, but also in subspecialties such as oncology, women's health, environmental medicine, and endocrinology.

CHAPTER EIGHT

The Original Conventional Holistic Healer

While CAM practitioners can point to 375,000 in their number, a more ubiquitous healer staffs the front lines of holistic health, the 3.2 million nurses in the United States. Working tirelessly, they are the eyes and ears, as well as the heart and soul of healthcare.

The modern-day roots of nursing can be traced back to Florence Nightingale, who in 1854 brought a team of 38 volunteer nurses to care for injured British soldiers during the Crimean war. More solders were dying of diseases spread by poor sanitation—typhus, typhoid, cholera and dysentery—than were being killed by wounds on the battlefield. Nightingale's attention to healing created the nursing profession, her emphasis on sanitation sparked the field of public health.

The essence of nursing; however, can be traced back to ancient Greek and Roman mythology in the persona of the goddess Hygeia. The daughter of Asclepius, the god of medicine, Hygeia stood for health, cleanliness and sanitation. She worked along with her four sisters, each of whom performed one or more facets of the healing arts. The word panacea is derived from the goddess of the same name who was responsible for universal remedies. Hygeia's other sisters were the goddesses of beauty, the healing process, and recuperation from illness.

It has only been in the last twenty-five years that the adjective 'holistic' has been added as a qualifier for a subset of nurses who seek to return the profession to its healing roots. The American Holistic Nurses Association (AHNA) is a non-profit membership association for nurses and other holistic healthcare professionals. The American Nurses Association recognizes the AHNA as an "official nursing specialty;" membership is now at 4,500.

Holistic nurses draw upon their nursing knowledge and combine it with expertise and intuition to become better therapeutic partners with people in their care. By definition, holistic nurses emphasize the interconnectedness of body, mind, emotion, spirit, social/cultural, relationship, context, and environment. The genesis of the profession is well explained in this adapted excerpt from *Implementing Visions of Health and Healing*, 2008:

> "In 1981 at our beginning, there was an unprecedented shortage of nurses. Working conditions meant long hours and minimal pay. Nurses were leaving hospital nursing to move

into areas where they felt appreciated and could give the depth of care they knew needed to be given. Today the nursing world is more complex. It moves faster, with technology becoming the master rather than the servant. Once again, there is an increasing nursing shortage. Nurses want to work in healthcare areas where self-healing and self-care are recognized and valued."[312]

Emphasizing the primacy of personal transformation, the AHNA states that, "Holistic nursing is not necessarily something that you do: it is an attitude, a philosophy, and a way of being." As the physical, mental and emotional demands on nurses escalate, these healers must define their own paths to Total Engagement. Similar to the model we have set out for physicians, the nurse's path begins with the journey of self-discovery and a willingness to confront the inherent discrepancy between knowing about health, and practicing a healthy lifestyle.

This gap was clearly revealed at the Preventive Cardiovascular Nurses Association meeting in 2012 dedicated to New Cardiovascular Horizons. Ninety-five preventive cardiovascular nurses underwent the Cleveland Heart Lab's Inflammation Testing consisting of traditional lipids and advanced cardiovascular biomarkers. Traditional markers were as follows:

- 44% had serum cholesterol >200 mg/dL
- 38 % of the females had HDL <50 mg/dL
- 46% of the males had HDL-C <40 mg/dL
- 65% had LDL-C >100 mg/dL

When compared with screenings of non-healthcare related participants, the results showed great similarity. Participants were also screened for three advanced inflammation markers: hsCRP, a generalized marker of inflammation, and two vascular specific tests, Lp-PLA2 and myeloperoxidase (MPO). Multiple elevated markers equate to greater near-term risk of a cardiovascular event; 56% of the nurses had one, and 19% had two markers elevated.[313] The gap between knowing better and doing better is obvious to all who are in healthcare.

No Substitute for a Healthy Culture

Multiple studies have documented burnout in all categories of nursing, as well as its link to organizational factors such as the nature and type of leadership, nursing communication between colleagues, physicians and administrators, and social support. These are some of the factors that shape the nursing culture and affect not only nurses' satisfaction but also patient satisfaction and outcomes.

In the inpatient setting dysfunctional relationships between staff nurses and nurse managers are a major contributor to burnout.[314] In one study of 1,780 RNs, a subset of 509 commented on the quality of supervision and several major issues. These included "(a) inadequate unit leadership and the frequent turnover of nurse mangers, (b) insufficient physical presence of the supervisor on the unit, (c) failure to address problems—too much sweeping them aside or not even being aware they exist, and (d) modest awareness of numerous staffing issues."[314] In fairness to the nurse managers, their stressors come not only from those they supervise, but also from their administrators, and this often puts them in a no-win position.

Other studies demonstrate the converse of dysfunction. In one study, nurses on units that have adequate staff, good administrative support for nursing care and good relationships with physicians reported lower levels of burnout. Patients on these same units were more than twice as likely as other patients to report high satisfaction with their care.[315]

The nature and quality of professional relationships, social support and the health of the organizational culture affect the decision of nurses to either stay in or leave conventional healthcare settings. However, a growing belief in holism and its rightful place in healing often catapults nurses in a new direction.

This was the case for Rauni Prittinen King, RN, Co-Founder and Executive Director of Guarneri Integrative Health Inc. at Pacific Pearl La Jolla and founder of the Miraglo Foundation (www.miraglofoundation.org). Prittinen King is the former Director of Programs and Planning at the Scripps Center for Integrative Medicine in La Jolla, California. She has over 20 years of experience in critical care nursing and served as the Nurse Case Manager for the Scripps Dean Ornish Program for Reversing Heart Disease.

Her philosophy of integrative health was born over her two decades in the conventional system. "When I teach workshops, I have slides on healing versus curing models. Surgery is a perfect example of a curing model: removing a tumor. But how does the wound heal? With integrative medicine we take both models, curing and healing, and this is when you get the best results," said Prittinen King.

Prittinen King can trace her integrative health awakening to a workshop she took in the early 1990s on energy healing. She states, "When I came back from this workshop, I started doing energy healing on my patients. They were so calm, they loved it, and that was my cue that the healing piece was what was missing in conventional care. I began doing Healing Touch at Scripps in 1993 and have now trained thousands of healthcare professionals."

The National Center for Complementary and Alternative Medicine (NCCAM) defines Biofield or "energy healing therapy" as "the channeling of healing energy through the hands of a practitioner into the client's body to restore a normal energy balance and, therefore, health. Energy healing therapy has been used to treat a wide variety of ailments and health problems, and is often used in conjunction with other alternative and conventional medical treatments."

Three schools of energy healing are practiced in the United States. These include Healing Touch, Therapeutic Touch and the ancient healing practice of Reiki. Each has its corresponding association and training programs: the Healing Touch International (www.healingbeyondborders.org), The Healing Touch Program (www.healingtouchprogram.com), and the International Center for Reiki Training (www.reiki.org). These energy practices can increasingly be found in multiple healthcare settings including hospitals, long-term care facilities, cancer treatment centers and hospice. In an excellent review of "Energy Medicine Advances in the Medical Community,"[324] Jane Hart, MD, a clinical instructor in internal medicine and chair of the Integrative Medicine Committee at Case Western Reserve University School of Medicine, in Cleveland, Ohio, points to how organizations are making energy medicine an employee benefit. For example, she notes "Planetree™ facilities offer Therapeutic Touch training to their employees, therefore making it a very accessible energy medicine modality to their patients."

Research is beginning to validate the clinical effectiveness of therapies such as Healing Touch. This was shown in a study addressing the challenge of healing returning combat-exposed active duty military with significant PTSD symptoms. A randomized controlled trial was conducted

CHAPTER EIGHT

on 123 active duty military with PTSD comparing the combination of Healing Touch and Guided Imagery versus a control group of treatment as usual. Over a three-week period, the Healing Touch/Guided Imagery group received 6 sessions.

As compared to the control group, the treatment group showed a statistically and clinically significant reduction in PTSD symptoms, depression and cynicism as well as significant improvements in mental quality of life.[316] Studies have shown that Healing Touch is also effective in reducing anxiety associated with a variety of health conditions,[317] and may aid in recovery from coronary artery bypass surgery.[318]

What Goes Around Comes Around

A unique attribute of energy is its ability to flow bi-directionally. In Prittinen King's case, her energy medicine energized her.

> "I realized through the energy healing workshop, that I could move towards holistic nursing. That was what my heart desired to do, but I didn't even know there was a possibility. I met Mimi in 95-96 when we were creating the research program for reversing heart disease. She was the head of program; I was a nurse case manager. So it's always like connecting the dots, one dot leads to another."

Fueled by a desire to work globally, Prittinen King left Scripps and started the Miraglo Foundation, a non-profit, 501c3 dedicated to providing healthcare and education and research to the underserved locally and globally. Some months later, she and Mimi started Pacific Pearl La Jolla, an integrative health center staffed by medical physicians, naturopathic doctors, psychologists, an acupuncturist, and a massage therapist.

Prittinen King teaches and practices Healing Touch and hypnosis within Pacific Pearl La Jolla, as well as in the Greater Los Angeles VA hospital, and other healthcare systems. She notes that Healing Touch addresses body, mind, spirit and emotions and is not aligned with any form of religion. However, she notes, "Many times the person finds his or her own spirituality in this process."

For Prittinen King, energy medicine has allowed her to touch the deep roots of nursing, healing, and return to the holistic state of nature that the ancient gods of Greece and Rome envisioned and Florence Nightingale shed light upon.

Mysticism finds its Mechanism

Conventional allopathic physicians have long been influenced—for good and bad—by the science of drug discovery and its narrowly focused rifle shot mechanisms of action. Internists place their faith in proton pump inhibitors or ACE inhibitors because they understand the biochemical blocking mechanisms of these substances. Our beliefs are intertwined with our tools. Surgeons find comfort in the tangibles of forceps and 4-0 catgut; radiologists in the pixels on the screen. Many physicians dismiss some complementary practices because science has not fully proven the mechanism behind their actions. The gap in the believability of CAM practices; however, is rapidly closing as advances in our understanding of genetics grows.

Concurrent with the sequencing of the human genome and the dramatic drops in costs for genetic analysis, the emerging science of epigenetics, is providing evidence that lifestyle, metabolic and holistic practices can prevent disease and extend the lifespan. The term epigenetics describes cellular modifications caused by the environment that do not change DNA sequence. Changes are effected by the activation or suppression of epigenetic tags that turn genes on or off without affecting their basic structure.

These changes may be heritable. Examples of heritable epigenetic changes come from studies of children and grandchildren of pregnant women who endured hardship and starvation during the Second World War, and from studies of women in China during the 1950s. These children and grandchildren tend to be smaller and more prone to diabetes and psychosis.[319]

However, the most substantial evidence for epigenetics can be found in twin studies. Professor Tim Spector, PhD, head of twin research at King's College, London and author of *Identically Different: Why You Can Change Your Genes* (Phoenix Publishers) has shown that monozygote twins (who share the same genome) rarely die of the same disease. At some point in the lives of the twins, their environmental paths diverge. They become subject to different diets, environmental pollutants, stressors, etc. Spector has studied 3,500 pair of siblings, half of whom have had their entire genome sequenced. Pointing to the influence of epigenetics, he notes that if one identical twin gets heart disease, there is only a 30% chance that the other will as well. For rheumatoid arthritis this figure drops to only about 15%.[320]

At present, DNA methylation and histone modifications are the two most well studied epigenetic mechanisms affecting protein synthesis. Ongoing research is documenting how factors such as diet, illnesses, ageing, chemicals in the environment, alcohol use, drugs and medicines are affecting methylation. In his review of Epigenetics in Twin Studies[321] professor Jeffrey M. Craig, PhD, at the University of Melbourne, Royal Children's Hospital, notes positive associations "on the effects of in vitro fertilization on DNA methylation in placenta and cord blood; plasma homocysteine and methylation in cord blood; institutionalisation at an early age with methylation in whole blood; early life parental stress and, in adipose tissue, response to exercise in adults." However, he cautions that results have not been replicated in multiple, independent studies. Well-replicated studies support the association "between smoking and methylation at the *AHRR* (aryl hydrocarbon receptor repressor) gene either during pregnancy or in adult smokers." In addition, Craig notes that systematic reviews and meta-analyses of cancer studies have demonstrated consistent associations of methylation with disease.

Spector has shown differences in twin's methylation in pain tolerance, depression, diabetes and breast cancer and concludes that differences in genes being switched on or off between the twins increases the likelihood of disease.[322]

Individuals have the power to influence their methylation pathways through activity and diet, thus blunting or even thwarting the disease influencing effects of genes and the single-nucleotide polymorphisms. The Fat-Mass and Obesity Associated (FTO) gene has been linked to obesity, diabetes, hypertension and metabolic syndrome. Researchers analyzed genotype data from 21,674 Caucasian women who participated in the Women's Genome Health Study, for whom data on *FTO* rs8050136 genotype, BMI and physical activity were available. They showed that the carriers of the FTO risk allele have a higher BMI and an increased risk of cardiovascular disease; however this increase in risk only occurs in less active women. More active women do not show this association.[324]

Another study of FTO and BMI in Old Order Amish individuals looked more closely at the effect of exercise on 26 BMI associated single-nucleotide polymorphisms (SNPs). Shunning modern time and labor-saving advancements, the Amish walk extensively and engage in strenuous activities of daily living. Their active lifestyle was able to blunt the effect of the SNPs that were most strongly correlated to increases in BMI.[323]

Dean Ornish, MD, has produced one of the first randomized studies showing that cancer can be slowed and even reversed by dietary and lifestyle changes. Ornish's treatment program involves strict adherence to a low-fat diet with emphasis on mostly plant-based foods such as grains and beans, fruits, and vegetables. Participants agree to walk a minimum of half-hour per day, take stress management programs, do yoga or meditation, and attend a weekly support group.

Ornish enrolled a group of 93 men with Gleason scores under seven indicating a well-differentiated or low-grade cancer. The men had all elected to undergo watchful waiting and were randomized into the Ornish program or usual care. At the conclusion of one year, six of the control patients underwent conventional treatment for an increase in PSA and/or progression of disease as demonstrated by magnetic resonance imaging. None of the treatment group underwent surgery or radiation. PSA decreased 4% in the experimental group but increased 6% in the control group (p = 0.016).

The study also examined the serum collected from the participants for its ability to inhibit the growth of LNCaP prostate cancer cells in culture. The serum from the Ornish group inhibited growth almost 8 times more that serum from the control group. (70% vs 9%, p <0.001). Those participants with the most rigorous adherence to the treatment plan showed the greatest decreases in serum PSA and inhibition of LNCaP cell growth. Peer reviewed commentary about the Ornish study highlighted the importance of staging, adherence to the program, and continual physician monitoring for patients who adopt a lifestyle program in conjunction with their watchful waiting course of action.[323]

The Tale of the Telomeres

Additional support for how lifestyle and holistic practices can affect longevity can be found in the pioneering work of Nobel Prize winning scientist Elizabeth Blackburn, PhD, and her work on telomeres. These appended ends of our 46 chromosomes have been shown to be the equivalent of a biological clock. They are markers of biological aging that reflect the amount of cellular turnover taking place in our bodies. Telomeres exhibit individual variations in length and also in the rate and timing of shortening. Erosion of telomeres has been linked to oxidative stress and inflammation.[325, 326] Countering the shortening process, the protein-RNA enzyme telomerase lengthens the telomere through the addition of TTAAGGG sequences.

Blackburn began her research at the University of California, Berkeley and is now at the University of California, San Francisco where she works with a team of scientists examining the link between shortened telomeres and telomerase, and multiple chronic diseases and psychological states. In addition to the association with cardiovascular disease, telomere shortening has also been linked to osteoarthritis[327] and osteoporosis,[328] vascular dementia,[329] pulmonary fibrosis,[330] major depressive disorders,[331] and some cancers,[332] as well as infertility, type 2 diabetes, and CNS diseases, among others. Telomere shortening is also associated with other lifestyle related behaviors such as smoking, obesity, stress and sedentary habits. Studies have shown that women who have been subject to violence exhibit significantly shorter mean telomere length than women who had never been abused. Those women who suffered the longest had the greatest degree of telomere shortening.

Telomere research is also showing that violence and abuse in childhood creates a long tail on one's health in later life. One study examining childhood adversities showed that the abused children had elevated IL-6 and TNF-α levels, as well as shorter telomeres as compared to a group of non-abused children. The researchers estimated that this telomere difference could equate to a 7–15 year difference in lifespan.[333]

Blackburn's work is also shedding light on how integrative health practices may extend the lifespan, beginning with the halting and reversal of cardiovascular disease through exercise, diet and stress reduction. Her study on mindfulness meditation demonstrated increase telomerase activity after a meditation retreat in comparison to well-matched controls.[334]

Much of her cardiovascular data has been derived from The Heart and Soul Study, a prospective cohort trial of patients in the San Francisco bay area that is examining the influence of psychosocial factors on cardiovascular events in a population with stable coronary artery disease.

Leucocyte telomere length has been shown to be an independent predictor of coronary heart disease.[335] A recent study in the *British Medical Journal* involving over 44,000 individuals confirmed this.[332]

Blackburn and her team also found a strong association between physical fitness and telomere length in 944 patients who had provided DNA samples and underwent exercise treadmill testing. There was a significant association between lower exercise capacity and a shorter mean telomere length. "Participants with low exercise capacity (<5 METS) had a 94% greater odds of having short telomere length than those with high exercise capacity (>7 METS)."[336] Additional telomere data from the Heart and Soul Study showed a positive correlation with levels of marine omega-3 fatty acids docosahexaenoic acid (DHA) and eicosapentaenoic acid (EPA). The researchers obtained serial omega3 levels and conducted telomere analysis on a group of 608 ambulatory patients, followed for six years. The study showed an inverse relationship between blood level of marine omega3 fatty acids and the rate of telomere shortening. Those individuals in the lowest quartile for omega3 levels had the fastest rate of telomere shortening.[337]

Telomerase research is adding to the epigenetic evidence from the Ornish Gleason 6 study noted above. In an examination of 30 men, 49-80 years old with slow growing prostate cancer, the Ornish program of a low-fat nutrient rich vegan diet, stress management and exercise was shown to increase telomerase.[338] Another study showed that participants who completed a three-month meditation retreat, scored higher on positive mental health, and had increased telomerase as compared to a group on the waiting list for the retreat.[339]

This emerging science is providing possible mechanistic evidence to support benefits for some of the less easily quantified aspects of mental, emotional and spiritual health. In an article entitled "An intricate dance: Life experience, multisystem resiliency, and rate of telomere decline throughout the lifespan." UCSF researchers Eli Puterman, PhD, and Elissa Epel, PhD, make a strong case for a holistic approach to creating multisystem resilience to modify the effects of stress and shape the rate of biological aging. They note that:

> "Telomere length captures the interplay between genetics, life experiences and psychosocial and behavioral factors. Over the past several years, psychological stress resilience,

healthy lifestyle factors, and social connections have been associated with longer telomere length and it appears that these factors can protect individuals from stress-induced telomere shortening."[340]

Telomere measurement, particularly the sensitive and unique assay available from Life Length (www.lifelength.com), a leader in the field and now in partnership with the Cleveland HeartLab, is a diagnostic assay that physicians should consider adopting in their clinical practice.

Clarifying Your World Viewpoint

If we were to keep scores in integrative medicine, the points would be in units of meaning, not in minutes. Tieraona Low Dog, MD, explains her take on physicians' perspectives:

> "Integrative medicine doesn't require you to be with a patient for ninety minutes. It can be done in a routine ten-minute appointment. Integrative medicine is a philosophical approach, a framework for seeing the world. When physicians see their patients as broken souls in need of repair, medicine can be an incredibly heavy burden. If not careful, one can become bitter, as well as arrogant, for not only can physicians not 'fix' everything; but the truth is that patients often hold the keys to their own healing already within them."

In Part Two, *Heal Your Patients*, we have touched on the basic tools of Integrative Medicine. In working with unfulfilled physicians to find their calling, Low Dog encourages them to first embrace their discomfort and define their frustrations. One of the frustrations, she notes, "is not having enough tools in the toolbox." If this is your situation, we encourage you to delve deeper into lifestyle, functional, and holistic medicine.

Low Dog also notes that when there is a great discomfort, something else may need to shift; physicians may need to embrace new business models that allow them to rekindle their passion for care. An examination of these emerging models of care reflects the creativity and ingenuity inherent in United States healthcare practitioners. In Part Three: *Heal Your Practice,* we have profiled a very small sample of some of the best innovators, who in the words of Tim Gunn from *Project Runway*, "Make it work."

THE HOLISTIC PARADIGM

PART THREE
HEAL YOUR PRACTICE

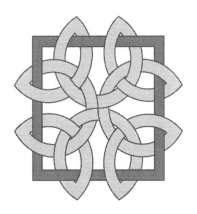

Every time you are tempted to react in the same old way, ask if you want to be a prisoner of the past or a pioneer of the future."

— Deepak Chopra, MD

9
Apply Tinctures of Time and Passion

When we prepared our applications for medical school, our counselors urged us to make certain that two themes ran through our personal stories: a passion for some aspect of science and a desire to help others. These are the two pillars that uphold the medical profession and drive our desire to fix that which is broken and to find cures for patient's ills.

With idealism in mind, as medical students, most of us never gave much consideration to what it would be like to actually practice medicine. For an older generation, the baby boomers, this was not necessary. At the end of training, there would be a lucrative career with stability and prestige. Today's younger physicians labor under no such illusions. Many boomer physicians no longer harbor these idyllic visions, as well.

In our work with physicians, public health educators, and healthcare policy makers we have heard the common refrain that our healthcare system is "broken." Some physicians have drawn a parallel to the paradigm shifts in Isaac Asimov's Foundation Trilogy. For a new order to emerge, the old order must fall apart and die. We must enter a period of chaos before a new, more stable structure emerges.

We are certainly in a period of chaos, but there is much to hold onto as we move forward as Tieraona Low Dog, MD, reminds us:

> "Just imagine waking up tomorrow in a world with no hospitals, no surgery, no diagnostic equipment, no trauma care, no medications. If we ever doubt how valuable our current system is, just imagine what it would look like if it were not there."

Low Dog lives in rural New Mexico where scarcity can be a fact of life and self-reliance is a necessity. She points to the material overabundance in our society as one of the factors that is creating a "soul sickness" in Americans.

CHAPTER NINE

"There is a reason that alcohol is called spirits, for its abuse is often driven by the desire to heal something within." Low Dog points to the importance of finding your calling. Her path to medical training was a winding one. She entered medical school at the age of 34 after pursuing careers as an herbalist, mid-wife, massage therapist, and martial artist. She counts herself fortunate to have entered training with a different perspective, and believes in the importance of finding your passion. "Just think where we would be if the world renowned medical illustrator Frank Netter, MD, had not found his calling and had the courage to follow it."

Fortunately, many other physicians are identifying their passions and are creatively recreating their professional lives within medicine. These trailblazers are changing a broken system, one patient at a time.

Be the Best Doctor You Can Be

From the age of 10, Alan Reisinger, MD, a Baltimore based internist knew he wanted to become Dr. Marcus Welby, the warm hearted, idealized, early 1970's television personification of the primary care physician. After going through medical school and residency with his classmate, the two went into primary care practice in the early 1980s, and the practice was everything Reisinger had hoped for. He remarked,

> "We had a few offices; we made house calls. There was enough time in the system to be a medical detective, to do preventive care and to understand our patients' lives." Reisinger found deep satisfaction in this arrangement until managed care hit the East Coast in the mid to late 80s when. "We were just overwhelmed by the contract agreements, the discount fees for service, the capitated life concept and we didn't have the business sense to handle that."

Reisinger and his partner sold their practice to one of the large local hospitals where, early on, they reaped the advantages of financial backing, consultants and administrative support. Reisinger became president of the primary care medical group of FPs, OBs, IMs and PEDs, a group that is successful to this day. But the pressures within the healthcare system started taking their toll.

"As the years went by, I would look across my desk at my

partner and we would both shake our heads. We had gone from loving our practice to hating it. We were always rushed, always late; we never felt we had enough time to handle patients' problems. At one point it got so bad that we handed the patients a form in the waiting room asking them to list three problems they would like to discuss with the doctor. If they had more than three they were asked to make another appointment. I wondered: what else could we do? How can we survive another 15-20 years practicing medicine this way?"

Along with his partner and wife, Reisinger attended a weekend workshop on how to survive the next millennium in medicine. The presenters, all very bright well-trained physicians, with 120 years of clinical experience between them, reaffirmed that things were bad, and were going to get worse. Their solution revolved around efficiency. Reisinger was told that the average doc at that time spent 8 minutes of actual face-to-face time with the patients; they would help cut that down to four. This would be accomplished with multiple triage-type forms and the use of a midlevel practitioner attached to every exam room. The midlevel practitioners would do everything that didn't require a physician. The doc would just need to come in and give the pronouncement; the prescriptions would be prepared and ready for signature.

"The selling point of their system was that we could see twice as many patients and make twice as much money. While this might be a great system for someone who wanted to churn patients through, it was far from the solution I had hope for. The last thing they covered in the seminar, however, caught my attention. They mentioned that there was something called retainer based or concierge medicine and that a small percent of physicians were doing this. They provided some examples. At the time I was under the assumption that the model would only work for physicians with wealthy patients. Our practice was in a mid-upper level blue-collar community. I left thinking our patients will never go for this; we are dead in the water."

Around that time Reisinger saw an advertisement for MDVIP and their personalized, smaller practice, membership model. Along with his partner, he attended a MDVIP program for physicians where he learned that MDVIP physicians had the freedom to do a 90-minute physical and

CHAPTER NINE

a 30-minute office visit. Commenting on that occasion, Reisinger said:

"There were about a dozen MDVIP doctors in attendance and what struck me was how happy they seemed. I was ready to join; my partner was much more skeptical. He said he couldn't take the risk. He had kids he had to put through college and suggested we would have to go our own ways.

My partner's fears were assuaged after MDVIP conducted their analysis of our practice and utilized their predictive model to determine whether our practice was a good fit with them." MDVIP routinely does extensive due diligence on the physician, the market and the practice, before accepting a physician into their network. "They were able to predict, with 97% accuracy, just how many patients we would be able to convert from our existing practice of 4,000 patients. They helped with all aspects of recruitment including teaching us how to explain the process to patients, providing communication tools, assisting us with legal requirements and creating town hall meetings for us. MDVIP also provided our EMR software along with a very responsive in-house support team that coached us on how to use it to best advantage. They also have a team to guide the physicians and staff through Meaningful Use and PQRS requirements, and a seasoned VP who interacts with the commercial payors on our behalf."

Reisinger goes on to note that there were some unexpected, pleasant surprises.

"The first was that most of the patients who came over to the practice were working class people. They were school teachers and bus drivers who value their health and are willing to spend the equivalent cost of a cup of Starbucks a day for longer appointments, preventive care, 24/7 access, and same day appointments."

Describing the recruitment process, Reisinger commented:

"The initial membership patients are the ones who love you, value your care and don't want to lose their relationship and history with you. Most people, however, are skeptical at first. They may decide to try it for a year. We retain more than 92% of these patients. We have about 8% turnover, and a replacement rate equal to that. Many of the patients who were in our conventional practice, and who elected not to join initially, have found their way back to us.

Reisinger smiles when he notes one of the "loses" in his current setting.

"We no longer have the telephone tree. The phone gets answered within two rings by somebody that has a smile on their face. This was really remarkable for our patients. Everybody knows the job of the front desk person is to protect the doctor and keep the patient from getting through. Instead, patients got someone genuinely interested in helping them."

Reisinger was also pleasantly surprised by MDVIP's interest in documenting outcomes and cost savings. A peer-reviewed study comparing the MDVIP personalized health model to conventional care found a 79% reduction in hospital admissions for Medicare patients, and a 72% decrease for those with commercial insurance between the ages of 35-64 in MDVIP-affiliated practices. This translated into a one-year healthcare system savings in excess of $300 million.[341]

MDVIP Medicare patients also had lower readmission rates for such conditions as acute MI, CHF, and pneumonia as compared to non-MDVIP Medicare patients. MDVIP readmission rates are below 2% for these conditions compared to the national averages that range from a low of 16% to a high of 24%.[341]

Another study, conducted by MDVIP's chief medical officer Andrea Klemes, DO, and cardiologist Marc Penn, MD, Director of the Summa Cardiovascular Institute in Akron, Ohio, showed improved cardiovascular risk detection in more than 95,000 patients who had undergone a multi-marker metabolic screening as part of their annual physical exam. Based on a lipid-only wellness panel, approximately 30% of patients presented as being at risk. When a multi-marker panel was used, 70% of patients were found to be at risk, with 40% having more than one marker positive.[342]

MDVIP has no sign up fee for physicians. Patients pay a $1,650 a year membership fee directly to MDVIP of which the physician gets two-thirds parceled out bi-weekly according to the number of active members in the practice. MDVIP physicians continue to accept commercial insurance and work within Medicare guidelines. Reisinger currently has 430 patients, his partner 330. MDVIP caps practices at 600 members.

CHAPTER NINE

Reisinger is happy at how his patient visits end.

"The last thing I ask every patient before we leave each other is whether there is anything we haven't talked about that is on their mind. I ask that because I actually have the time to address anything that comes up. I am making my living doing what I love, what I am trained to do, practicing real medicine and making a real difference in patients' lives."

Other Ways to Transition

Concierge care has its detractors. Some physicians and public health officials worry that by providing an upgraded experience for those who can afford it, care will be worse for those in the back of the plane. These critics also point to the additional strain placed on the providers of conventional care. For example, in a small or mid-sized town, if two physicians elect to embrace the membership model, this can set loose several thousand patients who have to now obtain care elsewhere, adding to the burdens of the physicians in that community.

While MDVIP is the largest and most well known of the membership models, there are other types of models and other consultants to which interested physicians can turn.

Specialdocs Consultants, Inc. (www.specialdocs.com) is a boutique consulting firm that helps physicians make the transition from the traditional model into concierge or personalized care practices. Roberta Greenspan, a seasoned healthcare executive whose experience spans both hospital and private practice settings, founded the company in 2002. Specialdocs has assisted more than 150 physicians in 31 states make successful transitions into concierge care.

According to Greenspan, "Physicians seek our help in achieving two primary goals: a better lifestyle for themselves and more time to provide comprehensive quality care for their patients. Ideally, they also want to exceed their current income." Specialdocs provides personalized, custom-designed models for their physicians. Their financial arrangement involves a one-time initial start-up fee and a sliding payment scale over their two and a half year contract.

Greenspan points out that the transition into concierge care is not for every physician. Her team does extensive due diligence on the practice and the physician including data analysis, references, site visits, and interviews with physicians, staff and their spouses. Greenspan notes that, "Sometimes the most stellar credentials belie lackluster interpersonal skills." To assess this, her team sits in on patient visits to determine whether the patients "love and truly connect with" their physician. Historically, Specialdocs has turned down more clients than they have engaged. For example, Greenspan stated their philosophy has always been to "reject any physician who is only looking for a way to generate more income without any expressed desire to improve the patient care experience."

Specialdoc's personalized and individualized attention provide the rationale for their two and a half year contractual agreement. "We brand the physician, not Specialdocs. To the best of our ability, each practice is individually tailored to that particular physician's desires and the needs of his or her specific patients," she said.

Overcoming Limitations of the Concierge Model

Tom Blue, Chief Strategy Officer of The American Academy of Private Physicians (www.aapp.org), is creating a different type of concierge consultancy in his role as co-founder of n1Health (www.n1health.com). For one thing, the emphasis at n1Health is squarely on functional or "root cause" medicine. For another, n1Health is structured to help physicians create concierge practices that avoid plateauing at a sub-optimal patient volume. Blue discusses what he terms the "concierge conversion conundrum:"

> "Until now the industry model has been conversion focused. Companies are helping physicians primarily target their existing semi-affluent Medicare patients who are willing to pay money to avoid having their care disrupted. The standard arrangement involves 1/3 of the fees going to the company, and the other 2/3 staying with the practice.
>
> Business resources are almost totally directed toward conversion, and practice promotion post-conversion is unfunded and generally overlooked. This is one of the reasons that most concierge practices hover at about 280 members, essentially operating at 50%-70% of capacity.

CHAPTER NINE

> We designed the n1Health model to provide marketing dollars to drive new patients into practices. The important thing is to appeal to patients outside of the practice that have no prior relationship with the physician."

Blue sees an issue with how membership based physician services are delivered today. He states, "Concierge medicine is a business model and not a value proposition."

Blue believes that great value can be created by establishing concierge practices built on functional medicine as the selling point for patient enrollment. Reflecting this approach, n1Health has adopted the tagline 'The Power of Personalized Medicine.' In his research, Blue often asks existing concierge doctors what they are doing.

> "Many are practicing the same medicine, only slower. Yes, there is greater access for patients, and higher levels of satisfaction for both patients and physicians, but there is too little attention paid to how to put the added time and money to the best possible use."

Blue believes n1Health addresses another critical issue: creating enterprise value for the practice.

> "Physicians who wish to retire are often extremely disappointed to learn that the value of their business is their accounts receivable and the depreciated value of their equipment. At n1Health we have created a model that allows for the transferring of a vessel of value, based upon the patient base. This is similar to what we see in other fields such as insurance or financial planning."

It is clear that the concierge model is being manifest in a number of forms and that physicians interested in exploring this business model now have more options and choices than ever before.

Fishing in a Different Pond

The concierge model, as practiced by companies such as MDVIP or Specialdocs is built upon helping a self-identified interested physician, with strong clinical and interpersonal skills, mine their current practice to obtain a base of membership patients. The companies use their marketing skills to bring new patients into the practice with the goal of limiting the total number to under 600 patients.

Paladina Health (www.paladinahealth.com) has taken a different route to acquiring what they term, belly buttons. They provide their primary care medical home (PCMH) approach primarily for mid- to large-sized self-funded companies. Features of the model include personalized care and 24/7 access to the physician by phone, email or in-office at a conveniently located clinic. While the concierge model first identifies the doctors and then recruits patients, Paladina first identifies an interested employer then actively recruits the physicians for that location.

Jami Doucette, MD, MBA, Leader at Paladina uses the term belly buttons to cut through the confusing array of employer-base health insurance terms such as members, subscribers, dependents, active employees, claimants, retirees, patients, etc. While attending Tufts' joint MD-MBA program, Doucette served as an advisor on concierge-type practice transformations in New England and was active in establishing Tufts' concierge practice, one of the earliest academic hospital concierge practices.

While Doucette was originally attracted to the surgical specialties, his interest in business led him to eschew residency for a career in investment banking. He went to work for a Nashville-based boutique investment bank focusing on mid-market health care mergers and acquisitions. Doucette moved to Arizona, raised some capital, and started a private concierge model business called ModernMed, which did reasonably well for the first year and a half, before changing emphasis and becoming one of the first companies in the country to sell its unique configuration of PCMH services to businesses. A little less than five years after inception ModernMed was acquired by the dialysis company DaVita in 2012 and merged with DaVita's homegrown Direct Primary Care company, Paladina Health. As part of their larger acquisition strategy, during that year, DaVita also acquired the California based physician group HealthCare Partners LLC in a $4.42 billion transaction.

Occupational physicians have long functioned in larger, mainly manufacturing companies where they are responsible for worker health and safety. Onsite, these physicians work to recognize and resolve workplace hazards and reduce absenteeism. They are involved in the formulation of health policies, the management of illness and disability, and preventive medicine. The American College of Occupational and Environmental

CHAPTER NINE

Medicine (www.acoem.org) is comprised of 4,500 physicians and is welcoming of physician membership.

The Paladina Health PCMH brings the personalized care model to the worksite, and in doing so not only benefits employer and patient, but also the physicians who provide the care. Doucette notes the freedom afforded the practitioners:

> "The physician is free to provide the care at the place and time that is right for them and the patient. We are location agnostic, care can be provided onsite or nearsite. The physicians can choose to do a home visit or use their time researching the best care for their patient. By changing the way in which Paladina is paid, namely through a flat-fee engagement with employer, the physician that is not accountable to a volume-based incentive driven by fee-for-service, but rather to a quality of care and service incentive that benefits the patients tremendously."

Physicians employed by Paladina receive a salary and bonuses tied to clinical metrics such as HbA1c for diabetes, or blood pressure control in hypertensives. Similar to the concierge companies, Doucette looks for physicians with not only great clinical abilities, but also the engaging bedside manner and service orientation that underlies a successful employer-based PCMH.

Doucette is impressed with how participants have reacted to the Paladina approach:

> "One of our earliest sites was with a diversified population of 1,200 employees in Dallas. I have never had any business endeavor received so positively. In phone calls and personal emails, the employees talked about the joys of easy access to 'my physician.' One employee whose husband didn't trust doctors, got quality care and follow up for a chronic illness. Another patient wrote how we saved her life with early diagnosis of a tumor."

Because of the variability in healthcare laws, Paladina operates on a state-by-state basis. They currently have about fifty clients drawn from the ranks of private companies, as well as state and municipal employees. While the sales cycle for adoption is long, Paladina continues to grow at an impressive rate matching their ambition for becoming a dominant national force. They invite physicians interested in their model to learn more about the company.

KISS Comes to Medicine

The voluntary simplicity movement is alive and well. From farm to table, from machine made to hand crafted, from big business to microenterprise, there is a trend to keep things simple and to find joy in a smaller scale. Many physicians have bought into this philosophy. Eschewing mountains of paperwork and complexity, they have streamlined their office practices to return to a simpler structure.

Jeff Gladd, MD, established a solo family practice outside of Ft. Wayne, IN, in 2004. Several years later, due to the "choking nature" of health insurance, he went to work as a salaried employee for the local hospital, again in conventional family medicine. It was at this point that his 15 pound weight gain ballooned to 50. He no longer had time for his young family. He began experiencing bouts of anxiety. Influenced by the work of Michael Pollan and Andrew Weil, MD, both of whom stress the importance of eating real, unprocessed food, Gladd transformed both his diet and his personal and professional outlook. He lost 50 pounds and shed SSRIs for good. From then on, at the conclusion of his 30-40 encounters, he would ask his patients if they were interested in a more natural, less pharmaceutically oriented approach to health. Gladd noted that, "Eighty percent just wanted the medications, but the other twenty percent lit up at the possibility."

Gladd was able to convince the hospital system to allow him to spend two days a week doing Integrative Medicine. When demand grew, he transitioned to full time. Sparked by his appearances in local media and community outreach, the IM practice soon had a six-month waiting list. Patients were coming from near and far. It was at this point that the idealistic ran smack into the realistic. As measured by traditional performance indices such as revenue and referrals for more sophisticated testing, IM practices within hospital systems often operate at a loss. When the administration informed Gladd that he would need to step up production in order to maintain the practice as currently configured, he made the choice to set out on his own. Parting on amicable terms, Gladd was able to continue leasing his office space from the hospital at a favorable rate.

CHAPTER NINE

Without any formal business training, Gladd decided instead to rely on a basic principle. He would structure his practice around a time-based model that eschewed insurance reimbursement. He established an hourly fee for his time, and those of the two nurse practitioners, dietician and health coach who joined him. Gladd describes his current financial model:

"I bill patients for the time I spend with them. My current rates are $300 an hour; the nurse practitioners bill at $200 an hour, and health coaches $50 an hour. We use the HelloHealth (www.hellohealth.com) platform as our personal health record system in which we are able to share labs, interact, videoconference or track email. Patients' credit cards are on file. A typical short email 'visit' is billed out at $40.

We generate some revenue on specialty labs such as microbiome testing, digestive and salivary analysis to cover the costs of administration; we also derive minor revenue from several lines of pharmaceutical-grade physician-only supplements. We don't push patients to purchase from us; in fact, we are not very good salespeople. We try to provide higher quality products at prices similar to the lesser quality products available from health stores. As a convenience to patients we also offer some of the healthy foods and snacks that my family eats and make them available to our patients."

Gladd sees patients two and a half days a week and is "as busy as I want to be." He has plenty of time for himself and his family. Gladd makes a strong case that small can be beautiful:

"The healthcare system has tried to make practice so complex, with HIPPAA, Meaningful Use, and ICD-10, it has us thinking that the only way we can practice is under a big umbrella in which a larger entity takes care of all of this for us. A medical practice can become successful by appreciating the simplicity of a transaction. Patients are used to being consumers. They are used to paying money for things that have value. So let it be simple, allow it to be about relationships."

As for breaking away from the conventional, high-volume insurance based model and opting for a lower volume, lower stress practice, Gladd encourages fellow physicians to take the leap of courage by employing the following model: "Ready, Fire, Aim. Just go ahead and put something out there. Maybe it's a day a week. See how your patients engage with you."(www.gladdmd.com)

Much like the difference between hothouse and heirloom tomatoes, each 'micro' practice is unique in terms of shape and flavor. The practitioners are free to focus on and incorporate the tools they are most comfortable with and those that will meet their patient's needs. It is the uniqueness of the practice and its hand crafted focus that allows the clinician to attract the kinds of patients who believe in their approach. These are the kinds of patients that the practitioner most enjoys treating. Below are examples of some types of hand-crafted 'micro' practices.

- Steve Knope, MD, one of the earliest concierge physicians in the US to adopt a membership model, provides pro bono care, including physical rehabilitation to injured Navy seals. The probono work makes up about ten percent of his practice, and according to Knope "is the most rewarding part of my career, thankfully the concierge work allows me to do this." Knope has a strength and conditioning coach on staff as well as space for rehabilitation to take place.

- Craig Koniver, MD, a family practice physician in Charleston, whose practice is called Primary Plus Organic Medicine, LLC, has pared back even further. Koniver sees 5-8 patients a day without any staff support. His patients come via word of mouth. Koniver offers his patients a variety of follow up options and payment plans. This includes a direct fee for the first visit followed by a range of costs depending upon upon the complexity of the patient's needs, the amount of time required and the method of communication. One of the most common follow up plans includes a fee for four visits and unlimited emails.

- Brad Jacobs, MD, ABIHM, has the most 'micro' of practices, catering to an exclusive group of approximately 100 patients. Jacobs, a nationally recognized IM physician, has served as Endowed Professor and Founding Medical Director for the UC-San Francisco Osher Center for Integrative Medicine. He specializes in treating many of the highly driven Silicon Valley and Bay Area executives. As a proponent of lifestyle medicine, and walking his talk, it is not unusual for Jacobs to bike, swim or hike with his patients. Jacobs is one of the first US physicians to utilize telomere testing in his practice and has demonstrated the profound impact that lifestyle can have on telomere length and quality of life.

- Susan Blum, MD, an early pioneer in Functional Medicine, has established the Blum Center for Health in Rye Brook, NY. What distinguishes the practice is the BlumKitchen, featuring classes and programs to teach patients how to incorporate a whole-foods, plant-based diet into their lives. Patients may engage with the practice through a consult, a cooking class or a workshop. Blum not only has a nutritionally oriented staff, but also a Feng Shui and body mapping expert on her team.

- Brian Alman, PhD, a clinical psychologist in Del Mar, CA, demonstrates that physicians are not the only ones with creative approaches to patient care. In the crowded field of positive psychologists, Alman stands out two ways. The first is his ability and willingness to take on the difficult cases few other psychologists are able to handle. Alman has been a key consultant for Kaiser Permanente who sends him patients who have failed tradition therapy. Alman's cases have included multiple generations of sexual perpetrators and their victims, priests who have molested children, the morbidly obese, and patients with bulimia and anorexia. As unique as the patients he counsels, is Alman's approach. Rather than seeing patients on a weekly basis, Alman spends an entire day with them. And rather than being confined within the office, that day is spent outside, walking and talking on the nearby beach. He has followed patients for 5-10 years via email, text, phone, and Skype. He also provides follow-up videos via the Internet.

We will discuss branding in greater detail in the next chapter, but it is worth noting the unique face to the marketplace that each practitioner has created.

- Knope positions himself as "Tuscon's Only Retainer Medicine Practice," and stresses his long-standing roots as a founder of the concierge movement. He is the author of a book entitled, *Concierge Medicine* (Praeger). (www.conciergemedicinemd.com)

- GladdMD is more than a practice. It is "a movement dedicated to empowering individuals." His is clearly an Integrative Medicine practice along with supplemental products available through his store. Gladd is upfront with his personal transformation of weight loss and health promotion through whole foods eating. The small team approach is evident with bios of two Nurse Practitioners, a Certified Health Coach, an Integrative Dietician and a Project Manager prominently displayed.

- Koniver has created www.organicmedicinenow.com and an outreach program called 'Break Free' that includes a weekly newsletter and comprehensive guide.

- Jacobs provides "Integrative Medicine for mind, body and soul." In his presentations he draws upon his personal experience of his father and sister's life threatening illnesses and his challenges and successes in utilizing conventional and alternative treatments, as well how to incorporate his 6 Pillars of Healthy Living to optimize quality of life and manage health conditions. He recounts stories on surfing, tai chi, yoga, and more to bring to life customized approaches to help people achieve what he calls "your best life." (www.drbradjacobs.com)

- Blum teaches 'Food as Medicine' in the BlumKitchen where she also makes products available for participants. Her corporate wellness programs emphasize teamwork through a group cooking process. Blum has been able to leverage her food-based functional approach, along with her charisma and proximity to the New York media market. She is a member of the Medical Advisory Board for The Dr. Oz Show and is frequently featured on national television and magazine publications. (www.blumcenterforhealth.com)

- Alman is the author of *The Voice: Listen Inside...Your Truth Will Set You Free* (Archer Books). The book presents a simple but powerful self-help method for overcoming stress and resolving stress-related issues. He offers multiple programs available for sale on his websites: www.drbrianalman.com and www.trusage.com.

Each of these practitioners is available to speak to groups, do keynotes, workshops and seminars. Just as Alman is able to make his environment work for both himself and his patients, and Blum has built a functional medical practice around a kitchen, so too are independent physicians able to create the environments they believe are conducive to health.

While the micro-practice provides benefits to the practitioner, it also affords macro benefits for the quality of patient care. Increasingly,

CHAPTER NINE

studies are supporting the 'smaller is better' approach. A recent study showed that practices of 1-2 physicians had 33% fewer preventable hospital admissions as compared to practices of 10-19 physicians. Practices with 3-9 physicians had 27% fewer admissions that the larger group. The study also showed that physician-owned practices had lower preventable admissions than those that were hospital-owned.[343]

Dip and then Dive in

The story of Lornell Hansen, MD, a family practitioner in Sioux Falls, South Dakota, is an increasingly popular one. It is a cautionary tale of first dipping one's toe in the aesthetic waters before fully diving in. In 2003, Hansen became intrigued with aesthetic lasers and the possibility of adding aesthetics to his hospital owned practice. Along with three partners, Hansen practiced primary care as part of Sanford Health. Hansen ran into resistance, first from his partners who did not want to spend the money, and then from the hospital that would not support his decision. Fortunately, he was able to work his way around a non-compete and in 2004 he opened LazaDerm Skincare Centre in a separate location from his primary care practice. He began by seeing aesthetic patients part time on his days off and evenings. His first employee was his sister, Denee Reinwald, who was willing to change her career direction and take a small salary while the practice grew. To this day, Reinwald manages all Hansen's clinics.

A decade ago, aesthetics was in its infancy. There was some demand on the East and West coasts and in Texas, but these places were far from Sioux Falls. Without dollars to invest in marketing, Hansen's cosmetic practice grew slowly, but steadily as the result of word of mouth. He used all the profits from LazaDerm to grow the Centre: getting more training, purchasing new equipment and adding new procedures and employees. As the Centre began to require more of his time, he moved from family practice to doing acute care for Sanford Health Systems on evenings and weekends, and continued to do so until he was able to break free and focus 100% of his time on LazaDerm. Even so, early on Hansen continued to moonlight about once a month in local small town emergency rooms and hospitals.

Today, Hansen operates three LazaDerm Centres, each staffed with a physician and a nurse practitioner. He also owns four clinics focused solely on vein care and operate as Physicians Vein Clinics. He speaks about the sacrifice and the ingredients for success in establishing an aesthetic practice in a smaller, Midwest market:

> "I think the most important thing other physicians need to understand is that this does not happen over night. It will take a lot of work and sacrifice. It took over 4 years for me to fully transition from family medicine to aesthetic medicine. There are too many companies willing to tell doctors to open a clinic and they will be busy immediately if they just buy that company's laser. That is why there are so many clinics with lasers and pieces of equipment that have become coat racks in a closet in the back of a clinic.
>
> It also takes a supportive wife. I have a wonderful wife and she was able to keep the household together and raise three wonderful children while I was working long hours and focusing on growing the business. She was 100% supportive even when our income had decreased during the transition.
>
> I started with caution. I jumped in but it took time to transition. I did not start within my old practice; I opened a completely different clinic in a different location. I did not want to have the two clinics associated with each other and wanted the aesthetic practice to be 100% independent of my family medicine practice. In my opinion this was the smartest thing I did when first opening the practice. At first, I was not sure how busy the practice would become but knew I wanted it to succeed and I was willing to do what was necessary."

Hansen continues to attend to deepen his knowledge base of the latest aesthetic techniques. He attends the American Academy of Cosmetic Surgery (AACS) and THE Aesthetic Show each year (www.aestheticsshow.com). He has trained with Jeff Klein, MD, in liposuction, and is a member of the American Society for Laser Medicine and Surgery (ASLMS).

Hansen had his sail up long before the winds of aesthetic desire strengthened. He survived the 2008-9 recession, and is now taking advantage of the rebound of interest and consumer spending.

In its 2013 survey, The American Society for Aesthetic Plastic Surgery (ASAPS) reported a 12% overall increase in cosmetic procedures performed in the United States over the previous year. Nonsurgical procedures such as neurotoxins, fillers, hair removal, skin rejuvenation and microdermabrasion increased by 13.1% to 9.5 million procedures. ASAPS estimates that at its member practices, more than $2.5 billion was spent on injectables alone. In addition, nearly $1.9 billion was spent on skin rejuvenation, a fast-growing sector of the aesthetic nonsurgical procedures.

The ASAPS statistics only report procedures done by board-certified plastic surgeons, dermatologists and otolaryngologists in the United States, and do not take into account the non-surgical procedures done by other specialties and non-physician practitioners. Given the growing adoption of these treatments, it is likely that the true market may be 50-80% larger.[344]

Diving into Aesthetics

Jay Shorr is the managing partner of The Best Medical Business Solution, Inc. (www.thebestmbs.com) a medical practice consulting firm specializing in the operational, administrative and financial health of the business entity. Shorr went into the business with his daughter after the untimely death of his wife, a renowned dermatologist in South Florida, whose practice Shorr had managed. Shorr leverages his skills and knowledge to guide physicians in practice transformation. Coming from an aesthetic background, he has advised thousands of physicians who want to incorporate aesthetics into their practice. He provides these guidelines for the new entrant into the field.

- Check with the state regulations to determine what procedures the physician and/or their staff are allowed to perform. What a medical assistant, aesthetician or RN can do in one state may be a violation just across the state line. Physicians are allowed to perform most procedures in all states. Depending upon the degree of invasiveness, also check with your malpractice carrier, particularly if you are considering doing liposuction.

- Establish your business structure carefully—and this holds true for IM practices as well. Make certain you don't run afoul of laws relating to kickbacks, fee splitting, or—in California—the corporate prohibition on the practice of medicine. (Become acquainted with attorney Michael H. Cohen's excellent blog www.camlawblog.com.)

- Get training, and then more training. Just because you have an MD/DO degree does not mean that you have familiarity with procedures that are performed in the aesthetic/med spa practice. It is imperative that you and your staff take specialized training to learn how to avoid the complications associated with the various treatments you want to perform. Lasers can cause severe burns and skin damage; neurotoxins can lead to lid ptosis; poorly placed fillers can produce deformities and in rare cases blindness; and various chemical peels can cause blistering and secondary infection. Specialty-trained aesthetic physicians in your area are often looking to denigrate the skills of non-residency trained physicians, so always err on the side of safety and conservatism in treatment.

- Several aesthetic conferences hold annual and periodic meetings throughout the year; they have primary and advanced training courses as an adjunct or as part of the curriculum. Other for profit groups hold trainings year round. A list of organizations that provide aesthetic training can be found in the Appendix.

- Most of the major vendors are more than willing to provide training when you purchase their equipment. If you did not purchase the equipment directly from the manufacturer, there are professional trainers who hold classes for nominal fees. All of the major filler companies have injector trainers in your area, and they can schedule the proper training needed. Many experienced nurse injectors, such as Sylvia Silvestri, RN, (www.beverlyhillsrn.com) offer training both locally and nationally.

- Create a business plan to include financials, staffing, supplies and equipment, procedures, advertising and marketing. Your marketing spend should be approximately 10% of your annualized revenue. Do not expect your current patient base to know about your new services so make certain you constantly remind them. Avoid the temptation to get caught up in daily deal discounts. These rarely work in medicine and only bring in patients who are looking for the next best deal; some states have deemed them illegal as well. These bargain shoppers have low return and referral rates.

- Do not be afraid to seek the advice of a consultant who specializes in this type of work. It may end up being cost efficient to seek the advice of an expert so you can focus on your core competencies.

CHAPTER NINE

A number of organizations provide in-house training on aesthetic devices as well as medical laser safety office training. The American Society for Laser Medicine & Surgery (www.aslms.org) provides a listing of reputable programs.

ASLMS also offers preceptorships that can provide more indepth training in the use of laser technology. Many aesthetic physicians offer similar opportunities as well. The Gateway Aesthetic Institute and Laser Center (www.gatewaylasercenter.com) offers preceptorships with their team. Tahl Humes, DO, of Vitahl Medical Aesthetics (www.vitahl.com) in Denver provides physicians with opportunities to spend anywhere from a day to a week learning techniques in her practice.

In addition to training, a good eye for beauty, a steady hand, and the willingness and capacity to deal with vanity and often unrealistic expectations are other prerequisites for success in this ever growing field.

The Path of Regenerative Medicine

Pardon the explicative, but we can't help but be amused by the title of a popular site that is heavily shared on Facebook entitled "I Fxxxing Love Science," (www.iflscience.com). This same enthusiasm is shared by many physicians who look forward to realizing the advances of the latest medical technology. One of these technologies involves the field of regenerative medicine, specifically both the promise and present use of stem cells. Before we describe how physicians are employing stem cell treatments today, a little background is in order.

There is much hype and confusion about the emerging field of regenerative medicine, a catchall term that includes both autologous and allogeneic cellular derived substances including stem cells and stem cell related products. On one side of the equation are researchers who point out that the field is promising, but provide the standard answer that "we're ten years away." Much of the scientific research is aimed at determining new types of stem cells along with their novel mechanisms of action, or devoted to the use of stem cells in drug discovery.

The stem cell research field was given a scientific turbo boost in 2006 with the discovery, by Nobel Prize winning scientist, Shinya Yamanaka, MD, PhD, a professor at Kyoto University, of a mechanism to create induced pluripotent stem cells (iPS). With the introduction of four genes, adult cells—most commonly skin—could be converted back into pluripotent stem cells, creating the equivalent of an embryonic stem cell but without the need to manipulate the embryo. These cells could then be differentiated along any number of tissue lines. While many issues need to be addressed before iPS cells can be safely used in patients, they are playing an important role in understanding the patient-specific basis of disease and personalizing the drug discovery process. This discovery, however, has diverted both scientific and media interest away from present and near-term clinical applications of stem cells.

On the clinical side of regenerative medicine are physicians who are either performing clinical trials with stem cells or who are actively doing autologous transplantation either with the patient's mesenchymal stem cells (MSCs) or platelet rich plasma (PRP). At the present time allogeneic stem cells are still in clinical trials and have not been cleared by the FDA.

The autologous MSCs are harvested either from the patient's adipose or bone marrow, or in the case of PRP from blood, isolated via centrifugation and the concentrate is reinjected into joints, soft tissue, or placed intravenously. Studies with autologous MSCs and PRP have shown that treatment is safe, with most AEs being related to the actual injection. We will confine our discussion in this section to MSC use.

The cellular benefits of MSCs have been well described in the literature. While MSCs have the potential of differentiating into other tissues, transplantation takes advantage of their abilities to regenerate tissue through paracrine effects including the production of growth factors that down regulate inflammation, mobilize other stem cells, prevent cellular apoptosis, rescue cells dying from ischemia, and enhance the stem cell niche.[345] MSCs display a wide array of genetic expression involved in cytokines and growth factors that affect the endothelium (FGF-2, FGF-7, VEGF-A, VEGF-B), smooth muscle (HGF, PDGF)), as well as migration and matrix differentiation (TNF-α, MCP-1).[346] Cardiac studies have shown that direct injection in infarcted myocardium can favorably affect patient functional capacity, quality of life, and ventricular remodeling.[347]

Intra-articular injection of MSCs are being extensively studied in osteoarthritis where they appear promising in mitigating pain and improving function.[348] While there has been an abundance of anecdotal evidence, RCTs are just beginning to examine therapeutic benefits of MSCs. There is much to learn about the type of cell, tissue effects on the condition being treated, the timing and route of administration, and the dosing of the cellular products.

The most common approach to harvesting MSCs involves isolating the stromal vascular fraction (SVF) from adipose tissue. When subjected to collagenase and centrifugation, the heaviest fraction of a lipoaspirate, the SVF, sinks to the bottom of the tube. This fraction contains not only the adipose derived mesenchymal stem cells, but other types of cells including pre-adipocytes (fat precursor cells), endothelial and pre-endothelial cells, stromal cells as well as non-cellular elements. When most clinicians discuss fat derived stem cell treatment with patients, they are really talking about the heterogeneic stromal vascular fraction. The largest body of scientific research, however, focuses on the actions of the MSCs within the SVF.

Harvesting MSCs from adipose has advantages over harvesting from bone marrow. It not only involves less discomfort, it also yields many more MSCs and obviates the need for expansion in culture. A typical lipoaspirate contains five hundred thousand to one million stem cells per cc of fat, or 10 to 40 million cells for a single treatment.

Increasingly, physicians are using the SVF fraction to complement autologous fat transfer in a procedure known as cell assisted lipotransfer (CAL). CAL helps improve the retention of the transplanted adipose. Autologous fat transfer is an alternative to facial fillers in aesthetic procedures; it is also used in repair after burns, trauma and post tumor resections as well as in lipodystrophies. An increasing number of physicians are taking advantage of the tissue regeneration abilities in MSCs beyond aesthetics.

Autologous Transplantation Today

Mark Berman, MD, traces his interest in the SVF back to 2010, when, as President of the American Academy of Cosmetic Surgery (www.cosmeticsurgery.org), he was exposed to CAL for breast augmentation. To better understand the science and the technique, Berman visited the two leading CAL surgeons in Japan, Drs. Yoshimura and Kamikura who were pioneering this technique. Upon his return from Japan, Berman started utilizing cell-assisted lipotransfer with his aesthetic patients.

Berman's first foray into SVF use outside of aesthetics occurred in collaboration with Los Angeles based orthopedic surgeon Tom Grogan, MD. The first few orthopedic patients experienced excellent results with improvement in mild to moderate osteoarthritis of the knee and hip. While improvement in these conditions is subject to the placebo effect, a number of patients with long-standing discomfort had markedly diminished discomfort and improved function well after any placebo effect would wear off. Along with Grogan, Berman started The California Stem Cell Treatment Center (www.californiastemcelltreatmentcenter.com), and began creating IRB protocols to guide their work. At this point, anecdotal evidence continued to point to clinical improvement as well as patient satisfaction. The Center began to attract a multispecialty team with interest in treating orthopedic, urologic, cardiovascular, pulmonary, autoimmune, wound care, and several other disease entities.

As Berman began to lecture at conferences and present his case studies, physicians from locations beyond Southern California became attracted to his work and wanted "to join his group." After doing an initial 20 cases with Grogan, Berman started working with urologist Elliot Lander, MD, on building out a business model that could scale with the guiding principles that the expansion would be fair and reasonable for the participating physicians, ensure patient safety, and as importantly, compile the data on all procedures done.

The new organization, The Cell Surgical Network (CSN) (www.stemcellrevolution.com), consists of affiliated member teams of multidisciplinary physicians. CSN emphasizes quality and is highly committed to clinical research and the advancement of regenerative medicine. Currently CSN operates in 22 states with multiple locations in the larger markets such as California and Arizona. Before being able to expand, Berman had to provide a satisfactory answer to the first question on the minds of all potential stem cell adopters: Is SVF transfer in violation of the FDA rules?

Berman is clear that the FDA does not prohibit this use. He notes:

> "The cells are autologous, they are taken from and injected back into the same patient and are not being manipulated, or expanded in any way, hence they do not fall under FDA 21 CRF part 1271. This code is directed toward laboratories that manipulate human cellular products and have the potential

CHAPTER NINE

of transmitting a communicable disease. California Stem Cell Treatment Center and all members of the Network use a completely closed sterile surgical procedure to isolate SVF (not pure stem cells). All supplies, devices and drugs are already FDA approved though not specifically for SVF or stem cell production."

Berman notes that SVF transplantation is a surgical procedure, outside of the jurisdiction of the FDA. As is typical of many surgical devices and drugs, it is completely legal, ethical and appropriate to use approved products off-label. Furthermore, Berman has submitted his IRB approved protocols to the FDA and has never had any communication from them that the protocols were not appropriate.

While Berman was excited about SVF use in medicine, he was put off by the high cost and complexity of the equipment being used for the procedure. He began work with Medikan, a Korean device manufacturer, on the creation of a less expensive collection device and with Roche on the development of a bovine-free collagenase to separate the lipoaspirate. The resulting device, The Time Machine, has brought costs down to affordable levels.

As interest grows in the Network, Berman's screening process has deepened as well. Physicians submit their credentials in the same way that they apply to be on a hospital board. While most of the physicians are cosmetic and orthopedic, primary care physicians and other specialists are increasingly coming on board. CSN has a very simple model. If a physician is accepted into the program, CSN trains the physician at no cost, provides all educational and marketing materials, IRB protocols and informed consent forms. The physician buys or leases the Time Machine, which sells in the range of $20,000 and orders the disposables from CSN. The CSN disposable fee, currently at $1,000 per case, covers medical malpractice, as well as the online database, research coordinators, administration, the documentation website and ongoing IRB protocols. To date, most of the applications for The Time Machine have revolved around aesthetics and orthopedics; however, under informed consent and IRB, patients are being treated for other conditions including neurological, wound care and metabolic. All physicians share a common treatment database that allows CSN to gather comprehensive data.

The Motivations for Now

Alan Wu, MD, is director of Priatas, Faculty at the UC, Riverside Stem Cell Research Center and a practicing cosmetic, reconstructive and regenerative surgeon. Wu has completed further specialty training in surgical molecular biology, molecular embryology and phlebology; he is a well recognized stem cell expert. Wu notes that there are two types of patients:

> "Some have heard of procedures currently being done for their condition. The second type doesn't know anything about regenerative procedures, but they are at their wit's end. I will ask them what they've tried, and to see how far they've gone in the current standard of care. I try to gauge their level of frustration. I let them know that are some alternative options we can look into. I provide them with some preliminary information and some websites to look at. I ask them to do some basic research, and then if interested, to return. It's important for them to understand the options and choices and to come to their own conclusions. Together we work to set reasonable expectations. This way if the procedure doesn't work, there are no hard-felt feelings."

Wu believes regenerative medicine holds the possibility for revitalizing both patients and physicians.

> "We're looking at patients having a difficult time going to terminus of standard care, and not achieving results. These are the patients we feel badly about; we are struggling to help them out. It is depressing and sad when you see a patient suffering. They get passed around because nobody has anything to offer. It gets to the point where the medical community avoids the patient."

Addressing the limitations of standard care, Wu discussed the case study of an 85-year-old man on anticoagulants whose cardiologist refused to clear him for a knee replacement. Wu asks:

> "What do we do with these people? Give them drugs to dull the pain. Money is spent accomplishing nothing; patients are still suffering. In this case, stem cell injections relieved the patient's pain. When I first saw the patient, he was able to ambulate minimally with use of a cane. Following one

intra-articular injection of SVF he was able to ambulate without use of the cane and experienced less pain, which was quite remarkable given his pre-procedure diagnosis of 'bone on bone' degeneration of the joint. Ancillary markers such as erythema, edema and range of motion were also considerably improved within just 4 weeks."

Wu notes that others using SVF with equivalent methods are reporting similar unpublished findings. Wu has an extensive caseload of patients he has successfully treated with autologous stem cells in a running case series. Among the most impressive results have been those achieved in wound healing, where he has treated approximately 25 cases of chronic unhealed wounds. He cites the case of a diabetic with a leg amputation and a chronic, non-healing would that resisted closure with standard grafts.

"Stem cell transplantation healed the wound. Using a combination of adipose derived stem cells for initial therapy (2 sessions, 6 weeks apart) and PRP (3 sessions, 4 weeks apart) we were able to revascularize and thicken compromised tissue and ultimately able to recruit additional regenerative cells to the chronic site at a cost well below current standard of care. So we have a choice, spend an inordinate amount of money on a non-effective standard of care or spend a mere fraction of this amount to fix what previously had been unfixable."

Wu is willing to treat patients now, even though all the evidence is not in on efficacy. He notes:

"Where we get in trouble, in all of medicine, is when we have this attitude that it's theory-animal model-clinic side, then proven. The problem is that we've seen that that methodological process is extremely expensive, and you can't always do that."

Addressing the challenges of quality and training, he states, "One of the challenges in a young field such as regenerative medicine is that there is no formal organization providing accreditation. A couple organizations are forming. Much like Emergency Medicine that didn't have certification 50 years ago, at some point there will be a recognized certification for regenerative medicine." In the interim, Wu has provided a list of conferences and training programs for physicians interested in learning more about stem cells. It can be found in the Appendix.

Wu believes regenerative medicine can help revamp and reinvigorate a physician's practice.

> "The overhead for starting something like this is not very high, the buy-in and the equipment is not like building a new surgery center or an operating room. What I hear back from actively practicing clinicians is that regenerative medicine is fun. It's interesting. Everybody is fascinated by stem cells. I have doctors looking at themselves and saying 'I might need this too, myself someday.' There's a natural curiosity within the scientific and medicine community. There's real science, real medicine here. Some of it doesn't work, admittedly. But that's what we're in it for, to find what is going to work for our patients."

When Illness Hits Home—Finding the Missing Piece

In 1997, Jen Landa, MD, then a newly minted 28-year-old OB/Gyn in Florida came face to face with her own chief complaint, one that was neither well documented, nor well understood at that time. More than a decade later, it is still rarely discussed with openness in clinical practice. Landa had lost her sex drive.

The recently married OB/Gyn knew something was wrong but didn't know where to turn for answers. Not only was the condition embarrassing, but as a woman's healthcare specialist Landa felt she was supposed to have the solution to her problem.

After the birth of Landa's first child, she developed other symptoms, among them a deep sense of exhaustion and fatigue no matter how much she slept. Her work, which had been the area of her life in which she excelled, no longer was providing satisfaction. In fact, it was creating just the opposite: fear. "I used to thrive on the emergencies like getting a baby out through C-section in two minutes flat. Now I was afraid to enter the delivery room. I was preoccupied with worries among them the phobia of being sued. I felt like a failure. I was a bad mom, wife and doctor. I entertained thoughts of giving up my career," she stated.

At this point, Landa had ruled out the most common causes of fatigue: her routine blood and serum chemistries were fine. Seeking to lower her

CHAPTER NINE

stress levels, she gave up OB and concentrated instead on an outpatient Gyn practice.

It was at this time that she started attending the American Academy of Antiaging Medicine (A4M) meetings and enrolled in The Fellowship for Anti-Aging and Regenerative Medicine.

> "I realized that years of birth control pills had screwed up my hormones. I no longer had any free testosterone. The BCPs contributed to adrenal fatigue. I started to see more and more published studies on adrenal fatigue and the cortisol awakening response. I dived into nutrition and hormone replacement therapy," said Landa.

Eight years ago, Landa gave up her Gyn practice and totally devoted herself to anti-aging and functional medicine. A major focus of her practice is bioidentical hormone therapy (BHRT), which she discusses below.

> "There is a lot of confusion in terminology. Bio identical hormones is a marketing term, used for patient convenience; it is not a scientific term," says Landa.

Like many physicians she relies on bioidentical hormone prescription products such as micronized estradiol and progesterone. Landa emphasizes that compounded products are neither safer nor more "natural" than available prescription products, many of which are derived from plants. She uses customized prescriptions from two compounding pharmacies—with which she has great familiarity—when she wants to provide hormones at lower doses than are available in prescription products, for customized vaginal creams and for off-label use of testosterone/progesterone compounds. She has provided patients with low doses of testosterone with progesterone for ten years with excellent results and without any complications. She believes that there is good safety data in terms of breast cancer and heart disease.

> "While I would love to have a randomized controlled trial, this may not happen in my lifetime. I don't feel that I can deny my patient access to these compounds. I thoroughly discuss the risks and benefits of the treatment and also make certain to note that they have not been 100% proven."

Landa is the Chief Medical Officer of BodyLogicMD (www.bodylogic-md) a franchise group of A4M fellowship trained physicians that focus on BHRT along with customized nutrition and fitness regimens, and stress reduction techniques. Each physician is free to practice in his or her own way.

The Take Home Message

If you are at the point where you are considering augmenting or restructuring your practice, you are not alone. Other physicians are in various stages of change. For those who are considering making these changes, we'd like to provide the following points to consider.

1. If you intend on making a radical change, make certain to honor the skills that got you to where you are now.

2. Keep your motivations as pure and patient-centered as possible. Len Wisneski, MD, counsels colleagues who want practice success to employ a simple formula, "The service to profit ratio has to be greater than one. If your efforts are more than 50% geared toward profit, you are unlikely to succeed."

3. Fully immerse yourself in the student experience. Attend conferences, seminars and take courses. Put aside inner doubts, criticisms, and comparisons and instead, approach educational experiences with what in Zen is called 'beginner's mind.'

4. See what other non-competitive colleagues are doing and ask their advice. Find some role models, pick up the phone and call them. You will find remarkable openness on the part of most of your peers.

5. Create a plan. Create a worst-case plan. Create a contingency plan. Recognize that you win over patients one at a time, and this often takes more time and money than you had originally planned to spend.

6. Carefully select consultants to guide you. Interview several, get references; make certain their deliverables are realistic and measurable. Consider doing a preceptorship. Call a physician whose skills and practice you admire and arrange to compensate them for visiting them and seeing patients together.

7. Recognize that the franchise/or collective marketing model can hedge your downside and get you out of the gate faster, but depending upon the structure, it can also limit your upside. Some physicians in these schemes become resentful of the parent organization at the point

CHAPTER NINE

where the practitioner feels she is doing all the work and the company is no longer delivering ongoing value for their share of profits.

8. Have courage. Reread Chapter 4.

9. Recognize that success takes a team effort. You need everyone in the practice aligned, positive, and present around the provision of exceptional quality care. Remember the patient defines quality, not the clinicians. To deliver on this promise, you will need to examine your leadership and team building skills.

10. Finally, decide who and what you want to be to your patients and the marketplace in general, in short what is your 'brand?' What mix of unique features and benefits, experience, knowledge and skills will allow you to attract the types of patients you would like to treat.

We will now direct our attention to these last two items, branding and leadership.

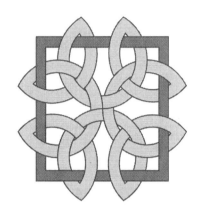

Whilst the technical tasks of medicine are important, it is at the level of the team, the service and the organisation that much good health care is generated. Achieving results through people and managing change is a universally difficult task and one which few are skilled in, trained or prepared for.

— Sir Liam Donaldson

10
Ingredients of a Successful Practice

Building a Brand

When you raise the subject of branding and marketing with some conventional physicians, the result is often a knee-jerk reaction accompanied by a bitter taste in their mouths. There is the belief, particularly among older physicians, that it is unprofessional to market one's services or to "toot one's own horn." Many medical and surgical specialists such as oncologists, neurologists, and vascular surgeons hold this opinion.

Allow us to put these arguments to rest. To begin with, let's substitute the word 'reputation' for 'branding.' Now the focus becomes clearer, and so does the relevance of the following questions:

- Do you want to allow your reputation (brand) to evolve with no guidance from you?
- Are you comfortable putting your reputation (brand) in the hands of others who then define you?
- Do you believe that you have carved your reputation (brand) in stone, and it cannot easily be eroded or upturned?
- How confident are you that the referrals you obtain from your colleagues, based upon your stellar reputation (brand) will always continue, despite ongoing changes in the healthcare marketplace in your community?

Many physicians also confuse branding with advertising or with the development of a new logo or identity for the practice. What is branding? It is the sum total of every experience the patient has with you. The identity of the practice is an element, but it is only one factor that collectively creates the impression of quality—or lack thereof—in the mind of the patient. Is the practice easy to find? How safe and well lit is the parking lot? What does the office look like? How clean are the

CHAPTER TEN

bathrooms, exam rooms and the reception area? How long is the wait to see the healthcare practitioner? Even more important, how friendly and relaxed are the front office staff? Do the physicians appear to value others in the practice? Is the environment conducive to learning and healing?

Creating a Healthy Practice is an Inside-Outside Game

The only way to create a totally healthy practice is to attend to all the little details that collectively color a patient's impressions of you and your practice. The best way to do this is to periodically survey a subset of patients on a repeated basis. This can be done as a follow up to an office visit either on paper visit, on an Internet enabled tablet, or online at the patient's convenience. Companies such as Survey Monkey (www.surveymonkey.com) allow for easy customization and data collection. In the Appendix we have provided a list of potential questions as a guide to formulate your own surveys. They are organized into eight categories:

1. Telephone Inquiry
2. Building Exterior
3. Check In/Reception/Common Areas
4. Prescreen (Initial Services) if Applicable
5. Exam Room
6. Exam/Consultation by Practitioner
7. Patient Coordinator/Check Out/Billing
8. Overall Impression

In and of themselves, attending to these critical areas will not guarantee practice success, but it can lessen the likelihood of poor performance.

Healthcare Change is Changing

Stewart Gandolf, is co-founder and CEO of Healthcare Success Strategies (HSS), a healthcare marketing company that has helped 5,000 hospitals, physicians groups and corporations over their 20 years in business. HSS provides education and training via live and online advanced practice seminars, as well as consulting services that include branding, internet marketing and SEO, media buying, staff training, and doctor referral building. For some smaller organizations, the company functions as their offsite marketing department. HSS produces an insightful newsletter and multiple white papers that can be referenced on their site. (www.healthcaresuccess.com)

In his years in business Gandolf continues to be amazed by the Toffleresque future shock increase in the rate of change in the healthcare industry.

> "I liken it to the polar bear standing on the ice flow and watching it melt beneath one's feet. You have to always be alert to find the next ice flow to jump to. This is clearly exemplified by changing referral patterns in healthcare. We first started seeing this 15 years ago, when one of our clients, an OB/Gyn was recruited by the local hospital to move to a rural area and establish his independent practice in this underserved area. Several years later the hospital hired their own OB/Gyn to compete with him. Today we are seeing healthcare changing as small physician groups turn into super groups that are then bought by hospitals that are bought by insurance companies. The bottom line is that this restructuring can cause long standing referral patterns to dry up overnight."

Many of HSS's physician clients share the common desire to remain independent despite the handwriting on the wall. They are initially drawn to marketing as a defensive strategy, not because they intend to grow rich. "Usually there is an instigating factor, a new competitor emerges, or a change in referral patterns, or their motivation may simply stem from the desire to not die by 10,000 paper cuts," said Gandolf. He notes that many medical and surgical specialties are now allotting substantial dollars for practice promotion. He points to an oncology practice that just hired a senior marketing executive from Apple to brand and market the group's services.

Gandolf reinforces the importance of positioning one's practice to stand out amidst the sea of competition. He defines positioning as the rationale or argument for why a patient should come to you. Are you the most affordable, convenient, best trained, most exclusive, most integrative, etc.? Positioning, he notes, "provides a reason or theme that the entire practice can get behind." Gandolf shares an interesting story:

CHAPTER TEN

> "We once positioned a dental practice with a series of cartoon ads all about being gentle. We were all a bit worried about how this would be received. Not only did the campaign drive more patients into the office, the dental staff all started to actually treat their patients more gently."

One of HSS's long-standing clients, Jonathan Calure, MD, is clear about his positioning. He states, "No one wants the second best doctor treating them." A cardiothoracic surgeon by training, in 2005 Calure founded the first of his vein-only therapy centers in the Baltimore area. Hiring only board certified surgeons, Calure has expanded to six Maryland Vein Professionals (MVP) centers. The ambulatory surgery facilities are Joint Commission approved. MVP has done more than 30,000 vein treatments since inception.

In part, Calure selected this practice niche based upon the incidence of venous disease. "By age 60," he says, "70% of women and 40% of men will have varicose vein issues." Maryland Vein Professionals conducts between 300-400 radiofrequency ablations each month, and an equal number of sclerotherapies. The vast majority of treatments are insurance based.

According to Calure, the biggest challenge was to learn how to be a businessperson.

> "In medical training, they teach you how to be a good doctor, but they don't teach you how to feed yourself and your family. If you were to go out and ask fifty physicians to define the word 'business,' probably only one or two would give the proper definition: an entity that provides goods or services in which income exceeds expense. In the beginning I was doing everything from IT and accounting to marketing."

Calure points to the importance of marketing for his business.

> "We connect directly with patients. We get our leads through Google, television and magazine advertising, but much of it is word of mouth. Satisfied patients refer three or four friends to us.
>
> In our area we compete with many of the large hospital systems such as University of Maryland, Johns Hopkins, MedStar, and LifeBridge. The physicians in these settings

are often working 9-5 and getting a paycheck. The institution dictates all aspects of their practice, from staffing to policies, and payment structures.

I am privileged and lucky that I can control the way our staff and patients are treated and how the space looks. We run a busy practice, but have an empty waiting room. I can remove the inefficiencies from the system. We have handpicked a great staff of some 40 individuals. We have had minimal turnover; however I am always sensitive to the effects of how one bad fish can spoil the water for the entire group. I have the power to change this."

Calure helps teach other physicians who want to learn the business of establishing a vein center.

"My advice for my colleagues is to sit down with a piece of paper and go back to what they thought life was supposed to be like when they entered medicine and then realize that when they have their own practice they control their reputation and their lives."

The Positioning Process

Positioning begins by identifying the following: Who are you to your patients? How are you representing yourself? You have the option of focusing the practice individually on you as a provider, or on your business/center in which you practice with others. If you intend to build the practice identity around yourself, you will want to determine just how much personal information to share with your patients. How comfortable are you disclosing your story of change, warts and all? For some physicians, this information is front and center, and is a factor that resonates with their patients who may be going through similar issues. This level of openness lets patients know you will be sensitive to their needs. Other physicians draw boundaries between their personal and professional lives.

Increasingly, we are seeing physicians adopting two online 'brands:' a personal brand that focuses on their books, newsletters, and speaking engagement; and a second that relates to their practice and the healthcare team with whom they are associated. For example Mark Hyman,

MD, a leading functional medicine authority aligns www.drhyman.com with his personal promotion; the Ultra Wellness Center is the brand for his team approach to functional medicine. Mimi's site www.mimiguarnerimd.com is focused on her books, charitable foundation and role within AIHM; her Pacific Pearl site (www.pacificpearllajolla.com) offers patients multiple opportunities to connect with the center's integrative healers. Articles, publications, and personal philosophy about Scott Shannon, MD, a holistically-oriented psychiatrist in Colorado, and past president of ABIHM, can be found at his personal site www.wholenessmd.com; the expansive integrative team's services are explained at www.wholeness.com. The philosophy of wholeness is the common theme among the practitioners.

Many physicians get creative with their branding and taglines to emphasize their unique emphasis. Romila Mushtaq, MD, promotes, "Medicine meets mindfulness," Daniel Friedland, MD, offers "SuperSmart Health." Ron Hoffman, MD, an early pioneer in holistic and functional approaches to health, brands his work as "Intelligent Medicine." Creative taglines and program names are becoming more common as many of the descriptive urls are already taken in fee-for-service disciplines.

Support for Practice Promotion

From the marketing perspective, the field of IM is a bit late to the fee-for-service game. Dentists and aesthetic physicians have been honing their techniques for decades and have the art of patient recruitment, service, and retention and referral down to a science. Increasingly, consultants are coming into the integrative and functional medicine markets to help with practice promotion skills. These skills are discussed in greater detail in the next chapter.

In the same way that physicians determine which preceptorship opportunity might be best for them, so too, must they determine which practice promotion consultant might be the best fit. Each consultant brings a unique perspective to help your practice; their point of view is based upon their beliefs, experience, and orientation in the field. This orientation can vary, on the one hand, from a very patient-centric approach, to one that is physician centric and designed to build the physician's media presence.

Glenn Sabin, Founder of FON Therapeutics (www.fontherapeutics.

com) developed his practice marketing skills after a 25-year career running a media, marketing and business development company. He sold his company in 2009 to launch FON, and began applying these skills to the field of integrative medicine, which follows his narrative with and passion for integrative oncology. Sabin was diagnosed with chronic lymphocytic leukemia, still considered an "incurable" cancer, and was able to achieve multiple remarkable clinical outcomes, including a complete pathological remission (he cleared his marrow) without conventional therapies.

Sabin started FON Therapeutics—standing for Force of Nature—as both a consulting firm and a comprehensive online business resource for physicians interested in keeping up with the latest developments in IM.

Sabin works with a wide range of integrative health businesses in the US and overseas, from small clinics to large hospital based systems. He understands the profound power of self-efficacy and 'whole person' integrative care because he has lived it. Drawing upon his own personal transformation has made him sensitive to the pain of his clients. He describes his consulting philosophy:

> "I use a thoughtful step-back approach. It begins by looking at what's happening with the business and what's happening in the life of the proprietor. Is there a good fit between how the physician is leading his or her life and how this matches up with their mission, goals and vision for the organization? Many practitioners of IM are not walking the talk. They can lose sight of what they need to do as individuals and physicians in order to succeed. Only after assessing the practitioner in the context of her enterprise can strategy be set and implemented."

Sabin works with clients on a project, time and/or retainer basis. The majority of his clients are independent physicians whose businesses are under $5 million in revenue. His book, *N-of-1*, co-authored with oncologist Dawn Lemanne, MD, MPH, will be published Spring 2015.

Go Big or Go Home

JJ Virgin's practice-promotion emphasis is much more outer directed (www.jjvirgin.com). It is oriented toward helping physicians succeed by

CHAPTER TEN

making better use of multiple media. Her approach is consumer-centric. "I am tired of my physicians using terms like 'optimal wellness' or 'life balance' or 'wellness' to describe their practices. Consumers want to lose weight fast and look younger," she says.

Virgin has a decade of experience helping physician practices grow, especially beyond the walls of their practices. Her current methodology rejects incremental improvement and instead focuses on ways to help physicians' businesses expand by 10X as quickly as possible. For physicians who want to take this quantum leap, she helps them hone their messages, establish partnerships, build networks, define best practices and utilize coaches.

Virgin shares her method in her bi-annual mindshare summit conferences (www.mindsharesummit.com) that attract 100-150 health care professionals. She invites leading experts such as Brendon Burchard on messaging, Dan Sullivan on strategic coaching, Michael Fishman on branding, and Mike Koenigs on technology to automate marketing.

Much of Virgin's credibility rests on her personal success. She is now a major consumer presence—a twice NY Times bestselling author with *The Virgin Diet: Drop 7 Foods, Lose 7 Pounds, Just 7 Days* and its companion *The Virgin Diet Cookbook.* (Harlequin and Grand Central Publishing). She has a top rated podcast, appears regularly in the media, speaks internationally and has a regular column on the Huffington Post.

If you determine that you could use the services of a practice promotion consultant, consider taking these steps:

1. Identify several potential vendors.
2. Send out a RFP (request for proposal). In the proposal see if you can clarify your objectives, the deliverables you are seeking and possible metrics for success. If you have difficulty determining these, have the vendors cover them in the scope of work.
3. Encourage the vendors to come into your office and do presentations. This can be a great way for you to learn about their marketing approach, as well as their personal promotional abilities.
4. In addition to asking for referrals, ask about clients who have not been successful and why. Identify the types of clients the vendor has had difficulty working with. Do you present any of these same elements?

5. Recognize that there is most likely a great deal of cushion built into the cost estimate for the vendor's services. So don't hesitate to push back and negotiate a better rate.

The Physician as Rock Star

One of our colleagues recently returned from a several day personal transformation retreat conducted by Deepak Chopra, MD, a healer whose work we deeply respect. The retreat was geared toward healthcare professionals and there were many physicians in attendance. When we queried our colleague as to how the physicians fared during the weekend, her impression was that a number of them were less interested in healing themselves, and more interested in figuring out how they could have Chopra's level of success, fame and fortune.

We have yet to perfect the treatment whereby we extract the enlarged physician ego, remove the metastases of comparison, and bring down the harmful biomarkers of competitiveness and jealously.

In interviews I (Mark) have conducted with some baby boomer and Gen-X physicians, there is a palpable resentment directed towards younger physicians who more naturally capitalized on social media and have built a bigger network of followers. These feelings are both unhealthy and misplaced.

In the long run you will do best if you focus on the work of healing patients for the right reasons. There are many outlets for media appearances and self-promotion, and many physicians dream of doing TED talks, appearing with Oprah, and becoming the next Dr. Sanjay Gupta. These are all worthy goals if you retain both your humility and professional ethics in the process of chasing fame. Just as in decades past, when some physicians "sold out" to pharmaceutical companies and pitched the company's products without qualification, today a small group of physicians are falling under the exaggerated influence of nutraceutical, cosmeceutical, and medical device companies. All of these products have a place in the therapeutic armamentarium; however they should take a back seat to honestly doing that which is best for your patient.

CHAPTER TEN

The Seven Tools of Practice Promotion

Regardless of the clinical direction in which you choose to move, there are some common areas in which you will want to excel. Below, we have provided some helpful hints to improve in some of the more important areas.

1. The Live Presentation

There is no shortage of venues at which physicians can deliver their message in the flesh; professionally at meetings in which you present research, teach techniques, or impart clinical wisdom; or directly to the consumer in groups both small and large. We will not discuss the professional seven-minute research or literature review PowerPoint presentation replete with its graphs, charts, and references that fly past the viewer often at speeds beyond comprehension; instead we will focus on the tools of engaging consumers and colleagues (who are consumers as well). Here are some tips:

- **Resist the temptation to put two hours of slides into a 30-minute talk**. Less is more. Better yet, reduce your talk to a handful of slides that are designed to either keep you on track, or illustrate (usually with a visual) one of your key points. Speak more directly to the audience.

- **Know thy audience.** Why are they attending? What do they expect of you? If you are uncertain, ask. Depending upon the nature and formality of your presentation, it is always helpful to be able to relate personally to one or more participants and acknowledge them in the course of your talk.

- **Use humor.** You can borrow liberally from pictures and jokes on the Internet to lighten the tone in the room. (Be aware of copyright issues.) Clever remarks and visuals also allow you to drive home your points. For example, a recent Internet posting pointed to the bipolar nature of health advice in women's magazines: half of each issue is devoted to loving and accepting yourself just the way you are, the other half is devoted to losing 20 pounds in 3 weeks! This type of joke helps women understand ambivalence in the change process.

- **Tell stories**. People remember stories. As a healthcare practitioner, you have many of them. Make certain to not violate patient confidentiality. Many physicians will obtain permission from their patients to use the patient's story with identifying demographics removed from it. Other physicians will tell composite-type stories that combine aspects of several cases into one.

- **Don't should on your audience**. Resist the temptation to preach and prescribe by saying, "You must…you have to …you should." Instead, focus on creating participant engagement in your talks. Throw reflective questions or direct queries out to the audience to gain their attention.
- **Watch your body language.** Avoid getting trapped behind a podium. Feel free to move around. Always look calm and relaxed and above all happy. Relax the shoulders. Breathe early, deeply and often.
- **Think of your presentation as a symphony:** with an introduction and a series of movements culminating in a finale. Use the power, pitch and tempo of your voice to captivate the audience. Vary your tempo. Vary your volume periodically. Pause for emphasis. Feel comfortable in the moment of silence when your message hits home for the attendee.
- **Add interactivity:** in the form of short exercises; people remember best that which they do.

When starting out, take advantage of every opportunity to speak to groups. Hold open houses at your practice; speak to religious and civic groups. Hone your message. After each presentation, honestly critique how you did. Remember, you will be your harshest judge. If you have the opportunity to video your talk, use this for reference. What did you do well? In what areas could you improve? How well did you listen to, paraphrase, and answer participant's questions? Were there some awkward moments or stumbles? How might you overcome this the next time you present?

2. The Website Video(s)

Once you have identified what sets you apart from the competition it is a great idea to make your best statement on video and use this in your online promotion. Some helpful hints:

- Take some time to compose your message. Rehearse a basic script

CHAPTER TEN

with your staff, and close friends.
- Don't try to squeeze a video in between patients.
- Get some coaching. If you have voice issues, work with a speech coach.
- Have your video professionally shot.
- Forget about doing a video at one of the conventions.
- Keep in mind appearing open, trusting, friendly, caring and positive.
- Take the same care in the production that you would take in an operative procedure.
- A good video need not be costly. It must be well staged, well lit and well produced.

Once you have a solid online video describing your uniqueness, you can move on to producing educational pieces for distribution through multiple channels such as Youtube or Vimeo. Make certain to follow the same guidelines as noted above for live presentations. Local, cable and national television stations consider these videos your resume, and will turn to them to evaluate your potential as an on-camera expert.

3. The Book

Few industries have been hit as hard by change as traditional publishing. With the advent and ease of digital rendering, a vanity book is within the realm of every healthcare practitioner. Adoption by major publishers is still an option, but those of us who have worked with major publishers know that the days of the significant six-figure advance and paid book road tour are reserved for only the biggest selling authors.

The best way to land a major publisher is to obtain an agent and to obtain an agent, you will need to create a book proposal that sells you, your concept, your writing style and what you can and will do to promote the book. Today, publishers count on their authors to self-promote. In fact, they equate you to a large retail chain and provide similar discounts. After allowances for promotional copies, most authors will buy their books from the publisher at 30-50% off depending upon volume. These publishers will also contractually obligate the authors for future works.

On the other hand, you can always self-publish. If you choose to go this route, you should consider your book as an extended business card, one that sets forth your philosophy, tells your story, identifies your unique value proposition or the treatment/solution that you want to be know for. You can give the book away, or sell it in your practice or at talks and workshops where the attendees value obtaining your autograph and inscription. The book can deepen your connection with attendees. They get to take a little bit of you home with them.

Many healthcare providers don't have the skills and time to devote to book writing, yet these same providers are often quite eloquent giving talks. In this case, the easiest way to start a book is to transcribe one of your talks, and then hire someone to clean and organize the writing. This also allows you to overcome the writer's block that comes from staring at a blank screen.

You can find many freelancers online who can edit, design, and proof your manuscript. The cost of digital publishing has become quite reasonable, and you can start with quantities as low as 100 copies.

The difficulty of self-publishing is distribution. For this, you can turn to Amazon. Their CreateSpace group (www.createspace.com) can also help with the layout and publishing of the book.

Increasingly, authors are electing to e-publish either shorter pieces, or entire books. The later can be distributed in electronic version through sources such as Kindle or iTunes. For authors who do not envision themselves signing books at talks and workshops, solely publishing in an electronic version makes sense.

4. Radio/Audio

Just as publishing has changed, so too has radio; however, the parallel is much more akin to healthcare consolidation. Simply put, over the last decade, the big radio stations have gobbled up the smaller independents. This has changed the nature of the station's relationships with physicians who go on air.

Ron Hoffman, MD, is a holistic practitioner and author who started his practice in 1984 when holistic practitioners were few and far between and patients even scarcer. Hoffman related how in the early days of building his practice and national reputation, he would speak anywhere—on one occasion traveling from Manhattan to a suburban library in Queens to talk to eleven people. These early talks, however, allowed him to hone his craft and work on the power of the spoken word. Hoffman began his radio career in 1993, first with a short weekly show, then a longer weekly show, and finally for twenty years with a daily prime health program from 3-4 pm on WOR, New York City's top AM Radio show.

Today, radio access for healthcare practitioners is "pay to play." The cost to advertise varies greatly. A weekly one hour show can range from $1,000 a month in small markets to $6,000-$7,000 a month in larger ones. A focused radio show can promote one's practice or products. A weekly, one-hour program consists of roughly four, ten-minute segments. Usually these shows run on the weekends. They can either be pre-recorded or live, but to be successful each segment should have a call to action such as "visit my website," "make an appointment," or "download...." Some physicians are able to recruit sponsors to offset most, and sometimes the entire cost of the programming. Shows that offer viewer call-ins allow potential patients to develop comfort with your philosophy and treatment methods and can drive listeners to seek your services.

As for Hoffman, he has ported his content over to the audio medium over which he has the most control: the podcast. Hoffman records his topic, edits it as necessary, posts it on his website, iTunes and Stitcher (www.drhoffman.com) and links it to his social media accounts. Hoffman's following grows stronger each month.

5. Online & Social Media

Online promotion is always a moving target. It begins with a website that has been optimized for search engine optimization (SEO), that is easy to navigate, ideally has crisp video, and is updated with regular frequency. If you add valuable, free content in the form of blogs, podcasts, and other educational outreach opportunities, you provide a reason for patients to continually return to your site. While you will most likely turn to a local design firm for your site, bear in mind that many millennials have grown up quite familiar with online digital content and management. An office staff member with rudimentary online skills, for example, can easily update a site that is built on WordPress.

While your website is your base, outreach is increasingly involving social media such as Facebook, Linkedin, Twitter, Pinterest, Tumblr, etc.

As noted above, you will need to decide whether your accounts are more personally or more organizationally focused.

There is variability across the different specialties regarding the relevance of social media in attracting patients. Social media can be particularly valuable to distinguish your practice is a crowded field such as aesthetics in which practitioners tend to fight the commoditization battle and there is confusion over quality and price.

Integrative Medicine, at this stage in its development, appears to be a field that is less affected by commoditization. While there may be competition among medical, chiropractic, and naturopathic physicians, or among nurse healers, acupuncturists, and massage therapists, for the most part, patients hone in on wanting the services of a particular healer.

For the IM practitioner, social media has its greatest value on the backend as it allows patients to stay in touch with you and for you to keep your image, knowledge, and philosophy top of their minds.

6. Advertising & Outreach

Advertising and outreach are ways in which you let the larger community know of your presence. Ideally, these activities are designed to get the consumer to go to your website or call the practice to schedule an appointment. The traditional ways to build your reputation still have a valid place in an advertising strategy. These include magazine ads in the type of publications that resonate with your potential customers, sponsorship of community events tied to charities, and radio and television advertising; however more of the advertising dollar is moving online.

Online pay-for-click advertising may be an appropriate strategy to acquaint patients with your services. This can be done through Google AdWords in which patients who search for treatments in your location are presented with your information. Yelp offers a suite of services including targeted ads on Yelp Search. They will also remove competitor adds from your Yelp business page. Yelp has a variety of programs designed to enhance your profile through slide shows, videos and call to action buttons. Advertising costs range from $300-$2,200 per month.[349] Of growing importance is the area of online reputation management. This

CHAPTER TEN

marketing subspecialty got is healthcare start when physicians needed to counter negative reviews that appeared in search engine results, social media, or on rating sites. What began as a reactive strategy has turned into a proactive approach for generating higher customer reviews and more of them. There are hundreds of consulting groups that offer services to assist physicians with reputation management. However, there is also much you can do by yourself.

- **Be aware of what is out there on you.** Periodically conduct web searches on yourself. Scour the appropriate physician rating sites such as HealthGrades, Vitals, Rate MDs, Angie's List, Wellness.com, RealSelf, Google, and Yelp. Pay attention to the online discussions.

- **Recognize that you can neither acknowledge, nor respond directly to the patient.** This is a violation of HIPAA. However, if you can identify the patient you may be able to speak directly to them in person or on the phone where you can inquire as to the source of their dissatisfaction and apologize for causing any unintentional distress.

- **Determine if the patient has a legitimate reason for her complaint.** If the complaint is valid, you need to investigate it further. Determine whether the problem was with a staff member, the procedure or waiting time, or the cost, and whether there is a way to prevent this type of problem in the future. If you find that one individual in your practice is the source of patient dissatisfaction, you will need to have the appropriate performance discussion and take corrective action.

- **Get your message out there.** While you have less control of reviews written about you, there is much about your image that you can control. Make certain to create a comprehensive public LinkedIn profile noting your education, background and your philosophy of care. Take advantage of blogging once a week to let patients know the latest updates in your field, or in your practice.

- **Ask patients if you can post their 'thank you' notes.** Physicians often get kind letters from patients. These can be posted on your blog, on the rating sites, or attached to your LinkedIn profile. As part of a more comprehensive referral marketing strategy, you can also ask satisfied patients to post their positive reviews on the rating sites.

7. The Store

We have included this commercial component of your practice in the section on promotion, because product sales are a form of outreach; patients are taking your advice and bringing your recommendations into their home. Heated debates have recently taken place in the online physician services about the ethics of in-office selling of products. We agree with the naysayers to the extent that the profit motive is placed ahead of patient care. A balanced approach to this issue begins with a set of patient-focused questions.

- Based upon your research and experience, do you believe (and ideally have evidence) you are providing a helpful and potentially healing adjunct in the care of the patient?
- Will this nutraceutical product, book, CD, home device, etc. help the patient's condition or promote their health?
- Are you eliminating confusion by directing them to what you believe is a valuable resource?
- Are you making it more convenient for them to obtain the product in your office and at a time when your recommendations are fresh in their minds?
- Is the product—for any variety of reasons—superior to what they might obtain elsewhere?

Even with affirmative answers to these questions, there are still some roadblocks that must be navigated. Physicians in hospital owned practices may be prohibited from the selling of certain products. The road to getting approval for the product you value may be long and tortuous. Your practice may not be set up to inventory, sell, and account for products.

Reminiscent of the old pharmaceutical detailing days, a number of the quality physician-only nutraceutical suppliers will provide samples and discount codes for physicians to pass along to their patients. This removes the physician from the transaction process.

As to the issue of profit, this is simple to resolve. You are always at liberty to offer the products to patients without any markup or donate profits on product sales to charity. You should also be aware of potential backlash from patients who are able to find the identical product on the Internet at deeply discounted prices.

CHAPTER TEN

The Simple Axiom to Practice Happiness

You want to attract the type of patients you like to treat: those with whom you have good rapport, those with the kinds of problems you believe you can solve. You can elect to have an eclectic practice in which you treat all types of lifestyle and nutritionally related illnesses, or your practice can be laser-like in focus, as in the case of vein therapy.

As your interests deepen, and you gain greater skills in different disciplines you may elect to create 'silos' of treatment with the recognition that each can cross refer within the practice. The practice of James Mirabile, MD, an OB/Gyn in Kansas City, MO, illustrates this point. He dipped, dove and then delegated his way to practice success.

Burned out with obstetrics after 7,500 deliveries, Mirabile gave up OB to focus on his Gyn practice. Recognizing the interest and demand from his patients for cosmetic services, he was an early adopter of laser technology for skin rejuvenation and hair removal, and served as a KOL and trainer for several of the device companies. Today he prominently features aesthetics in the medspa component of his practice; however, treatments, including injectables, are done by his trained nurses. Mirabile attributes much of the financial success of his aesthetic practice to the use of the HydrafacialMD® (www.hydrafacial.com). This unique aesthetic device utilizes hydradermabrasion to exfoliate, cleanse and hydrate the skin, while also delivering antioxidants into the dermis. Mirabile notes that patients leave the treatment with the "wow factor" that encourages them to return for a package of visits. The added plus is that the modestly priced machine paid for itself in the first three months of use.

Having gradually gained 50 pounds over his years in practice, Mirabile came upon the physician-directed Medi-Weightloss program (www.medi-weightlossclinics.com). He lost the weight, started to feel great again, and began incorporating the program into his practice. Today, a skilled Physician Assistant runs the program out of his office.

Because so much of Gyn relates to hormonal dysfunction, Mirabile spent time learning about bioidentical hormone replacement and now uses SottoPelle pellet treatment (www.sottopelletherapy.com) with appropriate patients. Mirabile is very clear about his practice positioning

> "My love is my Gyn practice, but from a financial standpoint, I can't just do Gyn. As reimbursement continues to worsen, these other services balance out my revenue. I do very little

outside marketing, almost all my marketing is within the practice. A woman who has trusted me to deliver her children trusts me to manage her hormones, have her skin cared for by my office staff, or her weight attended to by my PA. This is good medicine, and I'm not doing anything crazy in my practice. We emphasize total health: looking good, feeling good, and preventing illness. I worked too hard to give up what I have and work for someone else. Rather than complain about reimbursement I decided to do something about it."

Focusing too narrowly on external marketing techniques can create the impression that marketing is an impersonal art. This is far from the truth. The best marketing is the quality of the one-on-one interaction you have with your patients. This focus on quality relationships actually sets you free to turn away patients. Ron Hoffman, MD, notes, " I don't accept everyone into my practice. I don't accept patients who are going to be difficult to work with, or who have unrealistic expectations, or who are not going to go along with my recommendations. Then there are some patients that I just don't know how to treat. By following these guidelines, I have more practice satisfaction, less aggravation and happier patients."

In the end, the process of marketing your practice boils down to some basics:

1. Decide on your treatment focus.
2. Gain the skills you need to best serve your patients.
3. Determine who you are in the local marketplace.
4. Create your brand.
5. Generate a plan to implement some or all of the seven practice promotion techniques.

Lead Well

During my ten-year sojourn into the world of aesthetics, I (Mark) probably visited more than 100 practices, and within minutes of walking in the door I could tell whether the practice was successful. I made this determination not by the size of the office, or the beauty of the facility, rather by whether the people behind the desk, the ones in the hall, and those scurrying between treatment rooms seemed happy, calm, and focused. Up close did they radiate warmth and caring? These emotions are difficult to fake. Whenever I came across a practice of contented staff, I knew that the doc in charge was well liked by co-workers.

No matter how and where you received your training, there is one thing we can say with great certainty. You didn't learn enough about practice leadership. The reality is, even if you or your staff has obtained MBAs and PhDs in organizational behavior, customer service, marketing or healthcare management, the reality is, it's not enough. Given the complexity of people, the stresses of life and work, and the market dynamics today, building and managing a team requires life-long devotion to continued analysis and modification of your leadership style.

Why? Because you don't do your practice alone, you are dependent upon the attitudes and behaviors of everyone in your office. Every day, the front office staff, your nurses, medical assistants, nurse practitioners, physician assistants, associates, or your business manager can either make or break your practice.

In our ABIHM/AHMA survey we asked the physicians to rate the relative strength of the business-related stressors in their practice. The results are shown below.

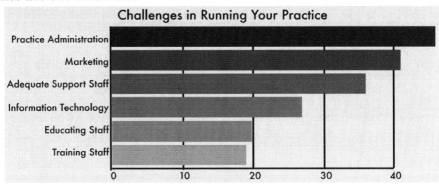

Figure 18: ABIHM/AHMA 2014 Practice Satisfaction Survey

Nature & Nurture Goes Against the Physician

By nature, and by training, most physicians tend to be very directive in their leadership style. By directive, we mean telling people what, when and how to do something. Physicians want their orders followed "Stat." In the operating room and emergency department, this type of behavior saves lives when time is on the line and decisions must be made quickly.

It is not uncommon for physicians to take their authoritative style too far. Nick Jacobs is a Fellow in the American College of Healthcare Executives and international director for SunStone Management Resources. An innovator in healthcare, in 1977, he was one of the earliest proponents for patient centered care (PCC) when he served as president of the Windber (PA) Medical Center. To his chagrin, the major barrier he faced instituting PCC was the behavior of a handful of physician bullies. He recounts how he went about creating a healthier culture.

"Our goal was to create a complete change in the environment. We identified the physicians whom the staff said were the worst bullies. They would scream at patients and staff, and throw objects in the OR. We let these physicians know this behavior would not be tolerated. When we took the bullying behavior away from them, they become desperate. They were like General Patton; they wanted me either dead or fired. Similar to the treatment of cancer, we had to systematically remove the bullying physicians from the organization. Ironically, the worst of the bullying docs came from the Ivy League medical institutions. We let quite a few of them go.

Well-crafted HR policies can help in dealing with bullying from healthcare practitioners, administration or staff. Physicians were brought before the Medical Executive Committee and offered two choices: 1. Resign from the staff without retribution, 2. Undergo anger management training and if they reoffended, they were removed from the staff and reported to the national physician data bank. For employees, with the first offense, the individual is counseled; for the second, it is 2-3 days off without pay, for the third, it can result in termination. Counseling and anger management, Disney and Ritz Carlton training can help prevent further incidents.

The result was HCAHPS scores that reinforce the importance of PCC. HCAHPS is a nationally standardized collective methodology to measure patients' perspectives on hospital care. It involves ratings on 21 patient perspectives of care including communication with physicians."

Overt bullying by physicians is less common today than in years past.

CHAPTER TEN

While it has no place in healthcare, elements of the directive style are important in practice. It is still your role to provide guidance and have your objectives fulfilled. This is particularly important when employees are just learning tasks and they need to be told exactly what to do and how to do it. But a directive approach can't be your only style; you must be flexible in dealing with others and able to adapt to the needs of your people. The behavior of your entire staff is a reflection of your leadership and the extent to which staff feel knowledgeable, understood, valued, included, and appreciated. In, short, the extent to which they feel part of a great team dedicated to providing great service.

What is Leadership?

There are many definitions of the word leadership. We'll work with the one that is most practical and relevant for your practice.

Leadership is a process of using your influence to obtain desired results.

If, for example, you want to influence your phone receptionist to answer the phone with a well-delivered script, you are attempting leadership behavior. If you want your physician's assistant to follow your protocol for treatment, you are attempting leadership behavior. In order to influence others, a leader must exert power, of which there are four basic types:

1. **Positional power:** Your positional power varies depending upon whether you are in a solo or group practice, independent or owned by a larger entity. In most cases the physician and/or the practice manager are the 'bosses' because they have the ability to hire, fire, reward and discipline. It's power inherent in the position. People do what you tell them because you provide their paycheck.

2. **Personal power:** Unlike positional power, this energy source comes from your personality and how you treat people. It is related to whether people care for you because you care for them. If you have personal power, people will go the 'extra mile' for you willingly. Great physician-leaders are also able to transfer the power of their presence in listening to and empathizing with their patients—over to staff members and others. This enables people to feel calm and comfortable when they are around you.

3. **Professional power:** This is related to specific knowledge and

task competency. For example, the 20 year old who fixes your computer has professional power because he knows more about computers than you do. Presenters at major conferences exhibit this type of power based upon their knowledge, research and teaching/presenting ability. Physicians acquire greater professional power through participation in societies, speaking at conferences, writing academic papers, or serving as KOLs for companies.

4. **Peer power:** This is power that is attributed naturally to an individual in a group setting. S/he is the person who seems to be the informal group leader to whom others turn for advice, guidance and direction—not because of rank or position—but because their opinions and behaviors shape those of others in the practice.

All of these powers come into play in your practice, but one of them stands out above the others. The best measure of your effectiveness as a leader is what happens when you are not around to supervise. When you are not directly supervising their work, is the phone being answered the way you want? Is your PA doing treatments according to your protocol? For these things to occur, notably in your absence, you must have a substantial degree of personal power. This is the people side of leadership, and understanding this power is the key to the issue of motivating others.

Unlocking Motivation

The first principle of motivation is "different strokes for different folks." In other words, people are motivated by different things. Some people value public praise, others written thanks, certificates, parties, or time spent with you. And, yes, people value money in the form of salary increases, bonuses and other incentives. The issue is, depending upon your financial situation and position, you may or may not be able to keep paying people more. You also don't want money to be the only motivator for doing a job well. On the other hand, you do want to incentivize people whose performance is exemplary, particularly if the practice is thriving. One of the motivational tools that is always at your disposal is to 'catch people doing something right.'

This phrase was popularized by Ken Blanchard, PhD, co-author of *The One Minute Manager* (HarperCollins). This classic text provides a very simple, easy to implement system of providing feedback for employees.

CHAPTER TEN

A universal truth is that most people on their jobs either get little or no feedback, or if they do, chances are it is negative. Their leader—the physician, or the office manager—shines the light on them only when they've 'screwed up.' The best feedback, of course, is positive, hence the concept of catching people doing something right. But there are some other rules to providing feedback. Specifically, feedback should be:

- **Immediate:** As close to the event as possible so that it is fresh in peoples' minds.
- **Task specific:** Your goal is to grow the competency of your staff and colleagues. The best way to do this is to give them specific information and guidance on how they are doing their tasks and what they can do to improve, in other words coach them.
- **For them:** Many physician leaders make the mistake of giving out praise when they are in a good mood, and forget to do so when the situation calls for it. Feedback is for the receiver, not the giver.
- **More positive than negative:** Ideally, you should find many more opportunities to praise behavior than to criticize it.
- **Focused on the event, not the person:** Avoid the temptation to make wholesale judgments of your people, i.e., "Jenny *always*," or "Sally *never*." This type of judgment does not help you improve performance; instead, focus on the tasks at hand.

Get in the habit of managing by walking around. As you do so, look for opportunities to catch people doing things well and then let them know, right then and there, how they are doing. Once you've praised them, then you can provide them with task specific feedback to help them get even better at their job.

Flexibility in Communication Style

Good physician leaders know they must tailor recognition and rewards to the unique needs of the recipient. They also know that they must deliver messages that the recipient deems meaningful and valid. One way to do this, with both staff and patients, is to orient the message to the recipient's personality type. Imagine that the only language the other person spoke was Russian. To build rapport with that person, it would be very helpful if you could learn a few words or phrases in that language. Flexibility of communication style is a key leadership attribute.

The concept of personality types and innate preferences was advanced by the pioneering Swiss psychologist Carl Jung, PhD, in the early twentieth century. Jung described a number of types—groups of individuals who shared a natural tendency to perceive the world and interpret information in a common manner. Jung's work forms the basis for a number of popular style-based assessments, the most well-known being the Myers-Briggs Type Inventory. The PowerSource Profile™ (PSP), developed by ChangeWell Inc. (www.changewell.com), is another Jungian-based assessment, but one that can be applied to worksite groups in a time-efficient manner. It also has the advantage of being specifically designed to help staff members deal with stress and become more resilient.

The PSP identifies people who may be high in four different types of energies.

- **Creative energy.** A preference for imagination and intuition, a forward sense of time, and a tendency to become stressed because of fragmentation, lack of attention to detail, and difficulty with follow-through. Creative individuals value variation. They are often drawn to more varied practices such as Integrative Medicine, wellness, and aesthetics because of the many types of activities in which they can participate, and the possibility of helping to transform others. These are the people who get easily bored by routine. Most are highly visual and imaginative.

- **Grounding energy.** A preference to use the senses, be practical and realistic, favor tried-and-true procedures and rules, and be stressed by changes to the predictable and orderly. Unlike more creative people, these individuals thrive on routine. They enjoy keeping things neat and organized and will naturally follow-through on details. They have a good sense for how long it takes to complete an activity .

- **Logic energy.** A preference for cause and effect, objective analysis, model building, and quantification; stressed by having to make decisions without enough data, and by situations (and people) with strong feelings. This energy type tends to be overrepresented by physicians, scientists, Wall Street analysts, bankers, business consultants, etc.

- **Relationship energy.** A preference to interpret information based upon how it will make others feel, keen attention to their own

CHAPTER TEN

emotions; stressors include having to say "no," getting burned out, and taking criticism personally. The greatest conflict comes into play with high–logic types who disregard their feelings and don't listen well. Many nurses, of both genders, have this as their dominant energy. They are drawn to the caring/helping aspects of medicine.

In order to tailor your communication to different types of energy, you need to abandon a one size fits all mentality and focus your communication on the recipient. The best way to do this is to have each of your staff take the PSP online and to share the results. The PSP can be sampled from Changewell Inc. through an email request referencing *Total Engagement.* (info@changewell.com).

Strengthening the Team

In the absence of the PSP, ask yourself, "Am I dealing with a high-creative, high-grounding, high-logic, or high-relationship individual?" It is true that all staff members share some common needs. They all have a need to know what is going on. They need to have their feelings acknowledged and validated. They need to understand how and where they fit into the practice. And they need to see themselves as a key contributor. But the different energy types differ in the degree to which they require these things. Specifically:

- **Creative people:** They are future- and possibility-oriented people who actually thrive on multi-tasking. You should engage their brainstorming abilities, encouraging and praising them for coming up with new ideas for the practice. Keep them challenged. If they are experiencing a lot of personal or organizational stress, watch out for fragmentation and scattering. If you notice these traits emerging, try to help them focus by identifying where best to apply their efforts.

- **Grounding people:** Keep your communication clear, simple, focused and time-based. Resist the temptation to overwhelm grounded people with too much detail, too many things at once, or frequent changes. These people can be among the most resistant to adapt to changes in the practice, often preferring "the way it was." Praise them often for their dedication, follow-through, attention to detail and throughput. Keep things neat and tidy.

- **Logic people:** Let high-logic individuals know that you value their analytical and decision-making skills. Praise them for their planning abilities. Give them activities in which they naturally excel such as gathering data, establishing flow charts and processes.
- **Relationship people:** Always attend to them with good eye contact and encouraging body language. Let them know that you have heard what they have said and that you value them for their concern and caring. Take enough time to hear them out fully. Try to use more *relationship* words such as *feel, believe, hope, trust, value,* or *share*. Be very careful of criticism. These people take things personally and can spend enormous amounts of energy, worry and sleepless nights obsessing over their interpretation of what you might have meant. Keep your eyes open for signs of burnout by frequently checking in with them.

While categorizing people according to their natural preferences can help you with your communication, you must remember, that *when it comes to task competencies, each individual is a combination of their natural tendencies and their acquired skills.* For example, a person who is highly relationship oriented by nature may well have acquired the skills of logic, analysis, and detail through education, training and work experience. Also, as you'll see from the PSP, individuals can be high in two areas at once, so this makes things a little more complicated. For example, a high creative person could also be strong in either logic or relationship energy (but not grounding). Conversely, a grounded person can also be strong in either of these energies (but not in creative energy). For the most part, you will be able to detect their dominant energy in their behaviors.

Your goal is to understand your staff, what makes them tick, and how to improve your leadership style to bring out the best in them. Understanding individual motivations, clarity of communication, and personality style all help you do just that. One additional overlay that you should consider is generational. You can't assume that your experience, values and beliefs are shared by older or younger generations with whom you work. If you are trying to understand the commonly held drivers of the different generations, we recommend an excellent resource, *Bridging the Generation Gap* (Career Press) by Linda Gravett, PhD, and Robin Throckmorton.

CHAPTER TEN

The Leadership Challenge

Clearly, there is no one prescription to follow to be a great leader. People are complex, and what motivates one person may not motivate another. Still, there are some common threads to knitting a strong team. You must focus more on praise than blame. It helps to adjust your style to better suit the personality and temperament of the recipient when you deliver a message. It's a good idea to frequently check for understanding, particularly when the pace is hectic. Finally, if you are able, creating financial incentives tied to specific measurables can make for happy, committed employees.

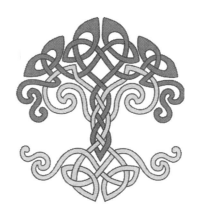

If somebody offers you an amazing opportunity but you are not sure you can do it, say yes – then learn how to do it later!

— **Richard Branson**

11
Life Beyond Clinical Practice

In 1975 Paul Simon had a number one hit entitled, "50 Ways to Leave Your Lover," whose lyrics included the advice to "Get out the back, Jack." There are an equal number of ways to get out the back door and either leave the clinical practice of medicine, or place an inordinate focus on non-clinical areas.

There are many role model physicians who have successfully made non-clinical change. While one set of stories revolves around older physicians who, after some years of practice, leverage their skills and interests into alternative areas, many medical students today are entering training with no intention of ever practicing clinical medicine. They see the value of gaining a medical education, but their interests are drawn to how to use this background to capitalize on health care trends; to settle down with an investment banking, private equity or venture capital firm; or to become the next healthcare entrepreneur of the year.

Ajay Major, a third-year year medical student and the co-founder of *in-Training*, the online magazine for medical students at www.in-training.org, describes one of the drivers of an entire cadre of emerging physicians as "medicine-plus." Major notes that this may be "medicine plus journalism, plus advocacy, plus entrepreneurship, plus technology, or anything else related to medicine." He continues:

> "With changing admissions pressures in modern medical education, students enter medical school from increasingly diverse backgrounds and with increasingly diverse interests. Medical students want to incorporate those interests into their education and into their future careers. These students see the ills of society, and they want to use their skills to help, skills that not too long ago may not have been considered integral to medicine: business, community building, writing."

CHAPTER ELEVEN

Major's own path is heavily grounded in his journalism skills, honed as the editor-in-chief of his undergraduate school newspaper. Today, his magazine *in-Training* has 25 medical student editors. The online publication has featured over 450 articles from 200 students at 84 institutions both domestically and internationally.

John Canady, MD, Medical Director at Johnson & Johnson, Global Surgery Group/Mentor WW, LLC, reinforces the importance of the "medicine" part of the medicine-plus equation. He makes the large industry case against coming out of medical school with a combined MD/MBA degree and foregoing further clinical experience. "I strongly encourage these young physicians to get several years of clinical practice under their belt. The big companies have rooms full of MBAs, but they hire people with clinical experience because of their medical insights into the marketplace. The level of respect afforded physicians is geometrically greater if they have clinical experience to back up their opinions," advises Canady, a former Professor of Plastic Surgery at the University of Iowa and past-president of the American Society of Plastic Surgeons.

SEAK a Career Outside Medicine

As a 44-year-old trial lawyer Steve Babitsky took the advice he now provides to many physicians: leverage your professional knowledge outside of its traditional field of practice. He started SEAK (www.seak.com), the largest resource for physicians to learn about non-clinical careers. SEAK has trained well over 25,000 expert witnesses, physicians, lawyers, nurses, and other professionals.

The company features an annual conference on non-clinical careers for physicians that is now in its eleventh year and attracts an audience of 300-400 healthcare professionals. In addition to listening to the lecturers, attendees have the opportunity to work on site with two dozen mentors, coaches, counselors, recruiters and employers.

Throughout the year SEAK conducts "how to" seminars nationwide, primarily related to six major non-clinical areas for physicians including:

- Medical Expert Witnessing
- Consulting for Physicians
- Writing

- File Review Consulting
- Inventing
- Independent Medical Examinations

A reaction common to attendees at SEAK functions, said Babitsky, is "the realization that the physician is not alone in his or her dissatisfaction." For many physicians SEAK provides a roadmap for getting started, and a methodology to counter what Babitsky notes is the largest impediment.

> "The big problem is inertia. Physicians think about making a change for years but they really don't take any action. We see medical professionals who are not ready to change jobs, but they can find what they need at our events. We have also seen physicians who meet the right people and, in the case of our conference, actually get job offers on the spot."

Babitsky points out that healthcare is roughly 1/6 of the United States economy, and emphasizes that physicians can ply their skills in the other 5/6 in careers as varied as becoming an astronaut to writing the next great medical detective television series. Babitksy is bullish on physician's skills and why these skills are in demand by organizations outside of clinical medicine. He states:

> "Physicians are the best and brightest in our educational system. You can't teach someone to be smart, trustworthy, dedicated, and possessed of a strong work ethic. When the snowstorm hits, it is the physician who walks to work to heal the sick. Physicians are used to getting up early in the morning and working hard. Many run their own businesses and have transferrable skills and experience that serve them well. For example, surgeons are often called upon by medical device companies to provide feedback on how products should be designed, and how they perform in the real world."

Each of the six major non-clinical career paths requires a different blend of personality and skills. He explains:

> "For example, for the physician who wants to go into independent consulting or to become an expert witness, he or she will have to be a self starter and have the ability to drum up business. Some consulting jobs require a great deal of travel,

as well. For the physician who joins an organization such an insurance company, while they start at a lower salary, they only work 40 hours a week, nine to five, usually in a nice, clean office. Other benefits often include an attractive bonus, 6-8 weeks of paid vacation and very little stress."

While Canady's job at J&J requires a great deal of travel, which he can do because his children are grown, he values the diversity of his current position. Canady remarks:

"My routine as a surgeon was very predictable. Mondays I had clinic, Tuesdays I operated, Wednesdays I had clinic in the afternoon and surgery in the morning, and so on. While I could have stayed in academic medicine for another 15 years, I wanted to do Version 2.0 of me and mix it up. In my role with J&J, no two days are the same. I interact with teams on clinical studies, regulatory issues, new business, as well as quality and safety. I sit in on companies pitching us ideas, products, intellectual properties and merger and acquisitions. I have served as Mentor's Medical Safety Officer for the last two years. Many individuals come to us with a great idea that they believe will be a great product but fail to consider the many off-ramps on the road to commercial success such as ease of manufacturing, supply chain and distribution."

Canady's advice for physicians interested in breaking into life sciences includes the willingness and ability to be a team player. He also advocates taking time to get to know the companies you are interested in working for, beginning with the local sales rep and then seeking introduction to higher levels of decision makers. It is best to keep expectations low and remain open to starting at an entry-level position such as a medical advisor.

While Canady's move was one of total immersion into corporate culture, Babitsky notes that many physicians can stay where they are but supplement their income with expert witness work, independent medical exams or file review services. He cites the benefits of each, "Some physicians will do expert witness work because the extra income affords them the opportunity to stay in clinical practice. Physicians may be paid $500-$600 or more per hour, and there is no overhead. These fees dramatically increase if a case goes to trial and involves the physician's testimony. For example, we are increasingly seeing radiologists, whose work is being outsourced, adopt expert witness work.

Independent medical exams are usually done in fields such as neurology, psychiatry, occupational medicine and orthopedics. These exams are usually related to worker's compensation or accident cases. Physicians can make $1,500-$2,000 per case.

File review for disability is ideal for the physician who has extra time in his or her schedule. This work involves no direct patient contact, no confrontation, and no malpractice."

The practice of Jonathan Rutchik, MD, MPH, exemplifies how diverse consulting and training activities can be knit together to provide a solid income. Rutchik is board certified in both neurology and occupational and environmental medicine. He sees patients in his five San Francisco bay area locations where he performs electromyography, California workers compensation medical legal evaluations, and IMEs. Rutchik also provides consulting services for industrial, legal, government, and pharmaceutical clients. Rutchik works three days a week seeing 4-5 new patients, performing 3-7 EMGs, and doing follow up. The remainder of his time is spent teaching at UCSF, doing depositions, or writing papers and articles. Rutchik feels that this work provides him with the balance he needs to pursue athletics, have free time, and travel with the family, all of which allow him to stay emotionally consistent and appreciative. Rutchik values the diversity of his work, but notes that he is at the mercy of the State of California that has recently cut fees for its medical evaluations.

Babitsky finds that many young physicians are drawn to the world of venture capital and private equity where they can apply their newly acquired MBA skills. Physicians with significant clinical and marketplace experience also vie for these jobs. The pay is high, but so is the competition. Physicians who want to move into the financial world may need to acquire or brush up some of their non-clinical skills such as communication, negotiation, writing and presenting skills. As Babitsky, notes, "It doesn't really matter how much you know if you can't communicate it. If you are presenting in front of a company's board of directors, you had better be able to rock n' roll."

Stephen Bochner, MD, is a Senior Client Partner with Korn/Ferry International. He is one of an approximate dozen executive recruiters

CHAPTER ELEVEN

nationwide who have medical degrees. Bochner helps major life science, device, private equity, and venture capital firms find physician talent. Trained as an OB/Gyn, Bochner was on clinical faculty at Stanford. He had built one of the largest practices in his Northern California area, but could not see doing OB/Gyn for the rest of his life. "At the same time, I saw many physicians doing interesting start up things in Silicon Valley," he said. This sparked Bochner to obtain an MBA from Stanford. Using his business knowledge, Bochner worked in consulting and venture capital, before moving into the executive search business.

Bochner discusses the skills he looks for in placing a job candidate:

"It depends on what the company is looking for. Many of the companies want a foundation of medical science background. For a device company, it is a major plus if the surgeon knows how to use their products and can evaluate current and new devices both from the eyes of the customer and from a regulatory perspective. Companies also look for a candidate with financial acumen and some management experience. These can be taught, but it is better if they are already in place. A lot of physicians are not sophisticated in their EQ (emotional intelligence) abilities. We evaluate them to see if they have developed an aptitude to cultivate relationship in their many forms."

Both Babitsky and Bochner emphasize that it takes time and planning, often over a 6 month to 2 year span to make a transition. Bochner also warns against considering business as a panacea to one's problems:

"Physicians know that their life is horrible now, and think that moving into business will solve all their problems. They can easily underestimate how hard it is to make money, to put up with all the travel, to deal with all the day-to-day realities. To get a job in the competitive labor market you have to be passionate about the field you want to enter. The upside is that the bureaucracy is less, there is no malpractice, and no one is telling you how much to charge for your time."

In searching for a non-clinical medical career, Babitsky finds that many physicians begin by asking themselves the wrong questions. "They start," he said, "by asking themselves how they are going to replace the money they are now making. The better question is, 'How much money am I losing as a clinical doctor?' Physicians often work 80 hours a week and twice as hard as most professionals. If they were out in the open market of business, and they found the right niche and position, how much could they command?"

Communicating and Consulting for Health

Today, thousands of physicians include in their Linkedin description or Twitter account the tagline, "author," and other descriptors such as speaker, retreat leader, or entrepreneur. More and more physicians are communicating via the written, online and spoken word. Taking advantage of this uptake, Basic Health Publications (www.basichealthpub.com), a niche publishing company, has created more than 300 titles in alternative medicine, health, and nutrition for an estimated 200 healthcare authors. Beyond book in hand, how can physicians take the next step by putting down the stethoscope and moving full time into media medicine and the potentially lucrative world of consulting?

Laura Jana, MD, (www.drlaurajana.com), a pediatrician/author/consultant in Omaha, Nebraska, discusses how she responds when people ask her what she does.

> "I reflexively answer that I am a pediatrician. Then comes the next inevitable question: Where is your practice? To which, when I reply that I am not in clinical practice, I get the follow-on question, So, what do you do? Then it becomes complicated."

What is simple, however, is Jana's passion for early childhood development and creation of healthy, caring responsible young people who turn into healthy, caring, responsible adults. Jana points out that, as defined by the American Academy of Pediatrics, she will always be a pediatrician whose professional work is aligned with their four child health priorities: poverty and child health; epigenetics; early brain and child development; and children, adolescents and media.[350]

Yet, rather than following the linear path of the pediatrician, Jana describes her journey in TED-talk terms as being "an intersect person," someone on the edge of major movements within healthcare who has been able to cobble together a unique approach. After a few years in private pediatric practice, Jana co-founded The Dr. Spock Company—one

CHAPTER ELEVEN

of the first online health sites in the late 1990's—and subsequently her own company, Practical Parenting Consulting. She has authored two books published by American Academy of Pediatrics, *Heading Home with Your Newborn: From Birth to Reality* and *Food Fights: Winning the Nutritional Challenges of Parenthood Armed with Insight, Humor, and a Bottle of Ketchup*, as well as three children books.

Her love of children started early, perhaps best exemplified by her "high school empire" providing babysitting services for 23 families. Her parents, both academic pediatricians, influenced her career path in medicine to a certain extent. Most notably, her mother, who served as Dean of the School of Public Health at the University of Michigan, head of the National AIDS Commission at the outset of the epidemic, and then went on to serve as President of the Josiah Macy Jr. Foundation (www.macyfoundation.org), an organization dedicated to fostering integration of academic health professionals, always encouraged her to follow her instincts and passions.

Jana's hands-on business skills were honed over a nine-year period as owner/operator of Primrose School of Legacy, a premier 200-student educational childcare center in Omaha. Her work was recognized by the community, earning her a "40 under 40" business award. Given the school's focus on the integration of early childhood education, development, safety and nutrition, the school provided high quality services to children primarily five years and younger.

> "I not only continued to manage fevers, rashes and behavioral problems on a daily basis in the child care setting, there was one month in which we had three children have anaphylactic reactions. I hadn't seen that number during my entire private practice. I also had to learn other skills not as common amongst pediatricians. I went out and got a commercial drivers license just in case I had to operate one of the school's three buses."

In her consulting work with companies, Jana is able to draw upon a rich background of skills including early work in cellular-molecular biology and neuroscience, conventional pediatrics, child passenger safety, early literacy, nutrition and strong communication skills. Her holistic self-view is represented by her belief that, "I am not defined by my profession, rather by what is useful for children." Jana encourages her professional audiences to become "the physician of the future," and stay keenly aware of the directions in which medicine is heading, which includes a major shift from a focus on illness to wellness. In addition to her longstanding involvement with the American Academy of Pediatrics, she has made it a point of attending such conferences as TED and TEDGlobal (www.ted.com), the mHealth Summit (www.iotinternetofthingsconference.com), STREAMHealth (www.stream.wpp.com), and Futuremed (www.futuremed.ca).

Jana utilizes her breadth of experience consulting with more than 40 companies which have included P&G, Lysol, car seat manufacturers and others. She gives this advice to physicians interested in going the consulting route.

> "I have always believed that good things could arise if we combine the powerful marketing arms of these companies with equally powerful, but accurate, evidence-based health messaging. The challenge is, when working with these companies, to not allow them to hijack your messaging. You always want to write your own talking points and not allow them to put words in your mouth. Sometimes we function under the impression that companies are intentionally misleading consumers, but in reality, I have found that the marketing people simply aren't aware of important information that is obvious to us as physicians.
>
> You also want to be aware of the subtle ways in which companies can influence your message. One of these is by omission. For example, in speaking for a company about the prevention of infection, I noticed that they had left out the importance of vaccines, which I reinserted into the message. Sometimes in contract negotiations, the big companies think that staying steadfast to your principles—like telling them all the things you can't do or won't say or that maybe it is just not a good fit—is just a negotiation ploy for more money. The reality is that you can't pay me enough to say things I don't believe in. Physicians are the best source of credible health information and we must stay ethical in this regard."

Jana's next consulting/promotion tip for physicians is one that is interwoven with patient engagement techniques and how these skills can be

CHAPTER ELEVEN

transferred into media, particularly video.

> "You can think of the video interview as a new form of public health education but it is not much different from the skills we use to engage patients and get behavioral change. You are transferring your bedside manner over to the camera. You want to really know your audience and where they are at. You also want to keep your message concise and easy to understand. I actually recommend media training for physicians. You learn how to convey a sense of caring and to give an answer that satisfies the viewer without getting into the realm of providing direct medical advice when it's not appropriate."

There is always a caveat to working in the world of intersection. You will always need to acknowledge and cope with the thoughts and feelings of the "imposter syndrome." In any given vertical tract of your work, there will always be individuals who have a much greater depth of knowledge. It is all too easy to become anxious and self-doubting if you focus on comparison. You can take refuge in the reality that no other person has your unique blend of experiences and knowledge, and your ability to synthesize, connect and provide valuable context.

If you plan on becoming a physician who delivers a synergistic message, drawn from multiple disciplines and either broadcast this via media, or take it into corporate consulting, consider the following:

- Create a plan to continually broaden your horizons. Subject yourself to learning some seemingly unrelated disciplines.
- Insert some down time in your life to allow your content synthesis to gel. Don't force it.
- The most challenging part of any synthesis is the model. Here's where a whiteboard, diagrams, and feedback from others can help you crystallize your thoughts.
- Once you have a model and a message, prune it back and reduce it to its essence. Simplicity is beautiful.
- Recognize that you will always have an edge of uncertainty when you do that which has not been done before.
- If you work with companies, keep your ethics intact. Turn down deals that put you into a position of compromise. You will sleep better at night.

- If you fancy a career in media, don't underestimate the importance of crafting the message, or the value of media training.

Work to Heal the System

Many physicians can find additional income and greater satisfaction in focused non-clinical activities such as expert witness review or IMEs. Others take a path that is more difficult to traverse. Driven by a more encompassing mission, they put down the stethoscope and direct their leadership skills toward healing the ailing US healthcare system.

Tim Stover, MD, MBA, is one of those physicians who is making a difference in how healthcare is being delivered today. Stover is President & CEO of Akron General Health Systems. His success creating a wellness oriented outpatient delivery model has been well chronicled. Under his direction Akron General has invested more than $110 million in three suburban facilities ranging in size from 140,000-217,000 square feet. As discussed earlier, the centers provide diagnosis, treatment and the full complement of clinical rehab services including physical therapy, sports medicine, sport performance and cardiopulmonary rehabilitation. Each facility has an associated health and wellness center. Stover comments:

> "We have a great hospital downtown, great docs, great technology; our investment is not to add beds but to develop wellness centers that help keep people out of those beds. We treat patients in an outpatient environment whenever medically appropriate. Our physicians recognize that we have created a community. People come to the center for a lot of different reasons."

Stover's personal path has been driven both by invention and by necessity. The invention path had its roots in Stover's West Virginia upbringing and early medical training.

> "In West Virginia the hospitals were basically a place to go to die. West Virginia was a different culture then and it still is today. The people wouldn't come to you. And when they did come to you it was because they had to. So we took health care to them. We would load residents and medical students in the back of trucks and take them into the hills to see patients in churches, schools and homes. This was in the days before nurse practitioners."

CHAPTER ELEVEN

From this early experience Stover gained an appreciation for the power of the community and the importance of "bringing the services to the people." The second leg of the invention trip came when Stover moved to Akron as an OB/Gyn.

> "I had to go downtown to do all my cases. One day a patient said to me that her husband got lost in the hospital trying to find a waiting room. I didn't connect with him after the surgery and he went nuts. He called me and said where the hell were you? The patient then asked me, 'Why do I need a hospital?' And I said 'Beats me, you don't.' I then realized I don't need an ICU, I don't need an emergency room; I need an operating room; I need anesthesia; I need a safe place but I don't need all this stuff to find out if my patient had endometriosis or not."

The year was 1993, and while there were a handful of outpatient surgical centers in operation nationwide, the concept had yet to make it to rural Ohio.

The third leg on the intervention journey is based on competitive athletics. Stover describes himself as "an old jock," having gone to college to play football. Yet in West Virginia there was a cadre of medical students who kept active. Stove was one of them. His early experience as an athlete allowed him to internalize the connection between exercise and health.

> "So I knew if we combined the outpatient delivery model with an exercise component that we could do both prevention and also treatment. I got a group of physicians together and went to the CEO of the hospital where we worked at that time and we said we wanted to build a facility but we don't want it on campus and we want to partner with you. After a long and tortuous path, after obtaining a certificate of need and completing complicated negotiations, the physician group entered into partnership with Akron General."

The necessity component that shaped Stover's life path is described below.

> "A seminal piece of my life is when I got viral myocarditis from a smallpox vaccination in the military. I had two constrictive episodes. I had to stop OB after my first one when

I ended up having a bilateral thoracotomy. When I stopped practice I didn't know what I was going to do. I call these occurrences 'God wings' as they are not coincidences; these things happen for a reason. Shortly thereafter I got a call from the University of Cincinnati and offered a job to create a department of care management. I was enrolled in my second MBA from the University of Tennessee's physician program, and felt I had something to contribute.

The skills I learned in my MBA program gave me the credibility to sit around the table with the finance guys and the attorneys. I understand when they are talking about NPV how they got the discounted rate. I don't make the spreadsheets anymore but I can if I needed to. Docs would always argue the data but often have no basis to do so if the issue wasn't clinical. I can argue financially now.

I think more docs should gain financial skills because when they get around the table, nobody except for the physician has touched a patient and this is a major advantage, because others often don't think about the patient. They say they do, but they can't. They've never done a physical exam or been in the room with a dying patient. We now have about 19 docs in some sort of MBA program."

Stove sold his Gyn practice in 2005. He was appointed CEO of Akron General Health Systems in early 2012. His illness, his wellness philosophy and his belief in the power of enabling others to do their work inform his management style to this day.

"When I took this job the board knew about my illness. I told them that I have been dealing with it for 12 years and if I have to rest I have to rest. And they said that's up to you; we just want you to do what needs to be done. And that's exactly what I tell the people who work for me. I don't check on them; I expect them to get their work done. I also expect them to have a life. Because I have a life, and I'm not going to give it up and I wouldn't expect it out of these guys either. They work better this way. And if we keep them well at work, which we do, they work even better.

We test that all the time. Since February of 2012 our

CHAPTER ELEVEN

physician satisfaction has more than doubled. What's even more gratifying to me is that our employee satisfaction has gone to the same level. We are a bottom up organization, we aren't top down."

Stover has partnered to create a division called Akron General Health and Wellness Innovations where his team helps other health systems plan, design, build, operate and finance health and wellness center projects. The division is working with organizations both domestically and internationally.

Working to Change the Culture

In contrast to Stover, Maia McCuiston Jackson, MD's approach to changing the healthcare system is narrower in scope. In addition to being a practicing pediatrician, two years ago she took on a position as Physician Director of Multicultural Services at the Mid Atlantic Permanente Medical Group. She dedicates some 20% of her time to this position in which one of her main objectives is helping to monitor and maintain the Culturally and Linguistically Appropriate Services (CLAS) standards. She is also a fierce advocate for health equity. She explains her role:

> "I love pediatrics, but now I am able to help on a broader scale and touch more lives. I learned to speak Spanish fluently while living in Florida and this has been a tremendous asset. In medical training programs we are dealing with a group of highly skilled and intelligent physicians, however, it takes more to be a good doctor. When a physician tells me he or she 'treats everyone the same,' this demonstrates a lack of cultural sensitivity and understanding of unconscious bias. It does a disservice to the patient.
>
> We do a great deal of training with our physicians around how to deal with our diverse patient population. As a result of the ACA we are now seeing a large population of people who have never received health care. They only know how to come to the ER when they have a problem. The concept that they can make an appointment and see a primary care physician is foreign to them. For many, this is their first exposure to preventive services and the first time they have had their

chronic conditions such as asthma or high blood pressure cared for in this setting. We are teaching our physicians how to work with these new patients."

In addition to her work within Permanente, Jackson serves on the regional Diversity & Inclusion council and helps both the health plan and the medical group with outreach into the community. She has received a grant to develop a culturally sensitive childhood obesity program in an underprivileged area.

For those of you who want to make a difference by taking on the system, there are some points to consider. While your clinical background and experience provides you a modicum of respect in the organizational world, for your efforts to be successful the changes you initiate will need to become institutionalized. The benefits of your work must extend beyond your term within the organization. It is best to approach this task by looking backward and asking yourself:

- What legacy are you creating?
- What is it you want to be known for?
- Do you have the organizational skills to move the mountain?
- Do you have the patience?
- How good are your interpersonal skills, because they will be called on to their maximum extent?

Become a (Passionate) Entrepreneur

There are no greater tales of passion and personal insight than those found in the reflections and writings of medical students and house staff as they go through their training. I (Mark) started my own healthcare writing career the day in gross anatomy when we were instructed to saw the cadaver in half and wrap the two sections in separate plastic bags. While our team had worked on "Willie" for weeks, the reality of mortality hit home. I went home, cried, and took out a pen and paper and started writing about my feelings. Unable to express them to others for fear of being misunderstood, or labeled as weak, the written word became the salve for my soul.

Today social media has allowed many young physicians (and older ones as well) to share their earliest emotional experiences of indoctrination

CHAPTER ELEVEN

into the healing arts. This ease of digital expression has unleashed a groundswell of medical students and residents discussing the painful—and arguably inhumane—process of medical education. Ajay Major of *in-Training* points to the popularity of the medical student voiced stories on his site in which the writers describe their visceral pain as they cope with the rigors of training and their confrontation of death and dying.

The system of medical education has changed little in the last five decades. To be fair, it is slightly better. In 2003, The Accreditation Council for Graduate Medical Education instituted standards for all accredited residency programs, limiting the average workweek to 80 hours (over a period of four weeks.). While the quantity of hours worked is down slightly, many other issues such as staffing ratios and patient complexity have not been addressed.

Every physician in training has stories of nearly—or actually—killing patients while sleep deprived or stressed by their patient load. Putting competency aside, these two factors alone combine to rob the physician in training of the necessary concentration, time and attention to detail to provide quality care.

Jennifer Joe, MD, a newly-minted Harvard trained nephrologist, two years out of her fellowship, relates an all too common tale of night float in which two interns and a third year resident have to care for 30-80 patients they have never met. For older physicians who were trained with these caseloads, and have little sympathy for the young physician's plight, we would encourage them to compare the thickness of their *Harrison's Principles of Internal Medicine* with the book of today. Medicine has become increasingly complex. Patients are sicker. And there are more of them.

Joe has been called upon by the Massachusetts Medical Society to participate in a cross functional meeting to examine the issue of humanism in medical training, the need of which was sparked by two incidents in New York. Weeks apart, two young physicians in their second month of residency jumped to their deaths in Manhattan.[50] While ignited in New York, social media spread the flames of concern to Boston, the nation's medical training capital.

Most good entrepreneurial ideas begin by trying to solve a problem; in this case the need for an online home for young physicians to share their thoughts and feelings, as well as to receive the necessary support to get their practice off on the right foot. Along with start up expert, James Ryan, Joe established Medstro.com (www.medstro.com) a social and professional networking site created by physicians for physicians. She hopes to capitalize on a $3B market opportunity.

Medstro.com brings together physicians and medical students into one online community. In addition to learning more about their colleagues, there are opportunities to participate in research activities, learn about job opportunities, and new treatment methodologies. Medstro pays the bills through a jobs database and opt-in job search program built into the site. Started in July of 2013, Medstro now has over 5,000 registered physicians, a database of 35,000 physician jobs and 100+ recruiter accounts. According to Joe, Medstro aims to "create a more open model than Sermo in which physicians hide behind pseudonyms—which encourages personal attacks, and a better experience than Doximity which serves more as an 'online Rolodex' offering HIPAA-compliant messaging and little to no social networking."

Solving the Big Problems in Healthcare

While Joe completed her medical training and pursued her grand idea, the lure of business and the possibility to solve one of the unmet challenges in healthcare can derail—or at least temporarily shelve—a medical career. Such was the case of Pelu Tran, a Stanford medical student who left med school in his third year to co-found Augmedix (www.augmedix.com) along with Stanford business graduate Ian Shakil.

The problem they tackled is as clear as the screen before your face: the pain of the EHR, which according to the latest Medscape Survey continues to infuriate physicians. Seventy percent of respondents state it decreases face to face time with patients, 57% report that it decreases ability to see more patients; for a quarter of the physicians it hinders their ability to respond to patient issues and effectively manage patient treatment plans.[351] Physicians using the larger systems like Cerner and Epic complain about the quality of their notes and the problems with interoperability. What's worse, they now have to be responsible for costing some of their services. The EHR related impediments to quality patient care continue to mount.

With an undergraduate degree in engineering, Pelu Tran was most closely drawn to biomechanics. His work on surgical devices as an

CHAPTER ELEVEN

undergraduate at Stanford led to patented products. After undergraduate he thought about either joining GE Healthcare or attending Stanford medical school, where he was initially drawn to reconstructive surgery. Attending medical school Tran applied his engineering problem solving skills to the environment in which he was placed:

> "As I continued to be exposed to medicine, I realized that the vast majority of the challenges we face in health care have little to do with improving therapies. I observed that the limitations, burnout, and frustration of my attendings were not due to inability to treat the patient, but were due to the processes in the medical system. As I worked in the different settings, I saw that the problem was how we deliver care. I realized that we will never be able to tackle the big problems of aging and cancer unless we fix the systemic problems in healthcare."

In his third year at Stanford Medical School, Pelu found his personal entry point into fixing a broken healthcare system.

> "In asking myself what are the core problems in medicine, I was struck by the idea that physicians are massively underutilized. A large percent of their time is spent not doing what they were trained to do. There is so much care that needs to be provided, but they spend their time doing paperwork and trying to communicate effectively."

It was when Tran learned about Google Glass from Shakil, that the solution was birthed.

By taking a streaming audio-video feed from Google Glass, Augmedix is able to populate—in real time and through a back-end powered by a combination of software and humans—the physician's EHR with encounter data. The physician reviews the record before accepting. Patients are educated that their physician will be using Google Glass and that streaming video will be taken, and they are given the opportunity to opt out. According to Tran, the "glass off" rate is less than 1%. The system can also add digital photos to the notes and serve up on-demand information to the Google Glass heads-up-display, much like Siri. Tran says that:

> "Pre-Augmedix, doctors spent 30-40% of the day on the EHR. Post Augmedix, they spend 1-5%. From an efficiency

standpoint, Augmedix saves a physician two hours a day, or alternatively, turns three doctors into four doctors. Physician satisfaction is very high. Patient satisfaction scores go up because doctors are literally spending more time—and more focused time—per patient. We have proven this with a high n-size sample in practices from multiple states."

As far as going back to medical school and completing his degree, Tran notes how fortunate he was to have attended Stanford Medical School, where, "I was not the first medical student to take a leave of absence and start a company. We will take it one year at a time. Stanford is encouraging me to keep learning, adding value and making sense out of healthcare. While I want to return to medicine, I am making a far greater contribution with Augmedix."

Great Ideas at 35,000 Feet

In listening to stories of how entrepreneurs came up with their big idea, these individuals often point to a spark of enlightenment that came to them from "out of the blue." For Gary Grosel, MD, an OB/Gyn in Cleveland, OH, the lightening bolt of creativity struck while he was reading the SkyMall section of his inflight magazine. Grosel was taken by the page that promoted summaries of the most important business books for executives. The summaries served as one-stop shopping for the busy executive who wants to keep up on current management trends.

At the time Grosel was facing his own need for recertification by the American College of Obstetrics and Gynecology (ACOG). According to Grosel, "OB/Gyns have to find and read 45 articles a year. What if I were to pull the articles together and summarize them? I could save the physicians time and effort; they could read the articles and take the test."

At this point in his professional life Grosel admitted to being burned out after 16 years in practice. While he was successful, he continually felt he had to put the needs of the practice above those of his family. The SkyMall idea rejuvenated Grosel. He founded EasyRecert, which he would later merge with another company to form Rapid Recert (www.rapidrecert.com) to serve the 57,000 OB/Gyns in ACOG. He states that, "Our goal is to make keeping up with the literature easier. We don't give physicians the answers. We provide the content in a way that allows physicians to retain more and in the meantime give them the ability to answer questions." Rapid Recert provides both print and online learning. Physicians can self-test and print their CME certificate that can provide them with up to 100 AMA PRA Category 1 credits.

Grosel's jump into business exemplifies some key entrepreneurial principles. Among them:

- First, identify a need. In this case Grosel identified a personal issue with broad applicability. Don't confuse an idea with a need.
- Do you have the capability to fulfill the need? The beauty of Rapid Recert is that it built upon a key physician skill: the ability to read and summarize the literature.
- Ask yourself: Is the market really large enough? In this case, the universe of 57,000 OB/Gyns was adequate.
- Determine what percent of the potential market you can capture and whether this is enough to make the business profitable. This also helps you determine your pricing.
- What does the competitive landscape look like? The ideal scenario is to be first to market.
- Identify your competitive advantage. Are you faster, cheaper, more comprehensive, easiest to use?
- Do you have enough resources to get the business to cash flow positive? You will most likely need at least twice the funding you project and at least twice the time.
- If you need to convene a team, make certain that you have legal representation; clear, distinct roles for team members, and expectations that are committed to writing.

The Problem with Being the Smartest Person in the Room

If you would like help with some of these issues, as well as the practical support of experienced entrepreneurs, fortunately there is a unique association that will exceed your expectations. Known as the Society of Physician Entrepreneurs (www.sopenet.org), it was started by Arlen Meyers, MD, MBA, Professor of Otolaryngology, Dentistry and Engineering at the University of Colorado Denver.

Ask entrepreneurs to share their stories and you will always find a force that initially drives them. Meyers embarked on the path to creating SOPE because of two powerful emotions: "anger and revenge." He explains:

> "I always knew I wanted to be an academic surgeon. However, I recognized early on that I had the entrepreneur gene. In the process of expressing this gene, I came to realize that most universities are anti-entrepreneur. I created four companies inside the structure of the University. Each one was like a breach delivery going through tech transfer, patent licensing— having to engage academic faculty who knew very little about the technology, and cared even less. So I decided on 'revenge' and the best way to do this was to start an association. The association would unite physicians around a common goal: to get an idea to a patient or to help someone else do it. In the process we have created a global association."

Meyers' method to guiding physicians in entrepreneurial change involves a frank, up-front assessment of personal values and self-worth. He comments:

> "How do you mentally divorce your self from being a doctor? You are special, entitled, smart, and deserving of success. To begin with, you have to let go of these thoughts and get over your external and intrinsic barriers. Instead, ask yourself, 'What is it that trips your trigger?' Any transition must satisfy a psychic need, one that is is not being satisfied as a practicing MD. While many physicians know they are unhappy, they are not sure what else they can do. They are immobilized by the fear that the only thing they know how to do is practice clinical medicine. I encourage physicians to look at their inner drivers such as fear, anger, greed or the need for love. To make a successful transition, physicians have to first figure this out."

He recommends that physicians create a personal SOAP note as if they were interviewing themselves. What is the chief complaint? The history of present illness—how did you get to this state?

Next, Meyers encourages physicians to do a Review of Systems including looking at their physical and emotional health, as well as their finances. How is the health of your balance sheet? What does your profit and loss statement look like? Do you have enough money to make the switch? For the financial examination he recommends "labs and imaging studies," such as speaking to a wealth manager, updating your will, and having a heart to heart financial talk with your significant other. For those who want to become entrepreneurs, Meyers also points to the need for referral to specialists.

> "What is going to get you where you want to go has nothing—or very little— to do with the skills that got you to where you are now. You need resources: people who will provide you with help, networks that create support, and mentors who can guide you and help you deal with some of the inevitable setbacks you will experience.
>
> Ultimately, the goal is to come up with a treatment plan that takes into account what makes you tick, clarifies why you are unhappy, and sets forth a plan to create a constructive chapter in your life that provides an opportunity to be happy. And entrepreneurship is just one path of the many that are possible."

The Doctor Will See You Now

For Alan Roga, MD, CEO of Stat Doctors (www.statdoctors.com), a telehealth company that offers patients 24/7 access to board-certified emergency medicine physicians, the lessons he learned as a practicing ER physician transferred well to the business world. The ER taught Roga the importance of teamwork and enabled him to feel comfortable making decisions when he didn't have all the information at hand.

Roga is an inner city kid from Queens, NY who eventually made it out to Arizona because he wanted a different life for his family. There he ran a large ER practice where he was committed to creating a great work environment. The practice did very well, patient care was great, he had no problem recruiting physicians, but over time his sense of meaning and purpose seemed to erode.

At the same time he caught the technology bug and came to the realization that with the right technology patients could gain better access to care as well as better outcomes at lower cost. That technology was telehealth; and it birthed his company, Stat Doctors.

Stat Doctors has a national network of emergency medicine doctors who provide services on the smartphone, phone, or over the internet, and includes video conferencing software for a face to face visit with the doctor. Stat Doctors is one of a handful of companies targeting their services to the growing corporate marketplace where the advantages are high member satisfaction, better access to care, and cost savings for the business. Some of the physicians in his network work full time, some part time. As far as the service, Roga notes:

> "We provide a virtual house call to diagnose and treat minor medical conditions in lieu of going to the physician or the ER. We connect any way the patient wants— via smart phone, computer or tablet. We see the patient within six minutes; the average eVisit lasts 12-15 minutes. However, it is a different house call for the physician. For one thing we had to retrain the physicians to slow down and ask more questions, in fact, to go back to history-taking 101. Physicians have practiced the same way for 90 years and are used to being in the room with a patient. They have ingrained diagnostic and treatment patterns they can do almost in their sleep. Now that they are not in the room, but are instead in front of a computer; it is a different experience and brings them back to those early days and focusing on history taking."

The physicians at Stat Doctors see up to three to four patients each hour for which they can make over $100 headache free with their malpractice covered. All they need is a computer and a smart phone. Roga sees the day when telehealth is its own specialty complete with certification for physicians who transact visits remotely. He also notes that while telehealth makes enormous business sense, it is a completely new business model and many organizations underestimate the degree of difficulty in making it work.

Research continues to support the explosive growth of telemedicine video consults. According to Harry Wang, Director, Health & Mobile Product Research, Parks Associates, "The number of doctor-patient video consultations will nearly triple from this year to the next, from 5.7 million in 2014 to over 16 million in 2015, and will exceed 130 million in 2018."[352]

CHAPTER ELEVEN

See One, Do One, Teach One

It's the phrase that represents how we were trained. We first observe, then we try, and when we have mastered a skill, we teach it. Fortunately a growing legion of once grumpy and burned out physicians have experienced and mastered the skills of personal and professional transformation and are now teaching them to their colleagues.

Ken Cohn, MD, is a board-certified general surgeon and CEO of Healthcare Collaboration, where he works with disgruntled doctors and healthcare leaders to improve clinical and financial performance. His journey of self-discovery began on the "Valentine's day massacre" the day the VA at White River Junction eliminated five part-time positions, his included. With his wife not wanting to move, Cohn enrolled in the MBA program of the Tuck School at Dartmouth. *USA Today*, in 1995, was able to identify only 75 MDs in the country with an MBA degree. After graduating, he thought that, armed with his new knowledge, he would teach fellow physicians the hard skills of accounting, financial spread sheets and project management.

It didn't take him long to realize that what really makes a difference in healthcare are the soft skills embodied in active listening, win-win negotiating, conflict resolution, and safe confrontation. Now, Cohn notes "A lot of physicians tell me that these should be called the hard skills because they are so difficult to do consistently well. They confess that it was easier to become a physician than to figure out what to do with their lives after being in practice for a few years. I help them keep their options open and learn what is out there."

Cohn has helped physicians rekindle passion for learning and teaching, change surgical residency training, and discover ways to apply hobbies, such as medical cartooning. Cohn is a frequent lecturer at the annual SEAK Non-Clinical Careers for Physicians Conference and is a co-instructor in the Physician Consulting Course with SEAK's founder Babitsky.

Another physician helping to heal wounded healers is Atlanta based, oculoplastic surgeon Starla Fitch, MD, creator of the Love Medicine Again program.

Fitch came to medicine in a roundabout manner. With a master's degree in sociology, she worked in rural Virginia going door to door doing surveys for the Virginia Center on Aging. Her subjects were the elderly and when it came to healthcare, they were confused. They didn't know the names of their diagnoses, and knew even less about why they were taking their different colored pills. Fitch began to lug a PDR to her visits to help identify the medications and explain their use.

Motivated by the sense that she was doing good, she went back to school and took the necessary courses to apply to medical school. She became an oculoplastic surgeon and married the man of her dreams. On the surface, all was going well. One day, as she pulled into her driveway after the ride home from work, she was listening to a silly country song on the radio when she burst into tears. Her husband opened the door and saw her in a state of distress; he didn't know what to do. The damn had burst and a torrent of feelings of frustration came pouring out.

Fitch decided she needed help. She loved taking care of patients but she was getting increasingly frustrated by the bureaucracy of the healthcare delivery system. She knew that it was common for executives to have business coaches, but she had never heard of physicians having them. She had to first address the misguided belief that it is a weakness if you have to ask for help and get a coach. She began working with a coach four years ago and has continued to seek various coaches since that time. Fitch began the inner work for mastering the skills of happiness.

Another pivotal moment came when she was leaving the hospital and one of the surgeons whom she highly admired remarked, "This would be a great job if it weren't for the patients." She was overwhelmed by his cynicism and concerned about the depersonalization that he later expressed. Fitch remarks that, "He was where I had been when I was in my garage. We joked about it, but I began to realize that perhaps I could help other physicians in the same way that I helped myself."

She began working with and interviewing colleagues, and writes a weekly blog at www.lovemedicineagain.com, as well as guest blogs at The Huffington Post and KevinMD.com. Her first book, *Remedy for Burnout: 7 Prescriptions Doctors Use to Find Meaning in Medicine*, was just released. In addition to her full-time oculoplastic surgery practice, she coaches physicians and other health care professionals, is a sought-after speaker, and leads weekend retreats on burnout prevention. Our profession needs more docs like Starla Fitch.

CHAPTER ELEVEN

Ten Take Homes Tips From Total Engagement

Before you read the last section of *Total Engagement*, we have one simple request of you. Go back through the book and identify a Dara knot—the embodiment of the roots of the oak tree—that resonated with you. Gaze at it for just a moment and then ask yourself: Which of my roots need to run deeper? Which need to be better connected to the earth? Where will I find nourishment for my physical, mental and spiritual development? In which directions must my roots grow to transform my practice? We will leave you with these ten tips to address these questions.

1. Look within. Take a deep dive. Identify your passions both inside and outside of medicine.

2. If you are on the edges of burnout, become a personal traveler on the road to wellness. Examine your diet and exercise patterns. Change your perspective. Turn toward gratitude, love, acceptance and service to others, and away from anger, hostility, and cynicism. Identify your personal support systems. Have a heart to heart talk with your significant other. Do this first, and everything else will come a bit easier.

3. When you shift the focus of your clinical interactions toward patient engagement and away from physician directing behavior, you also lighten the burden of care that you carry. It can feel good to offload some—not all—of the responsibilities of care.

4. Work on your motivational interviewing techniques. Start by learning more about how to empathize with patients. You can practice on staff. In the process you can be a source of positive energy that can become contagious.

5. Ask yourself, can I change my present practice structure by adding areas of interest? If not, should I consider taking the leap and going elsewhere, or perhaps adopting another structure of practice? Explore the membership and direct pay models.

6. Identify physician role models and learn more about their path to success. Buy some of their time and expertise. Hire a consultant or a coach. Create a plan. Identify a mechanism to hold yourself accountable for reaching your goals.

7. Join a club, better yet, become a member of a tribe. Tribes, like

AIHM have affirming cultures and systems of mutual obligation that can keep you on a positive and productive path.

8. Maybe you've had your run within medicine. You've paid your dues. Have the courage to find a path outside of the clinical realm. SEAK alternatives.

9. For the young physicians just out of training, don't just buy into the 'bigger is better model' without first considering all your alternatives.

10. Join us for our physician-centered weekend retreats at Pacific Pearl La Jolla. Take advantage of the healing breezes of the Pacific, the camaraderie of colleagues and the collected wisdom of our team.

Appendix

The Functional Medicine Matrix

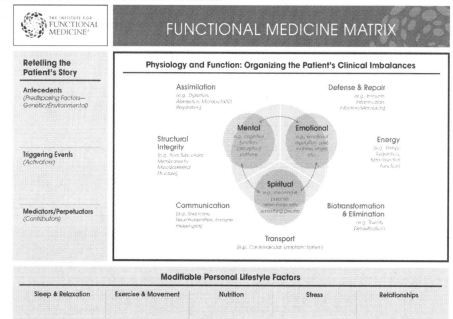

The Functional Medicine Timeline

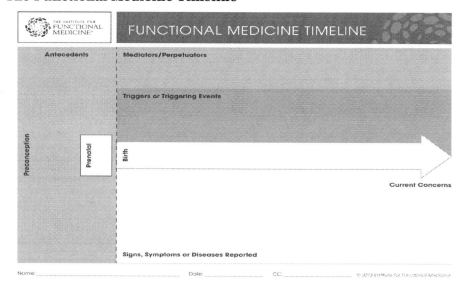

Appendix

The GO TO IT

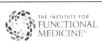

GO TO IT Steps: Practicing Functional Medicine

	Purpose	IFM Tools (examples)

GATHER	**GATHER ONESELF:** Mindfulness; optimizing the therapeutic relationship. **GATHER INFORMATION** through intake forms, questionnaires, the initial consultation, physical exam, and objective data. A detailed functional medicine history taken appropriate to age, gender, and nature of presenting problems.	• Mindful Meditation
		• Health History and Intake Forms
		• Medical Symptoms Questionnaire
		• Timeline
		    ◦ Chronological Story
		    ◦ ATMs and the Patient's Story
		    ◦ ABCDs of Nutritional Evaluation
		    ◦ Request and Report
		    ◦ Nutrition Physical Exam Forms

ORGANIZE	**ORGANIZE** the subjective and objective details from the patient's story within the functional medicine paradigm. Position the patient's presenting signs and symptoms, along with the details of the case history on the timeline and functional medicine matrix.	• Functional Medicine Matrix
		    ◦ Antecedents, Triggers, Mediators
		    ◦ Modifiable Lifestyle Factors
		    ◦ Clinical Imbalances

TELL	**TELL** the story back to the patient in your own words to ensure accuracy and understanding. The re-telling of the patient's story is a dialogue about the case highlights, including the antecedents, triggers, and mediators identified in the history, correlating them to the timeline and matrix.
	• Acknowledge patient's goals.
	• Identify the predisposing factors (antecedents).
	• Identify the triggers or triggering events.
	• Identify the perpetuating factors (mediators).
	• Explore the effects of lifestyle factors.
	• Identify clinical imbalances or disruptions in the organizing physiological systems of the matrix.
	Ask the patient to join in correcting and amplifying the story, engendering a context of true partnership.
		• The Patient's Story Reviewed & Shared with integration of the Functional Medicine perspective (i.e. ATMs, Timeline, and Matrix)
		• Personal Development Exercises to: Create and Strengthen the Therapeutic Relationship
		    ◦ Reflective Listening
		    ◦ Motivational Interviewing
		    ◦ Coaching & Behavioral Modifications

ORDER	**ORDER** and prioritization emerges from the dialogue of professional and patient. The patient's mental, emotional, and spiritual perspective is of primary importance for prioritizing the 'next steps.'	• Matrix

INITIATE	**INITIATE** further functional assessment and intervention based upon the above work:
	• Perform further assessment
	• Initiate patient education and therapeutic intervention
	• Referral to adjunctive care if needed
	    ◦ Nutrition Professional
	    ◦ Lifestyle Educator
	    ◦ Healthcare Provider
	    ◦ Specialist
		• Prescription for Lifestyle Medicine
		• Referral to Functional Nutritionist for
		    ◦ Additional Nutrition Evaluation
		    ◦ Biomarkers Laboratory Form
		    ◦ Dietary Interventions
		• Patient Education Handouts (examples)
		    ◦ Mindful Eating
		    ◦ Relaxation Response
		    ◦ Functional Nutrition Fundamentals
		    ◦ Core Food Plan and Therapeutic Suites

TRACK	**TRACK** further assessments, note the effectiveness of the therapeutic approach, and identify clinical outcomes at each visit—in partnership with the patient.	• Medical Symptoms Questionnaire • Body Composition Tracking

The three Institute for Fuctional Medicine documents above were reprinted with permission.

Appendix

Selected Learning Opportunities in Aesthetics

THE Aesthetic Show (www.aestheticshow.com)

American Academy of Anti-Aging Medicine (www.a4m.com)

American Academy of Cosmetic Surgery (www.cosmeticsurgery.org)

American Med Spa Association (www.amspa.site-ym.com)

American Society for Laser Medicine and Surgery (www.aslms.org)

American Society of Cosmetic Physicians (www.cosmeticphysicians.org)

Day Spa Association (www.Dayspaassociation.com)

International Association For Physicians in Aesthetic Medicine.(www.iapam.com)

International Master Course on Aging Skin (www.imcas.com)

The Institute for Functional Medicine (www.functionalmedicine.org)

Multi-Specialty Foundation (www.multi-specialty.org)

South Beach Symposium (www.southbeachsymposium.org)

Stem Cell Education Opportunities

World Stem Cell Summit (www.worldstemcellsummit.com)

International Society of Stem Cell Research (www.isscr.org)

The Clinical Translation of Stem Cells: Select Biosciences (www.selectbiosciences.com)

International Stem Cell Society (STEMSO) (www.stemso.org)

International Federation of Adipose Therapeutics (www.ifats.org)

Age Management Medical Group (www.agemed.org)

The American Academy of Cosmetic Surgery Section on Stem Cells (www.cosmeticsurgery.org)

THE Aesthetic Show Section on Stem Cells (www.aestheticshow.com)

Cell Surgical Network Webinars and Annual Clinical Meeting (www.ipscell.com)

Bioheart Webinars in Regenerative Medicine (www.my.brainshark.com)

The Ortho Biologics Group (www.prpseminar.com)

Sports Medicine Training Seminars (www.theandrewsinstitute.com)

PRACTICE QUALITY ASSESSMENT

1. Telephone Inquiry
- Was the phone answered in three rings or less?
- Was the name of the business used?
- Did the person identify him/herself?
- Were you put on hold?
- If yes, for how long (in minutes)?
- Was the phone answered by an automated system?
- If yes, please rate user friendliness.
- If on hold, did you listen to music or information about the practice and procedures?
- Please rate the politeness and professionalism of the person who answered the phone.
- Were you asked how you heard of the provider or who referred you?
- Were concerns or problem list and goals elicited?
- Was an effort made to schedule a convenient appointment?
- Please rate how well your questions were answered, with 5 being excellent and 1 being poor.
- Were you asked whether you had visited the clinic's website?
- Did you receive a reminder call, email or text message before your appointment?

2. Building Exterior
- Was the location easy to find and access?
- Could you find directions on the clinic's website?
- Was the location signage accurate and legible?
- Was the parking area clean and convenient?
- Was the exterior of the location well maintained?

3. Check In/Reception/Common Areas
- Were you acknowledged upon approaching the reception desk?
- Please rate the responsiveness and friendliness of the greeter.
- Was the greeter well groomed and professional in appearance?

Appendix

- Were all the employees in the reception area polite, friendly and professional in appearance and demeanor?
- Was your privacy and that of other clients protected?
- Was the paperwork you may have completed easy to understand and relevant to your visit?
- Please rate the comfort and cleanliness of the reception area.
- Please rate how the overall atmosphere inspired confidence.
- Was the restroom clean and well-stocked?
- How long was your wait before being escorted to the consultation room?
- Were there brochures or any written materials about treatment in the reception area?

4. Prescreen/Initial Services (If Applicable)
- Was the employee well groomed and professional in appearance and demeanor?
- Rate the level of confidence this employee instilled on a scale from five to one. (5=high, 1=low)
- Were you informed how long you may have to wait for the provider?
-

5. Exam Room
- Please rate the ambience and comfort of the consultation room.
- How long did you wait for the provider in the consultation room?
- Were there materials for you to look at while you waited?

6. Exam/Consultation by Practitioner
- Did the practitioner introduce himself?
- Did the practitioner wash his/her hands or apply gloves before examining you?
- Please rate how well the practitioner explained the exam procedure and insured your comfort.
- Please rate how comfortable the practitioner made you feel discussing your health issues.
- How thoroughly were treatment options described?
- For procedures: Did the practitioner discuss his/her experience/training with this procedure?

- How attentive and sensitive to your needs was the practitioner?
- Did the practitioner ask if you had any questions?
- Please rate how thoroughly your questions were answered.
- Do you feel that the practitioner spent enough time with you?
- Please rate the level of confidence the practitioner inspired.

7. Patient Coordinator/Checkout/Billing
- Were you acknowledged on approaching the checkout area?
- Please rate the responsiveness and friendliness of checkout personnel/patient coordinator.
- Was a follow-up appointment discussed?
- How comfortable were you discussing fees?
- Were you told what type of payments are accepted?
- Were financing options or other means to afford expensive procedures discussed?

8. Overall Impression
- Please rate your overall experience.
- Do you feel the practitioner treated the staff with respect and kindness?
- Would you return to this business?
- Would you recommend this business to others?

Bibliography

1. Holistic Primary Care. (2010) *An Executive report from Holistic Primary Care's first annual physicians survey*. New York, NY. Holistic Primary Care.
2. WebMD. (2014). *Medscape physician's lifestyle report 2014*. New York, NY. Peckman, C.
3. HIS. (2014). *Telehealth report 2014*. Englewood, CO. Roashan, R.
4. Tager, M. J., & Mulholland, S. (2008). *The Art of aesthetic practice: How to profit from the cosmetic boom*. Rancho Santa Fe: ChangeWell, INC.
5. WebMD. (2014). *Medscape physician compensation report 2014*. New York, NY. Peckman, C. & Kane, Leslie.
6. Chesanow, N. (2014, May 14). Cash-only practices: 8 issues to consider. *Medscape*. Retrieved June 18, 2014, from http://www.medscape.com/viewarticle/824543_2
7. The Physician's Foundation. (2012). *A survey of America's physicians: Practice patterns and perspectives*. Merritt Hawkins.
8. Historical. (2014). *Centers for Medicare & Medicaid services*. Retrieved June 18, 2014, from http://www.cms.gov/Research-Statistics-Data-and-Systems/Statistics-Trends-and-Reports/NationalHealthExpendData/NationalHealthAccountsHistorical.html
9. Tandon, A., Murray, C., Lauer, J., & Evans, D. (2013). *Measuring overall health system performance for 191 countries*. GPE Discussion Paper Series, 30, 18.
10. Retail prescription drugs filled at pharmacies (Annual per Capita by Age). (n.d.). *Kaiser Family Foundation*. Retrieved June 18, 2014, from http://kff.org/other/state-indicator/retail-rx-drugs-by-age/
11. 2007 statistics on CAM use in the United States. (n.d.). *NCCAM*. Retrieved June 18, 2014, from http://nccam.nih.gov/news/camstats/2007
12. Bormann, J. E., Thorp, S., Wetherell, J. L., & Golshan, S. (2008). A spiritually based group intervention for combat veterans with posttraumatic stress disorder: feasibility study. *Journal of Holistic Nursing, 26*(2), 109-116.
13. American Medical Association. *Increasing awareness of the benefits and risks associated with complementary and alternative medicine*. 1. (2006). available at www.ama-assn.org/ama1/pub/upload/mm/471/306a06.pdf.
14. Townsend, A. (n.d.). Cleveland Clinic to open Center for Functional Medicine; Dr. Mark Hyman to be director. *cleveland.com*. Retrieved October 3, 2014, from http://www.cleveland.com/healthfit/index.ssf/2014/09/cleveland_clinic_to_open_cente.html
15. Clinic. (2014, March 5). Cleveland clinic among first in U.S. to open hospital-based Chinese herbal therapy clinic. *Cleveland Clinic*. Retrieved June 18, 2014, from http://my.clevelandclinic.org/media_relations/library/2014/2014-3-5-cleveland-clinic-among-first-in-the-us-to-open-hospital-based-chinese-herbal-therapy-clinic.aspx
16. The Department of Defense. (2014). *Integrative medicine in the military health system report to congress*. Falls Church, VA. United States Government.
17. Gentilviso, C. (2014, January 22). Aetna CEO on health care system: 'The patient really isn't a person'. *The Huffington Post*. Retrieved September 7, 2014, from http://www.huffingtonpost.com/2014/01/22/mark-bertolini-davos_n_4636284.html
18. *Integrative medicine in America: How integrative medicines is being practiced in clinical centers across the United States*. (2012). Encinitas, CA: The Bravewell Collaboration.
19. Feldhahn, S. C. (2013). *The good news about marriage: Debunking discouraging myths about marriage and divorce*. Colorado Springs, CO: Multnomah Books.
20. Gallup. (2013). *State of the American workplace*.
21. Institute of Medicine. (2011). *Reliving pain in America: A blueprint for transforming prevention, care, education and research*. Washington, DC.
22. Rosch, P. J. (1991, May). Job stress: America's leading adult health problem. *USA Magazine*
23. Riddle, John. "Asthma and stress management." Asthma and Stress Management. *Health Central.*, n.d. Web. 6 May 2014. http://www.healthcentral.com/asthma/livingwithit-255364-5.html
24. The Physicians Foundation. (2010). Health reform and the decline of physician private practice. Merrit Hawkins
25. Seabury, S. A., Jena, A. B., & Chandra, A. (2012). Trends in the earnings of health care professionals in the United States, 1987-2010. The Journal of the American Medical Association, 308(20), 2083.
26. MedSynergies. (2013). *The Dynamic of physician alignment*. Media Health Leaders: A Division of HCPro.
27. Health insurance CEO pay skyrockets in 2013. (n.d.). *Healthcare-NOW!*. Retrieved September 30, 2014, from http://www.healthcare-now.org/health-insurance-ceo-pay-skyrockets-in-2013
28. Mathews, A. W. (n.d.). Same doctor visit, double the cost. *The Wall Street Journal*. Retrieved May 6, 2014, from http://online.wsj.com/news/articles/SB10000872396390443713704577601113671007448
29. The Physician's Foundation. (2010). *Health reform and the decline of physician private practice*. Merritt Hawkins.
30. Beebe, M. (2004). *CPT 2005: current procedural terminology* (4th ed.). Chicago, Ill.: American Medical Association.

31. Diamond, F. (n.d.). The pursuit of happy docs. *Managed Care Magazine Online*. Retrieved July 16, 2014, from http://www.managedcaremag.com/archives/0903/0903.planwatch.html

32. D. L. Nelson, B. L. Simmons (2004). P. L. Perrewé, D. C. Ganster, ed. *Eustress: an elusive construct an engaging pursuit* (First Edition ed.). Oxford, UK: Elsevier Jai.

33. Larsen, R. J., & Buss, D. M. (2008). *Personality psychology: domains of knowledge about human nature* (3rd ed.). Boston: McGraw Hill.

34. RM, Dodson JD. (1908). The relation of strength of stimulus to rapidity of habit-formation. *Journal of Comparative Neurology and Psychology, 18*: 459–482.

35. What is Stress Risk Assessment?. (n.d.). *What is a stress risk assessment*. Retrieved July 16, 2014, from http://www.mas.org.uk/stress-management/stress-risk-assessment/what-is-a-stress-risk-assessment.html

36. Gould, K. L. (1998). *Heal your heart: how you can prevent or reverse heart disease*. New Brunswick, N.J.: Rutgers University Press.

37. Smith, G. D., Harbord, R., & Ebrahim, S. (2004). Fibrinogen, c-reactive protein and coronary heart disease: Does Mendelian randomization suggest the associations are non-causal?. *QJM, 97*(3), 163-166.

38. Benatti, F., Lira, F., Oyama, L., Nascimento, C., & Jr., . L. (2011). Strategies for reducing body fat mass: effects of liposuction and exercise on cardiovascular risk factors and adiposity. *Diabetes, Metabolic Syndrome and Obesity, 4*, 141-154.

39. Prystowsky, E. N., Benson, D. W., Fuster, V., Hart, R. G., Kay, G. N., Myerburg, R. J., et al. (1996). Management of patients with atrial fibrillation : A statement for healthcare professionals from the subcommittee on electrocardiography and electrophysiology. American Heart Association. *Circulation, 93*(6), 1262-1277.

40. Nykamp, D., & Titak, J. A. (2010). Takotsubo cardiomyopathy, or broken-heart syndrome. *Annals Of Pharmacotherapy, 44*(3), 590-593.

41. Grundy, S. M. (2004). Definition of metabolic syndrome: Report of The National Heart, Lung, and Blood Institute/American Heart Association conference on scientific issues related to definition. *Circulation, 109*(3), 433-438.

42. Opasich, C., Rapezzi, C., Lucci, D., Gorini, M., Pozzar, F., Zanelli, E., et al. (2001). Precipitating factors and decision-making processes of short-term worsening heart failure despite "optimal" treatment (from the IN-CHF Registry). *The American Journal of Cardiology, 88*(4), 382-387.

43. Mäkikallio, T. H., Huikuri, H. V., Mäkikallio, A., Sourander, L. B., Mitrani, R. D., Castellanos, A., et al. (2001). Prediction of sudden cardiac death by fractal analysis of heart rate variability in elderly subjects. *Journal of the American College of Cardiology, 37*(5), 1395-1402.

44. Chen, G. Y., & Nuñez, G. (2010). Sterile inflammation: Sensing and reacting to damage. *Nature Reviews Immunology, 10*(12), 826-837.

45. Chandrasekaran, B., & Kurbaan, A. S. (2002). Myocardial infarction with angiographically normal coronary arteries. *JRSM, 95*(8), 398-400.

46. Yasgur, B. S. (2013, December 23). Are doctors suffering from compassion fatigue. *WebMD*. Retrieved March 31, 2014, from http://www.medscape.com/viewarticle/813967

47. Shanafelt, T. D., Boone, S., Tan, L., Dyrbye, L. N., Sotile, W., Satele, D., et al. (2012). Burnout and satisfaction with work-life balance among US physicians relative to the general US population. *Archives of Internal Medicine, 172*(18), 1377.

48. Orton P, Orton C, Pereira Gray D. Depersonalised doctors: A cross-sectional study of 564 doctors, 760 consultations and 1876 patient reports in UK general practice. *BMJ Open 2012*

49. Rose, K. D., & Rosow, I. (1973). Physicians who kill themselves. *Archives of General Psychiatry, 29*(6), 800-805.

50. Sinha, Pranay. (2014). Why do doctors commit suicide?. *New York Times*. Web. 2 Oct. 2014

51. Goebert, D., Schechter, J., Kunkel, M., Kent, A., Ephgrave, K., Bryson, P., et al. (2009). Depressive Symptoms In Medical Students And Residents: A Multischool Study. *Academic Medicine, 84*(2), 236-241.

52. Brodsky, L. (n.d.). Suicide in female physicians: Recognize, respond, reconsider. *KevinMD.com*. Retrieved July 16, 2014, from http://www.kevinmd.com/blog/2013/07/suicide-female-physicians-recognize-respond-reconsider.html

53. Spielberger, C.D., Johnson E. H., Russell, S.F., Crane, R.J., Jacobs, G.A., & Worden, T.I. (1985). "The experience and expression of anger: Construction and validation of an anger expression scale". In M.A. Chesney & R.H. Rosenman (Eds.), *Anger and hostility in cardiovascular and behavioral disorders*. New York: Hemisphere/McGraw-Hill.

54. Mcclelland, D. C. (1989). Motivational factors in health and disease. *American Psychologist, 44*(4), 675-683.

55. Mcconnell, M. M., & Eva, K. W. (2012). The role of emotion in the learning and transfer of clinical skills and knowledge. *Academic Medicine, 87*(10), 1316-1322.

56. Ofri, D. (2013). *What doctors feel: How emotions affect the practice of medicine*. Boston: Beacon Press.

57. Brancati FL. (1989). The art of pimping. *The Journal of the American Medical Association, 262*:89–90.

58. Wear, D., Kokinova, M., Keck-Mcnulty, C., & Aultman, J. (2005). Research basic to medical education: Pimping: perspectives of 4th year medical students. *Teaching and Learning in Medicine, 17*(2), 184-191.

Bibliography

59. Selye, H. (1956). *The stress of life*. New York: McGraw-Hill.
60. Epel, E., McEwen, B., Seeman, T., Matthews, K., Castellazzo, G., Brownell, K., et al. (2000). Stress and body shape: Stress-induced cortisol secretion is consistently greater among women with central fat. *Psychosomatic Medicine, 62*, 623–632.
61. Chiodini, I., Ambrosi, B., Adda, G., Arosio, M., Orsi, E., Beck-Peccoz, P., et al. (2007). Cortisol secretion in patients with type 2 diabetes: Relationship with chronic complications. *Diabetes Care, 30*(1), 83-88.
62. Dua, Y., Yang, C., Zhang, H., Liu, B., Wu, J., Dong, J., et al. (2014). Association of pro-inflammatory cytokines, cortisol and depression in patients with chronic obstructive pulmonary disease. *Psychoneuroendocrinology, 46*, 141-152.
63. Palacios, R., & Sugawara, I. (1982). Hydrocortisone abrogates proliferation of T-cells in autologous mixed lymphocyte reaction by rendering the interleukin-2 producer T-cells unresponsive to interleukin-1 and unable to synthesize the T-cell growth factor. *Scandinavian Journal of Immunology, 15*(1), 25-31.
64. Holmes, T. H., & Rahe, R. H. (1967). The social readjustment rating scale. *Journal of Psychosomatic Research, 11*(2), 213-218.
65. Adams, R. E., Boscarino, J. A., & Figley, C. R. (2006). Compassion fatigue and psychological distress among social workers: A validation study. *American Journal of Orthopsychiatry, 76*(1), 103-108.
66. Epel, E. S. (2004). From The cover: Accelerated telomere shortening in response to life stress. *Proceedings of the National Academy of Sciences, 101*(49), 17312-17315.
67. Kirschbaum, C., Pirke, K., & Hellhammer, D. H. (1993). The 'trier social stress– A Tool for investigating psychobiological stress responses in a laboratory setting. *Neuropsychobiology, 28*(1-2), 76-81.
68. Tomiyama, A. J., Blackburn, E., Epel, E., Kirschbaum, C., Wolkowitz, O., Dhabhar, F. S., et al. (2012). Does cellular aging relate to patterns of allostasis?. *Physiology & Behavior, 106*(1), 40-45.
69. Diener, E., Suh, E. M., Lucas, R. E., & Smith, H. L. (1999). Subjective well-being: three decade of progress. *Psychological Bulletin, 125*, 276-302.
70. Harker, L., & Keltner, D. (2001) Expressions of positive emotions in women's college yearbook pictures and their relationship to personality and life outcomes across adulthood. *Journal of Personality and Social Psychology, 80*, 112-124.
71. Estrada, C., Isen, A. M., Young, M. J. (1994). Positive affect influences creative problem solving and reported source of practice satisfaction in physicians. *Motivation and Emotion, 18*, 285-299.
72. Csikszentmihalyi, M., & Wong, M. M. (1991). The situational and personal correlates of happiness: A cross-national comparision. In F. Strack, M. Argyle, & N. Schwarz (Eds.), *Subjective well-being: An interdisciplinary perspective* (pp. 193-212). Elmsford, NY: Pergamon Press.
73. Aspinwall, L. G. (1998). Rethinking the role of positive affect in self-regulation. *Motivation and Emotion, 22*, 1-32.
74. Dillon, K. M., Minchoff, B., & Baker, K. H. (1985). Positive emotional starts and enhancement of the immune system. *International Journal of Psychiatry in Medicine, 15*, 13-18.
75. Danner, D. D., Snowdon, D. A., & Friesen, W. V. (2001). Positive emotions in early life and longevity: Findings from the nun study. *Journal of Personality and Social Psychology, 80*, 804-813.
76. Isen, A. M. (1970). Success, failure, attention, and reaction to others; The warm glow of success. *Journal of Personality and Social Psychology, 15*, 294-301.
77. Greenberg, M. (n.d.). Is money the secret to happiness?. Psychology *Today: Health, Help, Happiness + Find a Therapist*. Retrieved July 16, 2014, from http://www.psychologytoday.com/blog/the-mindful-self-express/201209/is-money-the-secret-happiness
78. Brickman, P., & Campbell, D. (1971). Hedonic relativism and planning the good society. In M. H. Apley (Ed.), *Adaptation-level theory: A symposium* (pp. 287–302). New York: Academic Press.
79. Tager, M., & Willard, S. (2014). *Transforming stress into power: The PowerSource Profile system*. Rancho Santa Fe, CA: Changewell, Inc.
80. Lyubomirsky, S., Sheldon, K. M., & Schkade, D. (2005). Pursuing happiness: The architecture of sustainable change. *Review of General Psychology, 9*(2), 111-131.
81. Botton, A. (2006). *The Architecture of happiness*. New York: Pantheon Books.
82. Goldman, S. L., Kraemer, D. T., & Salovey, P. (1996). Beliefs About Mood Moderate the Relationship of Stress to Illness and Symptom Reporting. *Journal of Psychosomatic Research, 41*, 2, 115-128.
83. Ashby, F. G., Isen, A. M., & Turken, A. U. (1999). A neuropsychological theory of positive affect and its influence on cognition. *Psychological Review, 106*, 3, 529-550.
84. Isen, A. M., Shalker, T. E., Clark, M., & Karp, L. (1978). Affect, accessibility of material in memory and behavior: A cognitive loop? *Journal of Personality and Social Psychology, 36*, 1–12.
85. Carnevale, P. J. D., & Isen, A. M. (1986). The influence of positive affect and visual access on the discovery of integrative solutions in bilateral negotiation. *Organizational Behavior and Human Decision Processes, 37*, 1–13.
86. Isen, A. M., Daubman, K. A., & Nowicki, G. P. (1987). Positive affect facilitates creative problem solving. *Journal of

Personality and Social Psychology, 52, 6, 1122-1131.

87. Wright, T., & Staw, B. (1994). *In search of the happy/productive worker: A longitudinal study of affect and performance.* Academy of Management Proceedings, 274.

88. Estrada C. A., Isen A. M., Young M. (1997). PA facilitates integration of information and decreases anchoring in reasoning among physicians. *Organizational Behavior and Human Decision Processes 72*, 117–135.

89. Lanza GA, Guido V, Galeazzi N, et al. (1998). Prognostic role of heart rate variability in patients with a recent acute myocardial infarction. *American Journal of Cardiology, 82*:1323–8.

90. Carney, R. M., Saunders, R. D., Freedland, K. E., Stein, P., Rich, M. W., & Jaffe, A. S. (1995). Association of depression with reduced heart rate variability in coronary artery disease. *The American Journal of Cardiology, 76*(8), 562-564.

91. Engs, R.C. (1987). *Alcohol and Other Drugs: Self Responsibility*. Bloomington, IN. Tichenor Publishing Company.

92. Randall, D. C. (2000). Towards an understanding of the function of the intrinsic cardiac ganglia. *The Journal of Physiology, 528*(3), 406-406.

93. Park, G., & Thayer, J. (2014). From the heart to the mind: cardiac vagal tone modulates top-down and bottom-up visual perception and attention to emotional stimuli. *Frontiers in Psychology, 5*, 278.

94. Darwin, C. (1965). *The expression of the emotions in man and animals*. Chicago: University of Chicago Press.

95. Wallace JE, Lemaire J. (2007). On physician well being-you'll get by with a little help from your friends. *Social Science and Medicine, 64*(12):2565– 2577.

96. Graham J, Albery IP, Ramirez AJ, Richards MA. (2001). How hospital consultants cope with stress at work: implications for their mental health. *Stress Health, 17*(2):85–89.

97. King MB, Cockcroft A, Gooch C. (1992). Emotional distress in doctors: sources, effects and help sought. *Journal of the Royal Society of Medicine, 85*(10):605– 608.

98. Weiner EL, Swain GR, Wolf B, Gottlieb M, Spickard A. (2001). A qualitative study of physicians' own wellness-promotion practices. *Western Journal of Medicine, 174*(1):19–23.

99. Lemaire JB, Wallace JE, Lewin AM, de Grood J, Schaefer JP. (2011). The effect of a biofeedback-based stress management tool on physician stress: a randomized controlled clinical trial. *Open Medicine, 5*(4), 154.

100. Randall, D. C. (2000). Towards an understanding of the function of the intrinsic cardiac ganglia. *The Journal of Physiology, 528*(3), 406-406.

101. Newsome, M., Pearsall, C., Ryan, T., & Starlin, P. (2014). Changing job satisfaction, absenteeism, and healthcare claims costs in a hospital culture. *Global Advances in Health and Medicine, 3*, Supply 1.

102. Friedland, D. (2014). Evidence-based medicine: A framework for emotional regulation, intuition, and conscious engagement. *Global Advances in Health and Medicine, 3*(2), 3-4.

103. Nidich, S. I., Grosswald, S., Gaylord-King, C., Tanner, M., Travis, F., Salerno, J. W., et al. (2009). A randomized controlled trial on effects of the transcendental meditation program on blood pressure, psychological distress, and coping in young adults. *American Journal of Hypertension, 22*(12), 1326-1331.

104. Eppley, K. R., Abrams, A. I., & Shear, J. (1989). Differential effects of relaxation techniques on trait anxiety: A meta-analysis. *Journal of Clinical Psychology, 45*(6), 957-974.

105. Sheppard WD II, Staggers FJ, John L. (1997). The effects of a stress-management program in a high security government agency. *Anxiety Stress Coping, 10*(4), 341-50.

106. Aron A, Orme-Johnson DW, Brubaker P. (1981). The transcendental meditation program in the college curriculum: a 4-year longitudinal study of effects on cognitive and affective functioning. *College Student Journal, 15*(2), 140-6.

107. Jayadevappa R, Johnson JC, Bloom BS, et al. (2007). Effectiveness of transcendental meditation on functional capacity and quality of life of African Americans with congestive heart failure: a randomized control study. *Ethnicity and Disease, 17*(1), 72-7.

108. Rainforth, M. V., Schneider, R. H., Nidich, S. I., Gaylord-King, C., Salerno, J. W., & Anderson, J. W. (2007). Stress reduction programs in patients with elevated blood pressure: A Systematic review and meta-analysis. *Current Hypertension Reports, 9*(6), 520-528.

109. Yamaoka, K., & Tango, T. (2005). Efficacy of lifestyle education to prevent type 2 diabetes: A Meta-analysis of randomized controlled trials. *Diabetes Care, 28*(11), 2780-2786.

110. Bormann, J. A "Burnout prevention" tool for improving healthcare providers' health and wellbeing: Mantram repetition. *Mental Health*. Retrieved July 16, 2014, from http://www.mentalhealth.va.gov/coe/cesamh/docs/Mantram_Repetition_for_Employees.pdf

111. Elder, C., Nidich, S., Nidich, R. & Moriarty, F. (2014). Effect of transcendental meditation on employee stress, depression, and burnout: A Randomized controlled study. *The Permente Journal, 18*(1), 19-23.

112. Ludwig, D. S., & Kabat-Zinn, J. (2008). Mindfulness in medicine. *The Journal of the American Medical Association, 300*(11), 1350-1352.

113. Krasner, M. S., Epstein, R. M., Beckman, H., Suchman, A. L., Chapman, B., Mooney, C. J., et al. (2009). Association of an educational program in mindful communication with burnout, empathy, and attitudes among primary care

Bibliography

physicians. *The Journal of the American Medical Association, 302*(12), 1284-1293.

114. Fortney, L., Luchterhand, C., Zakletskaia, L., Zgierska, A., & Rakel, D. (2013). Abbreviated mindfulness intervention for job satisfaction, quality of life, and compassion in primary care clinicians: A pilot study. *The Annals of Family Medicine, 11*(5), 412-420.

115. Ornstein, R. E., & Sobel, D. S. (1989). *Healthy pleasures*. Reading, Mass.: Addison-Wesley.

116. Hutchinson, J. C., & Sherman, T. (2013). The Relationship Between Exercise Intensity and Preferred Music Intensity. *Sport, Exercise, and Performance Psychology, 3*(3), 191-202.

117. Lescroart, M. (2011). The Healing Power of Touch. *Scientific American Mind, 22*(3), 7-7.

118. Martel, Y. (n.d.). Yann Martel on Life of Pi, Interpretation, Stillness, and Art. *Ann Kroeker Writing Coach*. Retrieved September 9, 2014, from http://annkroeker.com/2008/04/25/yann-martel-on-life-of-pi-interpretation-stillness-and-art/

119. Frankl, V. E. (2006). *Man's search for meaning*. Boston: Beacon Press.

120. Crujeiras, A. B., Parra, D., Milagro, F. I., Goyenechea, E., Larrarte, E., Margareto, J., et al. (2008). Differential expression of oxidative stress and inflammation related genes in peripheral blood mononuclear cells in response to a low-calorie diet: A Nutrigenomics study. omics. *A Journal of Integrative Biology, 12*(4), 251-261.

121. Physical Activity and Health. (2011, February 16). *Centers for Disease Control and Prevention*. Retrieved July 14, 2014, from http://www.cdc.gov/physicalactivity/everyone/health/

122. King, D., Dalsky, G., Clutter, W., Young, D., Staten, M., Cryer, P., et al. (1988). Effects of exercise and lack of exercise on insulin sensitivity and responsiveness. *Journal of Applied Physiology, 64*(5), 1942-1946.

123. Bogdanis, G. C. (2012). Effects of Physical Activity and Inactivity on Muscle Fatigue. *Frontiers in Physiology, 3*, 142.

124. Beetz, A., Uvnäs-Moberg, K., Julius, H., & Kotrschal, K. (2012). Psychosocial and Psychophysiological Effects of Human-Animal Interactions: The Possible Role of Oxytocin. *Frontiers in Psychology, 3*, 234.

125. Umberson, D., & Montez, J. K. (2010). Social Relationships And Health: A Flashpoint For Health Policy. *Journal of Health and Social Behavior, 51*(1 Suppl), S54-S66.

126. Park, W., Yu, J., Lee, M., & Kim, D. (2013). Effects of psychological distress and social support on mental fitness among patients of mental health services. *European psychiatry : the journal of the Association of European Psychiatrists, 28*(1), 1.

127. Holt-Lunstad, J., Smith, T. B., Layton, J. B., & Brayne, C. (2010). Social Relationships And Mortality Risk: A Meta-analytic Review. *PLoS Medicine, 7*(7), e1000316.

128. Parker-pope, T. (2010). Is Marriage Good for your HEALTH?. *The New York Times*. Retrieved September 11, 2014, from http://www.nytimes.com/2010/04/18/magazine/18marriage-t.html?pagewanted=all

129. Schwarzer, R., & Rieckmann, N. (in press). Social support, cardiovascular disease, and mortality. In *Heart disease: Environment, stress, and gender*. NATO Science Series, Series 1: Life and behavioral sciences, 327. IOS Press, Amsterdam.

130. Assad, K. K., Donnellan, M. B., & Conger, R. D. (2007). Optimism: An Enduring Resource For Romantic Relationships. *Journal of Personality and Social Psychology, 93*(2), 285-297.

131. Alviar, C. L., Rockman, C., Guo, Y., Adelman, M., & Berger, J. (2014). Association Of Marital Status With Vascular Disease In Different Arterial Territories: A Population Based Study Of Over 3.5 Million Subjects. *Journal of the American College of Cardiology, 63*(12), A1328.

132. Kiecolt-Glaser, J. K., Bane, C., Glaser, R., & Malarkey, W. B. (2003). Love, marriage, and divorce: Newlyweds' stress hormones foreshadow relationship changes. *Journal of Consulting and Clinical Psychology, 71*(1), 176-188.

133. McCraty, R., & Zayas, M. (2014). Intuitive Intelligence, Self-regulation, and Lifting Consciousness. *Global Advances in Health and Medicine, 3*(2), 56-65.

134. OECD Guiding Principles for Regulatory Quality and Performance. (2005). *Enhancing beneficial competition in the health professions*.

135. Canadian Mental Health Association. (2005). *Stress in the workplace: A general overview of the causes, the effects, and the Solutions*. Melanie Bickford.

136. Kobasa, S. C., & Puccetti, M. C. (1983). Personality and social resources in stress resistance. *Journal of Personality and Social Psychology, 45*(4), 839-850.

137. Leigh, J. P., Tancredi, D. J., & Kravitz, R. L. (2009). Physician career satisfaction within specialties. *BMC Health Services Research, 9*(1), 166.

138. Manojlovich, M. (January 31, 2007). Power and empowerment in nursing: Looking backward to inform the future. *OJIN: The Online Journal of Issues in Nursing, 12*(1), Manuscript 1.

139. RQ Health. (2012). A Roadmap for trust: Enhancing physician engagement. *Canadian Policy Network*. Kaissi, A

140. Senge, P. M. (2006). *The fifth discipline: the art and practice of the learning organization* (Rev and updated, ed.). London: Random House Business.

141. Kaiser Permanente. The health benefits of exercise. *Sports Medicine Winter Summit*. Sallis, R.

142. Jones, J., & Pfeiffer, J. W. (1973). *Annual Handbook for Group Facilitators*. San Diego, CA: Pfeiffer & Company.
143. Coleman, K. J., Ngor, E., Reynolds, K., Quinn, V. P., Koebnick, C., Young, D. R., et al. (2012). Initial validation of an exercise "vital sign" in electronic medical records. *Medicine & Science in Sports & Exercise, 44*(11), 2071-2076.
144. Bauer, J. J., Mcadams, D. P., & Sakaeda, A. R. (2005). Crystallization of desire and crystallization of discontent in narratives of life-changing decisions. *Journal of Personality, 73*(5), 1181-1214.
145. Colquhoun, D., & Novella, S. P. (2013). Acupuncture is theatrical placebo. *Anesthesia & Analgesia, 116*(6), 1360-1363.
146. Sierpina, V. S., & Frenkel, M. A. (2005). Acupuncture: A Clinical review. *Southern Medical Journal, 98*(3), 330-337.
147. Colquhoun, D. (2007). What to do about CAM?. *BMJ, 335*(7623), 736-736.
148. Senge, P. M. (2006). *The fifth discipline: the art and practice of the learning organization* (Rev and updated, ed.). London: Random House Business.
149. Pajouhesh, H., & Lenz, G. R. (2005). Medicinal chemical properties of successful central nervous system drugs. *NeuroRx, 2*(4), 541-553.
150. Press Release. (2013). High rates of unnecessary prescribing of antibiotics for sore throat and bronchitis observed across the United States. *Brigham and women's hospital*. Retrieved July 17, 2014, from http://www.brighamandwomens.org/about_bwh/publicaffairs/news/pressreleases/PressRelease.aspx?PageID=1566
151. Greenhough, A., Smartt, H. J., Moore, A. E., Roberts, H. R., Williams, A. C., Paraskeva, C., et al. (2009). The COX-2/PGE2 pathway: key roles in the hallmarks of cancer and adaptation to the tumour microenvironment. *Carcinogenesis, 30*(3), 377-386.
152. Bonetti, P. (2003). Statin effects beyond lipid lowering—are they clinically relevant?. *European Heart Journal, 24*(3), 225-248.
153. Muehlhan, M., Marxen, M., Landsiedel, J., Malberg, H., & Zaunseder, S. (2014). The effect of body posture on cognitive performance: a question of sleep quality. *Frontiers in Human Neuroscience, 8*, 171.
154. Berwick D. (2009). What 'patient-centered' should mean: confessions of an extremist. *Health Affairs (Millwood). 28*(4):w555-65.
155. Davis, K., Schoenbaum, S. C., & Audet, A. (2005). A 2020 vision of patient-centered primary care. *Journal of General Internal Medicine, 20*(10), 953-957.
156. Carroll, D. L. (1995). The importance of self-efficacy expectations in elderly patients recovering from coronary artery bypass surgery. *Heart & Lung: The Journal of Acute and Critical Care, 24*(1), 50-59.
157. Katz, D. (2014, May 2). A Holistic view of evidence-based medicine: Of horse, cart and whip. *The Huffington Post*. Retrieved July 21, 2014, from http://www.huffingtonpost.com/david-katz-md/healthy-living-news_b_5249309.html
158. Albert, R. S. (1992). *Genius and eminence* (2nd ed.). Oxford: Pergamon Press. (this should be the quote double check
159. Towers Watson. (2010). Raising the bar on health care: Moving beyond incremental change. *National Business Group on Health*. Helke S.
160. Albert, Robert S. Genius and eminence. 2nd ed. Oxford: Pergamon Press, 1992. Print.
161. Cooperrider, D. L., & Whitney, D. K. (2005). *Appreciative inquiry a positive revolution in change*. San Francisco, CA: Berrett-Koehler.
162. Stewart M. (2001). Towards a global definition of patient centred care. *BMJ. 322*(7284):444-5.
163. Stewart M, Brown JB, Weston WW, Freeman TR. *Patient-centered medicine: Transforming the clinical method*. 2nd ed. United Kingdom: Radcliffe Medical Press; 2003.
164. (2001). *Crossing the quality chasm a new health system for the 21st century*. Washington, D.C.: National Academy Press.
165. Scott, J. G., Cohen, D., Dicicco-Bloom, B., Miller, W. L., Stange, K. C., & Crabtree, B. F. (2008). Understanding healing relationships in primary care. *Annals of Family Medicine. 6*(4), 315–322.
166. Hsu, C., Phillips, W. R., Sherman, K. J., Hawkes, R., & Cherkin, D. C. (2008). Healing in primary care: A Vision shared by patients, physicians, nurses, and clinical staff. *The Annals of Family Medicine, 6*(4), 307-314.
167. Krumholz HM, Butler J, Miller J, et al. (1998). Prognostic importance of emotional support for elderly patients hospitalized with heart failure. *Circulation. 97*(10):958-964.
168. House JS, Landis KR, Umberson D. (1998) Social relationships and health. *Science. 241*(4865):540-545.
169. Mohammadi E, Abedi HA, Jalali F, Gofranipour F, Kazemnejad A. (2006). Evaluation of 'partnership care model' in the control of hyperten- sion. *Intwenational Journal of Nursing Practice. 12*(3):153-159.
170. Kaplan SH, Greenfield S, Ware JE Jr. (1989). Assessing the effects of physician-patient interactions on the outcomes of chronic disease. *Medical Care. 27*(3)(Suppl):S110-S127.
171. Greenfield S, Kaplan SH, Ware JE Jr, Yano EM, Frank HJ. (1988). Patients' participation in medical care: effects on blood sugar control and quality of life in diabetes. *Journal of General Internal Medicine. 3*(5):448-457.

Bibliography

172. Beecher, H. K. (1955). The Powerful Placebo. *JAMA: The Journal of the American Medical Association, 159*(17), 1602-1606

173. Kirsch, I., Moore, T. J., Scoboria, A., & Nicholls, S. S. (2002). The emperor's new drugs: An analysis of antidepressant medication data submitted to the U.S. Food and Drug Administration. *Prevention & Treatment, 5*(1).

174. Mayberg, H. S. (2002). The Functional Neuroanatomy of the Placebo Effect. *American Journal of Psychiatry, 159*(5), 728-737.

175. Tai-Seale MMcGuire TZhang W. (2007) Time allocation in primary care visits. *Health Services Research Journal. 42*(5) 1871- 1894

176. Ogden, C., Carroll, M., Kit, B., & Flegal, K. (2014). Prevalence of childhood and adult obesity in the United States, 2011-2012. *JAMA, 311*(8), 806-14.

177. Green, M., G. Makuos, and A. Zick. (2007). An Evidence-based perspective on greetings in medical encounters. *Archives of Internal Medicine, 167*: 1172-76

178. Beckman, H. B. (1984). The Effect of Physician Behavior on the Collection of Data. *Annals of Internal Medicine, 101*(5), 692.

179. Dyche, L., & Swiderski, D. (2005). The effect of physician solicitation approaches on ability to identify patient concerns. *Journal of General Internal Medicine, 20*(3), 267-270.

180. Pennebaker, J. W., & Chung, C. K. (in press). Expressive writing and its links to mental and physical health. In H. S. Friedman (Ed.), Oxford handbook of health psychology. New York, NY: Oxford University Press.

181. Pennebaker, J.W., & Keough, K.A. (1999). Revealing, organizing, and reorganizing the self in response to stress and emotion. In R. Ashmore and L. Jussim (Eds.), *Self and Social Identity: 2*: 101-121. New York: Oxford.

182. Klein, K., & Boals, A. (2001). Expressive writing can increase working memory capacity. Journal of Experimental Psychology: General, 130(3), 520-533.

183. (2009). Executive Summary: Standards of Medical Care in Diabetes--2010. *Diabetes Care, 33*(Supplement_1), S4-S10.

184. Eisenthal SE, Emery R, Lazare A, Udin H. (1979). "Adherence" and the negotiated approach to patienthood. *Arch gen psychiatry. 36*:393-398.

185. Hojat, M., Vergare, M. J., Maxwell, K., Brainard, G., Herrine, S. K., Isenberg, G. A., et al. (2009). The Devil Is In The Third Year: A Longitudinal Study Of Erosion Of Empathy In Medical School. *Academic Medicine, 84*(9), 1182-1191.

186. Kempe, C. H., Silverman, F. N., Steele, B. F., Droegemueller, W., & Silver, H. K. (1962). The Battered-Child Syndrome. *Journal of the American Medical Association, 181*, 17-24.

187. Reyes-Morales, H., Flores-Hernández, S., Tomé-Sandoval, P., & Pérez-Cuevas, R. (2009). A multifaceted education intervention for improving family physicians' case management. Family Medicine, 41(4), 277-84.

188. ISRN Psychiatry Volume 2014 Article ID 375439

189. Rakel, D. P. (2009). Number 406, "Standard". Family Medicine, 41(4), 289-290.

190. Rollnick, S., Allison, J., Ballasiotes, S., Barth, T., Butler, C.C., Rose, G.S., and Rosengren, D.B. (2002). Variations on a theme: Motivational interviewing and its adaptations. In W. R. Miller & S. Rollnick, Motivational interviewing: Preparing people for change (2nd ed. pp.). New York: Guilford Press.

191. Miller, W. R., & Rollnick, S. (2002). Motivational interviewing: preparing people for change (2nd ed.). New York: Guilford Press.

192. Pew Internet. (2012). Mobile Health 2012. Washington, D.C., Fox, S., and Duggan, M.

193. AAFP Policies. (n.d.). *AAFP.org.* Retrieved September 30, 2014, from http://www.aafp.org/about/policies

194. Virginia, A. (2004). Peripheral Arterial Disease in People With Diabetes. *Clinical Diabetes, 22*(4), 181-189.

195. Chobanian AV, Bakris GL, Black HR, et al. (2008). The Seventh Report of the Joint National Committee on Prevention, Detection, Evaluation, and Treatment of High Blood Pressure: the JNC 7 report. *JAMA. 289*: 2560–2572.

196. Steinberg BA, Bhatt DL, Mehta S et al. (2008). Nine-year trends in achievement of risk factor goals in the US and European outpatients with cardiovascular disease. *American Heart Journal. 156*(4): 719-27.

197. Number of Americans with Diabetes Projected to Double or Triple by 2050. (2010, October 22). *Centers for Disease Control and Prevention.* Retrieved September 15, 2014, from http://www.cdc.gov/media/pressrel/2010/r101022.html

198. Saydah SH, Fradkin J, Cowie CC. (2004). Poor control of risk factors for vascular disease among adults with previously diagnosed diabetes. *JAMA. 291*: 335–342.

199. Witters, D., & Agrawal, S. (2011, October 17). Unhealthy U.S. Workers' Absenteeism Costs $153 Billion. *Gallup Well-Being.* Retrieved September 15, 2014, from http://www.gallup.com/poll/150026/unhealthy-workers-absenteeism-costs-153-billion.aspx

200. Mokdad AH, Marks JS, Stroup DF, et al. (2004). Actual causes of death in the United States, 2000. *JAMA. 291*(10): 1238-45.

201. Katz DL. (2002). Effective dietary counseling: helping patients find and follow "the way" to eat. *The Journal of West Virginia State Medical Association, 98*(6): 256-9.

202. Senthilvel, E., Auckley, D., & Dasarathy, J. (2011). Evaluation of Sleep Disorders in the Primary Care Setting: History Taking Compared to Questionnaires. *Journal of Clinical Sleep Medicine, 7*(1), 41-48.

203. Dumitrascu, R., Heitmann, J., Seeger, W., Weissmann, N., & Schulz, R. (2013). Obstructive Sleep Apnea, Oxidative Stress and Cardiovascular Disease: Lessons from Animal Studies. *Oxidative Medicine and Cellular Longevity*, 1-7.

204. Greenberg, H., Ye, X., Wilson, D., Htoo, A. K., Hendersen, T., & Liu, S. F. (2006). Chronic intermittent hypoxia activates nuclear factor-αB in cardiovascular tissues in vivo. *Biochemical and Biophysical Research Communications, 343*(2), 591-596.

205. Roth, T. (2007). Insomnia: Definition, Prevalence, Etiology, and Consequences. *Journal of Clinical Sleep Medicine, 3*(5 Suppl), S7-S10.

206. Posnick, J. C. (2013). *Orthognathic surgery: principles & practice.* St. Louis, Missouri: Elsevier Health Sciences.

207. BCC Research. (2014). *Sleep Aids: Technologies and Global Markets.*

208. Ohayon, M. M., O'Hara, R., & Vitiello, M. V. (2012). Epidemiology of restless legs syndrome: A synthesis of the literature. *Sleep Medicine Reviews, 16*(4), 283-295.

209. Vogt, T., Ilis, . H., Lichtenstein, E., Stevens, V., Glasgow, R., & Whitlock, E. (1998). The medical care system and prevention: the need for a new paradigm. *HMO Practice, 12*(1), 5-13.

210. Cummings, N. A., Cummings, J. L., Johnson, J. N., & Baker, N. J. (1997). *Behavioral health in primary care: a guide for clinical integration.* Madison, Conn.: Psychosocial Press.

211. Westmaas, J. L., Alcaraz, K. I., Berg, C. J., & Stein, K. D. (2014). Prevalence and Correlates of Smoking and Cessation-Related Behavior among Survivors of Ten Cancers: Findings from a Nationwide Survey Nine Years after Diagnosis. *Cancer Epidemiology, Biomarkers & Prevention, 1*, Online.

212. Ashley, J. M. (2001). Weight Control in the Physician's Office. *Archives of Internal Medicine, 161*(13), 1599-1604.

213. Greenlund, K. J. (2002). Physician Advice, Patient Actions, and Health-Related Quality of Life in Secondary Prevention of Stroke Through Diet and Exercise * The Physician's Role in Helping Patients to Increase Physical Activity and Improve Eating Habits. *Stroke, 33*(2), 565-571.

214. McAvoy B, Kaner E, Lock C, et al. (1999). Our healthier nation: are general practitioners willing and able to deliver? *The British Journal of General Practice, 49*;187-190.

215. Potter M, Vu J, Croughan-Minihane M. (2001). Weight management: what patients want from their primary care physicians. *The Journal of Family Practice, 50*: 513-518.

216. Ruggiero L, Rossi J, Prochaska J, et al. (1999). Smoking and diabetes: readiness for change and provider advice. *Addictive Behaviors, 24*: 573-578.

217. Thomas R, Kottke T, Brekke M, et al. (2002). Attempts at changing dietary and exercise habits to reduce risk of cardiovascular disease: who's doing what in the community? *Preventative Cardiology, 5*: 102-108.

218. Sciamanna, C. N. (2000). Who Reports Receiving Advice to Lose Weight?: Results From a Multistate Survey. *Archives of Internal Medicine, 160*(15), 2334-2339.

219. Mehrotra C, Naimi TS, Serdula M, Bolen J, Pearson K. (2004). Arthritis, body mass index, and professional advice to lose weight: implications for clinical medicine and public health. *American Journal of Preventative Medicine, 27*(1):16-21

220. Loureiro, M. L., & Nayga, R. M. (2006). Obesity, weight loss, and physician's advice. *Social Science & Medicine, 62*(10), 2458-2468.

221. Abid A, Galuska D, Khan LK et al. (2005). Are healthcare professionals advising obese patients to lose weight? *A trend analysis. Medscape General Medicine, 7*(4):10.

222. Fontaine, K. R., Haaz, S., & Bartlett, S. J. (2007). Are Overweight and Obese Adults With Arthritis Being Advised to Lose Weight?. *JCR: Journal of Clinical Rheumatology, 13*(1), 12-15.

223. Halm J, Amoako E. (2008). Physical activity recommendation for hypertension management: does healthcare provider advice make a difference? *Ethnicity and Disease, 18*(3):278-82.

224. Wing, R. R., & Phelan, S. (2005). Long-term weight loss maintenance. *The American Journal of Clinical Nutrition, 82*(1), 222S-225S.

225. Tanoue, L. (2012). Quitting Smoking Among Adults — United States, 2001–2010. *Yearbook of Pulmonary Disease,* 2012, 72-74.

226. Prochaska, J. O., & Diclemente, C. C. (1986). *Toward a Comprehensive Model of Change.* US: Springer.

227. Department of Health. (2007). A Review of the use of the Health Belief Model (HBM), the Theory of Reasoned Action (TRA), the Theory of Planned Behaviour (TPB) and the Trans-Theoretical Model (TTM) to study and predict health related behavior change. *National Institute for Health and Clinical Excellence.* Taylor, D., Bury, M., Campling, N., Carter, S., Garfied, S., Newbound, J., and Rennie, T.

228. Healthcare 411. (n.d.). *Five Major Steps to Intervention (The "5 A's").* Retrieved September 16, 2014, from http://www.ahrq.gov/professionals/clinicians-providers/guidelines-recommendations/tobacco/5steps.html

Bibliography

229. Morris, J. N., & Crawford, M. D. (1958). Coronary Heart Disease and Physical Activity of Work. *BMJ,2*(5111), 1485-1496.
230. Centers for Disease Control and Prevention. (2012) Summary health statistics for U.S. adults: National Health Interview Survey, 2010. Hyattsville, MD: National Center for Health Statistics. *Vital and Health Statistics, 10.*
231. NIH. Clinical Guidelines on the Identification, Evaluation, and Treatment of Overweight and Obesity in Adults. *Obesity Education Initiative.* NHLBI.
232. Warren, T. Y., Barry, V., Hooker, S. P., Sui, X., Church, T. S., & Blair, S. N. (2010). Sedentary Behaviors Increase Risk of Cardiovascular Disease Mortality in Men. *Medicine & Science in Sports & Exercise, 42*(5), 879-885.
233. Laverty, A. A., Mindell, J. S., Webb, E. A., & Millett, C. (2013). Active Travel to Work and Cardiovascular Risk Factors in the United Kingdom. *American Journal of Preventive Medicine, 45*(3), 282-288.
234. Frank, E. (2000). Correlates of Physicians' Prevention-Related Practices: Findings From the Women Physicians' Health Study. *Archives of Family Medicine, 9*(4), 359-367.
235. Frank E, Schelbert KB, Elon LK. (2003). Exercise Counseling and Personal Exercise Habits of US Women Physicians. *JAMA, 58*:178-184.
236. Recio-Rodríguez, J. I., Gómez-Marcos, M. A., García-Ortiz, L., Rodriguez-Sanchez, E., Pérez-Arechaederra, D., Maderuelo-Fernandez, J. A., et al. (2014). Effectiveness of a smartphone application for improving healthy lifestyles, a randomized clinical trial (EVIDENT II): study protocol. *BMC Public Health, 14*(1), 254.
237. (2010). Tackling overweight and obesity. In Healthy weight, healthy lives: A toolkit for developing local strategies. *Faculty of Public Health. UK.*
238. Seven Day Physical Activity Recall (PAR). (n.d.). *PAQ database.* Retrieved September 30, 2014, from http://appliedresearch.cancer.gov/paq/q094.html
239. (2008). Creating a Clinical Screening Questionnaire for Eating Behaviors Associated with Overweight and Obesity. *Journal of the American Board of Family Medicine, 21.*
240. National Heart, Lung, and Blood Institute and North American Association for the Study of Obesity. (2000). The *Practical Guide to the Identification, Evaluation, and Treatment of Overweight and Obesity in Adults.* National Institutes of Health
241. Recio-Rodríguez, J. I., Gómez-Marcos, M. A., García-Ortiz, L., Rodriguez-Sanchez, E., Pérez-Arechaederra, D., Maderuelo-Fernandez, J. A., et al. (2014). Effectiveness of a smartphone application for improving healthy lifestyles, a randomized clinical trial (EVIDENT II): study protocol.*BMC Public Health, 14*(1), 254.
242. Senthilvel, E., Auckley, D., & Dasarathy, J. (2011). Evaluation of Sleep Disorders in the Primary Care Setting: History Taking Compared to Questionnaires. *Journal of Clinical Sleep Medicine, 7*, 41-48.
243. Cohen, S., Kamarck, T., & Mermelstein, R. (1983). A Global Measure of Perceived Stress. *Journal of Health and Social Behavior, 24*(4), 385.
244. Cohen, S., & Williamson, G. M. (1988). Perceived Stress in a Probability Sample of the United States.*The Social Psychology of Health* (pp. 31-67). Newbury Park, CA: SAGE Publications, Inc
245. McNair, D. M. (2012). Profile of Mood States, *POMS2* (Second ed.). North Tonawanda, N.Y.: Multi-Health Systems Inc.
246. Stress Management, Stress Management Tools, Stress Relief, Stress Reduction, Institute of HeartMath. (n.d.). *Stress Management, Stress Management Tools, Stress Relief, Stress Reduction, Institute of HeartMath.* Retrieved October 1, 2014, from http://www.heartmath.org/templates/ihm/applets/survey/index.php?data=84
247. RAND Health. (2013). *Workplace Wellness Programs Study.* RAND Corporation. Mattke S., Liu H., Caloyeras J.P., Huang C.Y., Van Busum, K.R., Khodyakov, D., & Shier, V.
248. Schneider, R. H., Grim, C. E., Rainforth, M. V., Kotchen, T., Nidich, S. I., Gaylord-King, C., et al. (2012). Stress Reduction in the Secondary Prevention of Cardiovascular Disease: Randomized, Controlled Trial of Transcendental Meditation and Health Education in Blacks. *Circulation: Cardiovascular Quality and Outcomes, 5*(6), 750-758.
249. Seifert, C. M., Chapman, L. S., Hart, J. K., & Perez, P. (2012). Enhancing Intrinsic Motivation in Health Promotion and Wellness. *American Journal of Health Promotion, 26*(3), TAHP-1-TAHP-12.
250. Family Practice Management. (2012). *Medicare Annual Wellness Visits: Don't Forget the Health Risk Assessment.* Hughs, C.
251. Lee, D., Pate, R. R., Lavie, C. J., Sui, X., Church, T. S., & Blair, S. N. (2014). Leisure-Time Running Reduces All-Cause and Cardiovascular Mortality Risk. *Journal of the American College of Cardiology, 64*, 472-481.
252. Ulrich, P. (2001). Protein Glycation, Diabetes, and Aging. *Recent progress in hormone research, 56*(1), 1-22.
253. Major Crops Grown in the United States. (n.d.). *EPA.* Retrieved September 29, 2014, from http://www.epa.gov/agriculture/ag101/cropmajor.html
254. Lianov, L., & Johnson, M. (2010). Physician Competencies for Prescribing Lifestyle Medicine. *JAMA: The Journal of the American Medical Association, 304*(2), 202-203.
255. Katz, D., & Meller, S. (2014). Can We Say What Diet Is Best for Health?. *Annual Reviews, 35*, 83–103.
256. Bazzano, L. A., Hu, T., Reynolds, K., Yao, L., Bunol, C., Liu, Y., et al. (2014). Effects of Low-Carbohydrate and

Low-Fat Diets: A Randomized Trial. *Annals of Internal Medicine, 161*, 309-318.

257. (2013). Mediterranean Diet for Primary Prevention of Cardiovascular Disease. *New England Journal of Medicine, 369*(7), 672-677.

258. Kris-Etherton, P. M., Harris, W. S., & Appel, L. J. (2003). Omega-3 Fatty Acids and Cardiovascular Disease. *Arteriosclerosis, Thrombosis, and Vascular Biology., 23*, 151-152.

259. (2013). On The Hunt For Personalized Medicine. *Nutritional Business Journal, Sample Issue*, 4

260. The Institute for Functional Medicine. (2009). *21st Century Medicine: A New Model for Medical Education and Practice.* IFM. Jones, D.S., Hoffman, L., Quinn, S.

261. IMS Health Incorporated. (2013). *Top 20 Global Products of 2013.*

262. Hadhazy, A. (n.d.). Think Twice: How the Gut's "Second Brain" *Influences Mood and Well-Being.Scientific American Global RSS.* Retrieved October 1, 2014, from http://www.scientificamerican.com/article/gut-second-brain/

263. Zhu, B., Wang, X., & Li, L. (2010). Human gut microbiome: the second genome of human body. *Protein & Cell, 1*(8), 718-725.

264. Jacob, A. (2013, February). Gut Health and Autoimmune Disease- Research Suggests Digestive Abnormalities May Be the Underlying Cause. *Today's Dietitian, 15*, 38.

265. Fasano, A. (2008). Physiological, Pathological, and Therapeutic Implications of Zonulin-Mediated Intestinal Barrier Modulation. *The American Journal of Pathology, 173*(5), 1243-1252.

266. Intestinal Permeability: regulation of the mucosal immune system and intercellular tight junctions.. (n.d.). *Saint James Hospital Malta.* Retrieved October 1, 2014, from http://www.stjameshospital.com/site1/intestinal-permeability-regulation-of-the-mucosal-immune-system-and-intercellular-tight-junctions

267. SUMMARY REPORT On Antimicrobials Sold or Distributed for Use in Food-Producing Animals. (n.d.). *Federal Drug Administration.* Retrieved October 2, 2014, from http://www.fda.gov/downloads/ForIndustry/UserFees/AnimalDrugUserFeeActADUFA/UCM231851.pdf

268. Mark, H. (2007). The Role of Mercury and Cadmium Heavy Metals in Vascular Disease, Hypertension, Coronary Heart Disease, and Myocardial Infarction. *Alternative Therapies in Health and Medicine, 13*, S128-33.

269. Leading Causes of Death. (2014, July 14). *Centers for Disease Control and Prevention.* Retrieved September 29, 2014, from http://www.cdc.gov/nchs/fastats/leading-causes-of-death.htm

270. Budnitz, D. S., Pollock, D. A., Weidenbach, K. N., Mendelsohn, A. B., Schroeder, T. J., & Annest, J. L. (2006). National Surveillance Of Emergency Department Visits For Outpatient Adverse Drug Events.*JAMA: The Journal of the American Medical Association, 296*(15), 1858-1866.

271. Routledge, P. A., O'Mahony, M. S., & Woodhouse, K. W. (2004). Adverse Drug Reactions In Elderly Patients. *British Journal of Clinical Pharmacology, 57*(2), 121-126.

272. Woolf, A. D., Goldman, R., & Bellinger, D. C. (2007). Update on the Clinical Management of Childhood Lead Poisoning. *Pediatric Clinics of North America, 54*(2), 271-294.

273. Alissa, E. M., & Ferns, G. A. (2011). Heavy Metal Poisoning And Cardiovascular Disease. *Journal of Toxicology,* 1-21.

274. 2006-2007 Pesticide Market Estimates: Usage | Pesticides | US EPA. (n.d.). *EPA.* Retrieved October 4, 2014, from http://www.epa.gov/opp00001/pestsales/07pestsales/usage2007.htm

275. Gulf War Veterans' Medically Unexplained Illnesses. (n.d.). *U.S. Department of Veteran Affairs.* Retrieved October 4, 2014, from http://www.publichealth.va.gov/exposures/gulfwar/medically-unexplained-illness.asp

276. Why You Shouldn't Love That 'New Car Smell'. (n.d.). *EverydayHealth.com.* Retrieved October 4, 2014, from http://www.everydayhealth.com/green-health/1120/why-you-shouldnt-love-that-new-car-smell.aspx

277. Regulatory Information. (n.d.). *Federal Food, Drug, and Cosmetic Act* (FD&C Act). Retrieved October 2, 2014, from http://www.fda.gov/regulatoryinformation/legislation/FederalFoodDrugandCosmeticActFDCAct/default.htm

278. (2009). *The Military Metaphors of Modern Medicine.* Inter-Disciplinary.Net. Abraham Fuks.

279. Ross, R., & Glomset, J. (1976). The Pathogenesis of Atherosclerosis Pt. 1 of 2. *New England Journal of Medicine, 295*, 369-77.

280. Black, PH & Garbutt LD J Psychosom Res. 2002 Jan;52(1):1-23.

281. Morrow JD et al. Increase in circulating products of lipid peroxidation (F2-Isoprostanes) in smokers. Smoking as a cause of oxidative damage. N Engl J Med. 1995; 332: 1198-1203.

282. Tappel A. Heme of consumed red meat can act as a catalyst of oxidative damage and could initiate colon, breast and prostate cancers, heart disease and other diseases. Med Hypotheses. 2007; 68: 562-564.

283. Shi M et al. (2007). Effects of anaerobic exercise and aerobic exercise on biomarkers of oxidative stress. *Environmental Health and Preventative Medicine,. 12*: 202-208.

284. Holvoet, P., Lee, D., Steffes, M., Gross, M., & Jacobs, D. R. (2008). Association Between Circulating Oxidized Low-Density Lipoprotein and Incidence of the Metabolic Syndrome. *JAMA: The Journal of the American Medical Association, 299*(19), 2287-2293.

Bibliography

285. Holvoet, P., Mertens, A., Verhamme, P., Bogaerts, K., Beyens, G., Verhaeghe, R., et al. (2001). Circulating Oxidized LDL Is a Useful Marker for Identifying Patients With Coronary Artery Disease. *Arteriosclerosis, Thrombosis, and Vascular Biology, 21*(5), 844-848.

286. Serruys, P. W., Hutchinson, T., D'amico, D., Birgelen, C. V., Garcia-Garcia, H. M., Buszman, P., et al. (2008). Effects of the Direct Lipoprotein-Associated Phospholipase A2 Inhibitor Darapladib on Human Coronary Atherosclerotic Plaque. *Circulation, 118*(11), 1172-1182.

287. Meuwese, M. C., Khaw, K., Boekholdt, S. M., Kastelein, J. J., Luben, R., Wareham, N. J., et al. (2007). Serum Myeloperoxidase Levels Are Associated With the Future Risk of Coronary Artery Disease in Apparently Healthy Individuals. *Journal of the American College of Cardiology, 50*(2), 159-165.

288. Goldstein, M. R., & Mascitelli, L. (2013). Do Statins Cause Diabetes?. *Current Diabetes Reports, 13*(3), 381-390.

289. Lipitor (Atorvastatin Calcium) Drug Information: Side Effects and Drug Interactions - Prescribing Information at *RxList*. (n.d.). RxList. Retrieved October 5, 2014, from http://www.rxlist.com/lipitor-drug/side-effects-interactions.htm

290. The science behind the Statin Induced Myopathy (SLCO1B1) Genotype. (n.d.). *Statin Induced Myopathy (SLCO1B1) Genotype*. Retrieved October 5, 2014, from http://www.bostonheartdiagnostics.com/science_portfolio_statin.php

291. Simpson, J. A., & Weiner, E. S. (1989). *The Oxford English dictionary* (2nd ed.). Oxford: Clarendon Press

292. Wenzel, S. E. (1998). Antileukotriene Drugs in the Management of Asthma. *JAMA: The Journal of the American Medical Association, 280*(24), 2068-2069.

293. Hui, K. K., Liu, J., Makris, N., Gollub, R. L., Chen, A. J., Moore, C. I., et al. (2000). Acupuncture Modulates The Limbic System And Subcortical Gray Structures Of The Human Brain: Evidence From FMRI Studies In Normal Subjects. *Human Brain Mapping, 9*(1), 13-25.

294. New Study Finds More Than 20 Million Yogis in U.S. - Yoga Journal. (n.d.). *Yoga Journal*. Retrieved October 5, 2014, from http://www.yogajournal.com/uncategorized/new-study-finds-20-million-yogis-u-s/

295. Diaz, A. M., Kolber, M. J., Patel, C. K., Pabian, P. S., Rothschild, C. E., & Hanney, W. J. (2013). The Efficacy of Yoga as an Intervention for Chronic Low Back Pain: A Systematic Review of Randomized Controlled Trials. *American Journal of Lifestyle Medicine, 7*(6), 418-430.

296. Okonta, N. R. (2012). Does Yoga Therapy Reduce Blood Pressure in Patients With Hypertension?. *Holistic Nursing Practice, 26*(3), 137-141.

297. Varambally, S., & Bangalore, N. (2012). Yoga therapy for Schizophrenia. *International Journal of Yoga, 5*(2), 85.

298. Yang, K. (2007). A Review Of Yoga Programs For Four Leading Risk Factors Of Chronic Diseases. *Evidence-based Complementary and Alternative Medicine, 4*(4), 487-491.

299. World Health Organization. (2000). *General Guidelines for Methodologies on Research and Evaluation of Traditional Medicine*. World Health Organization.

300. Ruston, J. (1971). Now, Let Me Tell You About My Appendectomy in Peking. *New York Times*, p. 1.

301. Redwood, D. (2010). Integrative Healthcare in Theory and Practice. *Pathways, 34*, 9.

302. Woolf, S. H. (2013). *U.S. health in international perspective: shorter lives, poorer health*. United States of America: the National Academy of Sciences.

303. Glucosamine/Chondroitin Arthritis Intervention Trial (GAIT). (n.d.). *NCCAM*. Retrieved October 5, 2014, from http://nccam.nih.gov/research/results/gait

304. (2002). Spinal Manipulation for Low Back Pain. *The Back Letter, 17*(8), 84.

305. 2012 Symposium. Cleveland HeartLab, Inc.. (n.d.). *Cleveland HeartLab Inc*. Retrieved October 5, 2014, from http://www.clevelandheartlab.com/2012-symposium/

306. Jennings, B. (2008). Work Stress and Burnout Among Nurses: Role of the Work Environment and Working Conditions. *Patient safety and quality: an evidence-based handbook for nurses* (pp. 671-682). Rockville, MD: Agency for Healthcare Research and Quality, U.S. Dept. of Health and Human Services.

307. Fletcher, C. E. (2001). Hospital RNs Job Satisfactions and Dissatisfactions. *JONA: The Journal of Nursing Administration, 31*(6), 324-331.

308. Vahey, D. C., Aiken, L. H., Sloane, D. M., Clarke, S. P., & Vargas, D. (2004). Nurse Burnout And Patient Satisfaction. *Medical Care, 42*(Suppl), II-57-II-66.

309. Galland, L. (2012). GERD as a Motility Disorder: A New Way of Thinking. *Alternative and Complementary Therapies, 18*(6), 292-296.

310. Naturopathic Medicine. (n.d.). *Corporate Wellness Programs*. Retrieved October 5, 2014, from https://www.mind-bodyexchange.com/disciplines/naturopathic-medicine/view

311. Compton, W. D., Fanjiang, G., Grossman, J. H., & Reid, P. P. (2005). *Building a better delivery system a new engineering/health care partnership*. Washington, D.C.: National Academies Press.

312. Mariano, C. (2007). *Holistic nursing: scope and standards of practice*. Silver Spring, Md.: American Holistic Nurses Association.

313. Miller, M., Mazzone, T., Bittner, V., Ballantyne, C., Stone, N. J., Pennathur, S., et al. (2011). Triglycerides and Cardiovascular Disease: A Scientific Statement From the American Heart Association. *Circulation, 123*(20), 2292-2333.

314. Hughes, R. (2008). *Patient safety and quality: an evidence-based handbook for nurses*. Rockville, MD: Agency for Healthcare Research and Quality, U.S. Dept. of Health and Human Services.

315. Vahey, D. C., Aiken, L. H., Sloane, D. M., Clarke, S. P., & Vargas, D. (2004). Nurse Burnout And Patient Satisfaction. *Medical Care, 42*(Suppl), II-57-II-66.

316. Jain, S., Mcmahon, G. F., Hasen, P., Kozub, M. P., Porter, V., King, R., et al. (2012). Healing Touch With Guided Imagery for PTSD in Returning Active Duty Military: A Randomized Controlled Trial. *Military Medicine, 177*(9), 1015-1021.

317. Wilkinson, D. S., Knox, P. L., Chatman, J. E., Johnson, T. L., Barbour, N., Myles, Y., et al. (2002). The Clinical Effectiveness Of Healing Touch. *Journal of Alternative and Complementary Medicine, 8*(1), 33-47.

318. MacIntyre, B., Hamilton, J., Fricke, T., Ma, W., Mehle, S., & Michel, M. (2008). The efficacy of healing touch in coronary artery bypass surgery recovery: a randomized clinical trial. *Alternatibe Therapies in Health and Medicine, 14*(4), 24-32.

319. Chronic Fatigue In-Depth Report. (2012, February 7). *New York Times*. Retrieved October 5, 2014, from http://www.nytimes.com/health/guides/disease/chronic-fatigue-syndrome/print.html

320. Olmos, P., A'hern, R., Heaton, D. A., Millward, B. A., Risley, D., Pyke, D. A., et al. (1988). The Significance of the concordance rate for Type 1 (insulin-dependent) diabetes in identical twins. *Diabetologia, 31*(10), 747-750.

321. Loke, Y. J., Saffery, R., Novakovic, B., Craig, J. M., Galati, J. C., Gordon, L., et al. (2013). The Peri/Postnatal Epigenetic Twins Study (PETS). *Twin Research and Human Genetics, 16*(01), 13-20.

322. Heyn, H., Spector, T. D., Gomez, A., Carmona, F. J., Esteller, M., Eyfjord, J. E., et al. (2013). DNA methylation profiling in breast cancer discordant identical twins identifies DOK7 as novel epigenetic biomarker. *Carcinogenesis, 34*(1), 102-108.

323. (2009). Errors in Funding/Support, Role of the Sponsor, and Additional Contributions in: Physical Activity and the Association of Common FTO Gene Variants With Body Mass Index and Obesity. *Archives of Internal Medicine, 169*(5), 453-453.

324. Ornish, D., Jacobs, F. N., Crutchfield, L., Dunn-Emke, S., Raisin, C. J., Pettengill, E. B., et al. (2005). Intensive Lifestyle Changes May Affect The Progression Of Prostate Cancer. *The Journal of Urology,174*(3), 1065-1070.

325. Samani, N. J., & Harst, P. V. (2008). Biological ageing and cardiovascular disease. *Heart, 94*(5), 537-539.

326. Mather, K. A., Jorm, A. F., Parslow, R. A., & Christensen, H. (2011). Is Telomere Length a Biomarker of Aging? A Review. *The Journals of Gerontology Series A: Biological Sciences and Medical Sciences ,66A*(2), 202-213.

327. Michou, L. (2011). Genetics of digital osteoarthritis. *Joint Bone Spine, 78*(4), 347-351.

328. Bartl, R., & Frisch, B. (2009). *Osteoporosis diagnosis, prevention, therapy* (2nd rev. ed.). Berlin: Springer.

329. Tollefsbol, T. O. (2007). *Biological aging: methods and protocols*. Totowa, N.J.: Humana Press.

330. Baughman, R. P., Carbone, R. G., & Bottino, G. (2009). *Pulmonary arterial hypertension and interstitial lung diseases a clinical guide*. New York: Humana Press.

331. Sturmberg, J. P. (2013). *Handbook of systems and complexity in health*. New York: Springer.

332. Gewirtz, D. A., & Grant, S. (2007). *Apoptosis, Senescence, and Cancer*. Totowa, NJ: Humana Press Inc

333. Epel, E., Daubenmier, J., Moskowitz, J. T., Folkman, S., & Blackburn, E. (2009). Can Meditation Slow Rate Of Cellular Aging? Cognitive Stress, Mindfulness, And Telomeres. *Annals of the New York Academy of Sciences, 1172*(1), 34-53.

334. (2014). Leucocyte telomere length and risk of cardiovascular disease: systematic review and meta-analysis. *British Medical Journal, 349*, g4227.

335. Kiecolt-Glaser, J. K., Gouin, J., Weng, N., Malarkey, W. B., Beversdorf, D. Q., & Glaser, R. (2011). Childhood Adversity Heightens the Impact of Later-Life Caregiving Stress on Telomere Length and Inflammation. *Psychosomatic Medicine, 73*(1), 16-22.

336. Krauss, J., Farzaneh-Far, R., Puterman, E., Na, B., Lin, J., Epel, E., et al. (2011). Physical Fitness and Telomere Length in Patients with Coronary Heart Disease: Findings from the Heart and Soul Study. *PLoS ONE, 6*(11), e26983.

337. Farzaneh-Far, R., Lin, J., Epel, E. S., Harris, W. S., Blackburn, E. H., & Whooley, M. A. (2010). Association of Marine Omega-3 Fatty Acid Levels With Telomeric Aging in Patients With Coronary Heart Disease. *JAMA: The Journal of the American Medical Association, 303*(3), 250-257.

338. Dansinger, M., Gleason, J., Griffith, J., Selker, H., & Schaefer, E. (2005). Comparison Of The Atkins, Ornish, Weight Watchers, And Zone Diets For Weight Loss And Heart Disease Risk Reduction: A Randomized Trial. *ACC Current Journal Review, 14*(2), 19-19.

339. Jacobs, T. L., Sahdra, B. K., Aichele, S. R., Zanesco, A. P., Bridwell, D. A., Wolkowitz, O. M., et al. (2010). Intensive Meditation Training, Immune Cell Telomerase Activity, And Psychological Mediators. *Psychoneuroendocrinology,306*, 1-18.

Bibliography

340. Puterman, E., & Epel, E. (2012). An Intricate Dance: Life Experience, Multisystem Resiliency, and Rate of Telomere Decline Throughout the Lifespan. *Social and Personality Psychology Compass, 6*(11), 807-825.

341. Klemes, A., Seligmann, R. E., Allen, L., Kubica, M. A., Warth, K., & Kaminetsky, B. (2012). Personalized preventive care leads to significant reductions in hospital utilization. *The American Journal of Mangaed Care, 18*(12), e453-e460.

342. Wald, D. S. (2013). The polypill and the prevention of heart attacks and strokes. *Future Cardiology, 9*(4), 465-466.

343. Casalino, L. P., Pesko, M. F., Ryan, A. M., Mendelsohn, J. L., Copeland, K. R., Ramsay, P. P., et al. (2014). Small Primary Care Physician Practices Have Low Rates Of Preventable Hospital Admissions. *Health Affairs, 10*, 1377.

344. ASAPS. (n.d.). *News Releases*. Retrieved October 1, 2014, from http://www.surgery.org/media/news-releases/the-american-society-for-aesthetic-plastic-surgery-reports-americans-spent-largest-amount-on-cosmetic-surge

345. Yang, W., Li, S., Weisel, R. D., Liu, S., & Li, R. (2012). Cell fusion contributes to the rescue of apoptotic cardiomyocytes by bone marrow cells. *Journal of Cellular and Molecular Medicine, 16*(12), 3085-3095

346. Marquez-Curtis, L. A., & Janowska-Wieczorek, A. (2013). Enhancing the migration ability of mesenchymal stromal cells by targeting the SDF-1/CXCR4 axis. *BioMed Research International, 2013*, 1-15

347. Patel, A. N., Geffner, L., Vina, R. F., Saslavsky, J., Urschel, H. C., Kormos, R., et al. (2005). Surgical treatment for congestive heart failure with autologous adult stem cell transplantation: A prospective randomized study. *The Journal of Thoracic and Cardiovascular Surgery, 130*(6), 1631-1638.e2.

348. Horie, M., Choi, H., Lee, R., Reger, R., Ylostalo, J., Muneta, T., et al. (2012). Intra-articular injection of human mesenchymal stem cells (MSCs) promote rat meniscal regeneration by being activated to express Indian hedgehog that enhances expression of type II collagen. *Osteoarthritis and Cartilage,20*(10), 1197-1207.

349. Yelp. (n.d.). *Advertising*. Retrieved October 3, 2014, from https://biz.yelp.com/support/advertising

350. Strategic priorities and AAP initiatives 2013-2014. (n.d.). *American Academy of Pediatrics*. Retrieved October 2, 2014, from http://www.aap.org/en-us/Documents/Strategic_Priorities_and_AAP_Initiatives.pdf

351. WebMD. (2014). *Medscape EHR report 2014*. Medscape. Kane, L., Chesanow, N.

352. Parks Associates: Doctor-patient video consultations will nearly triple from 5.7 million in 2014 to over 16 million in 2015. (n.d.). *Parks Associates: Doctor-patient video consultations will nearly triple from 5.7 million in 2014 to over 16 million in 2015*. Retrieved October 1, 2014, from http://www.parksassociates.com/blog/article/chs-2014-pr10

INDEX OF INDIVIDUALS AND ORGANIZATIONS

A

Ablon, Glynis 37, 38, 39
Abrams, Donald 19
Abramson, Paul 142, 143
Akron General Health System 167, 307
Alman, Brian 248, 249
Alpert, Richard 58
Alviar, Carlos 67
American Academy of Cosmetic Surgery 251, 256
American Academy of Private Physicians 241
American College of Occupational and Environmental Medicine 243
Academic Consortium for Complementary and Alternative Health Care 214
Academy of Integrative Health & Medicine 205
American Board of Integrative Holistic Medicine 20, 39, 205
American College of Sports Medicine 80, 166
American Holistic Medical Association 20, 39, 205, 210
American Holistic Nurses Association 222
American Institute of Stress 25
American Medical Association 17, 80
American Society for Aesthetic Plastic Surgery 251
American Society for Laser Medicine and Surgery 251, 254
Anatara 110
Augmedix 314

B

Babitsky, Steve 289, 299, 300, 301, 302, 320
Baker, Dan 46
Bale, Brad 190, 191, 192, 193
Bauer, Jack 92, 93
Baumeister, Roy 90
Beecher, Henry Knowles 128
Belasco, James 139
Bengelsdorf, Steven 91, 92

INDEX

Benson, Herbert 58
Berman, Mark 175, 176, 177, 178, 256, 257, 258
Bernard, Claude 53
Best Medical Business Solution 252
Blackburn, Elizabeth 38
Blanchard, Ken 290
Blanchard, Marjorie 76, 77
Bland, Jeffrey 181, 182
Blue, Tom 241, 242
Blum, Susan 248, 249
Bochner, Stephen 301, 302
BodyLogicMD 263
Bormann, Jill 56, 57
Brandman, Craig 108
Bratman, Steven 172
Bravewell Collaborative 18
Brooks, Phillips 69

C

California Stem Cell Treatment Center 257, 258
Calure, Jonathan 270, 271
Canyon Ranch Health Resort 46
Cell Surgical Network 257, 258
Center for Medical Weight Loss 159
Chandra, Amitabh 28
Chesney, Margaret 217, 218, 219
Chopra, Deepak 275
Cleveland Clinic 17
Cleveland Heart Lab 192, 223
Cohen, Michael H. 252
Cohn, Ken 320
Craig, Jeffrey M. 228
CreateSpace 279
Crossover Health 116, 119, 120

D

DaVita 243

INDEX

DiClemente, Carlo 156
Dill, Diana 108
Dodson, John Dillingham 30
Doneen, Amy 191
Doucette, Jami 243, 244
Dunn, Elizabeth 46
Dunn, Michael 46

E

Eatwell 160
Emmons, Robert 49
Epel, Elissa 38

F

Fairfield Medical Center 54
Fasano, Alessio 184
Fitbit 161
Fitch, Starla 50, 68, 321
FON Therapeutics 272, 273
Frank, Jerome 128
Frankl, Viktor 62
Friedland, Daniel 113, 114, 115
Friedman, Meyer 218
FuelBand 161

G

Gandolf, Stewart 268, 269
Gateway Aesthetic Institute and Laser Center 254
George, Penny 18
Gersh, Felice 165
Gilbert, Dore 99, 100, 101
Gladd, Jeff 245, 246
Goodman, Ira 188
Google 270, 281, 282
Gravett, Linda 294
Greenspan, Roberta 240, 241
Grogan, Tom 257
Grosel, Gary 315, 316

INDEX

Guarneri Integrative Health Inc. 224
Gumpert, Peter 108
Gunderson Health System 54
Gupta, Sanjay 275

H

Habit Change Company 140
Hall, Jack 163
Halpern, Jodi 135
Hansen, Lornell 250, 251
Hart, Jane 225
HeartMath 51, 52, 53, 54, 55, 69
HelloHealth 246
Herskowitz, Ahvie 109, 110
Hoffman, Ron 272, 279, 280, 285
Hojat, Mohammadreza 134, 135
Holmes, Jr, Oliver Wendell 93
Holmes, Thomas 36
Houston, Mark 174, 175
Hughes, Kristi 133, 189, 190
Humes, Tahl 254
HydafacialMD 282
Hyman, Mark 63

I

InMedica 7
Institute for Functional Medicine 133, 181
Institute of Medicine 125, 213, 215
Itamar Medical 192

J

Jackson, Maia McCuiston 310, 311
Jacobs, Brad 247, 249
Jacobs, Nick 287
Jana, Laura 303, 304, 305
Joe, Jennifer 312, 313

Jones, C. Jessie 166
Jones, David 182, 190, 195
Jung, Carl 291

K

Kabat-Zinn, Jon 58
Kaplan, Jeff 140, 141
Katz, David 109, 171, 172, 173
King, Rauni Prittinen 224, 225
Kirsch, Irving 128
Klein, Jeff 251
Klemes, Andrea 239
Knope, Steve 247, 248
Kobasa, Suzanne 74
Kofman, Fred 77
Koniver, Craig 247, 249

L

Landa, Jen 261, 262, 263
Lander, Elliot 257
Lawson, Karen 146, 147, 148, 149
LazaDerm 250
Lemaire, Jane 54, 55
Lemanne, Dawn 273
Life Length 232
Linkner, Edward 47, 48
Lipsenthal, Lee 24, 89, 114
Loomis, Evart 205
Looney, Jerry 205
Low Dog, Tieraona 155, 169, 232

M

Mack, Christy 18
Maddi, Salvatore 74
Major, Ajay 297, 312
Manojlovich, Milisa 74
Mantra 55, 56, 57, 58
Martel, Yann 62

INDEX

Maryland Vein Professional 270
Meeker, William 219
McCraty, Rollin 69, 70
McCullough, Michael 49
McEvoy, Larry 85
McGarey, Gladys 205
MDVIP 237, 238, 239, 240, 242
Medical Fitness Association 166, 167
Medikan 258
Medi-Weightloss 284
Medstro 313
MedSynergies 28
Meller, Stephanie 172, 173
Meyers, Owen 159
Miller, William R. 137
Mirabile, James 284, 285
Miraglo Foundation 224, 226
ModernMed 243
Mushtaq, Romila 35, 36
Mymee 143

N

n1Health 241, 242
National Consortium for Credentialing of Health and Wellness Coaches 149
National Health Interview Survey 206
National Institutes of Health 105
Nightingale, Florence 222, 227
Noffsinger, Edward 144, 145

O

O'Donnell, Michael 69
Offit, Paul 16
Ofri, Danielle 33
One Medical Group 175, 178
Ornish, Dean 225, 229, 231
Osher Center for Integrative Medicine 217

P

Pacific Pearl 224, 226
Paladina Health 243, 244
Pasteur, Louis 188
Patient Centered Medical Home 107
Pearl, Robert 29
Pennebaker, James 134
Penn, Marc 239
Permanente Medical Group 29
Pew Research 142
Pollan, Michael 64
Porter, Michael 118
Primary Care Medical Home 125
Prittinen King, Rauni 225, 226, 227
Prochaska, James 156
Puterman, Eli 231

R

Rahe, Richard 36
Rakel, David 136, 137
Randall, David 53
Reisinger, Alan 236, 237, 238, 239, 240
Rapid Recert 316
Reston, James 211
Ribley, Douglas 167
Rikli, Roberta E. 166
Robbins, Lewis 163
Roberts, Molly 212
Roga, Alan 318, 319
Rollnick, Stephen 137, 138
Rosenman, Ray 218
Ross, Russell 191
Rutchik, Jonathan 301

S

Sabin, Glenn 272, 273
Sallis, Robert 80, 81, 82
Saxena, Shilpa 199, 200, 201, 202

INDEX

Scott, John Glenn 126, 129, 127, 128, 131
SEAK 298, 299, 320, 332
Seligman, Martin 50
Selye, Hans 30, 34
Senge, Peter 77
Shakil, Ian 313
Shannon, Scott 272
Sharp HealthCare 83
Sharp Rees-Stealy Medical group 83
Shealy, Norm 205
Shorr, Jay 252
Shreeve, Scott 116, 117, 118, 119, 120
Silvestri, Sylvia 253
Smuts, Jan 205
Snider, Pamela 214, 215, 216
Sobel, David 59, 60, 61
Society of Physician Entrepreneurs 20
SottoPelle 285
Spector, Tim 228
Stat Doctors 318, 319
Stauth, Cameron 112
Stayer, Ralph 139
StepOne Health 108
Stewart, Moira 125
Stitcher 280
Stone, Leslie 195, 196, 198, 199
Stone, Michael 195
Stover, Tim 307, 308, 310
SuperSmartHealth 113
Survey Monkey 268

T

TED talks 275
Teisberg, Elizabeth 118
Telehealth 7, 8
The Integrator Blog News & Reports 216
Throckmorton, Robin 294
Tran, Pelu 313
Tygenhof, Bob 165

V

Veterans Administration 17
Virgin, JJ 274, 275

W

Weeks, John 214, 215, 216, 217
Weil, Andrew 243
Wisneski, Leonard 111, 210, 211, 212, 213, 214
Women's Health Initiative 160
Wong, Hansie 42
World Health Organization 209
Wrzesniewski, Amy 79, 80
Wu, Alan 259, 260, 261

Y

Yale University Prevention Research Center 109
Yamanaka, Shinya 254
Yelp 281, 282
Yerkes, Robert 30
Yoga Journal 208
Yogi, Maharishi Mahesh 56

Z

Zayas, Maria 70
Zink, J. Gordon 211

About the Authors

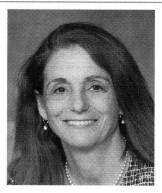

Mimi Guarneri, MD

Dr. Guarneri is board-certified in cardiovascular disease, internal medicine, nuclear medicine and holistic medicine, Dr. Guarneri is President of the American Board of Integrative Holistic Medicine, the Academy of Integrative Health and Medicine, and is Senior Advisor to the Atlantic Health System for the Center for Well Being and Integrative Medicine. Dr. Guarneri also is founder and director of Guarneri Integrative Health, Inc at Pacific Pearl La Jolla. Her medical degree is from SUNY Medical Center in New York, where she graduated number one in her class. Dr. Guarneri served her internship and residency at Cornell Medical Center, where she later became chief medical resident, and then cardiology fellowships at both New York University Medical Center and Scripps Clinic.

Dr. Guarneri began her career at Scripps Clinic as an attending in interventional cardiology, where she placed thousands of coronary stents. Recognizing the need for a more comprehensive and holistic approach to cardiovascular disease, she founded the Scripps Center for Integrative Medicine where state-of-the-art cardiac imaging technology and lifestyle change programs are used to aggressively diagnose, prevent and treat cardiovascular disease. Dr. Guarneri served as SCIM's Medical Director for 15 years.

To mention just a few of Dr. Guarneri's recognitions, awards and acknowledgements, she was honored in 2009 as the ARCS scientist of the year and in 2011, she won the Bravewell Leadership Award, which honors a physician leader who has made significant contributions to the transformation of the U.S. healthcare system. She was honored in 2008 by Project Concern International for her work in Southern India. In 2012, she received the Linus Pauling Functional

Medicine Lifetime Achievement Award from the Institute for Functional Medicine and the Grace A. Goldsmith award from the American College of Nutrition acknowledging a scientist for significant achievements in the field of nutrition.

Dr. Guarneri is the author of *The Heart Speaks* (Simon & Schuster 2007), a poignant collection of stories from heart patients who have benefited from integrative medicine. *The Heart Speaks* and Dr. Guarneri's clinical work were featured in a two-part PBS documentary, The New Medicine, on NBC's Today Show, and in PBS's To the Contrary and Full Focus. *The Heart Speaks* also was optioned for a scripted television series.

Dr. Guarneri is a much sought-after speaker who lectures internationally. Twenty four of her lectures were published as a Great Course, The Science of Natural Healing, in 2012.

Dr. Guarneri also has authored many articles that have appeared in professional journals such as the Journal of Echocardiography and the Annals of Internal Medicine and she is regularly quoted in national publications such as the Yoga Journal, Body+Soul, Trustee magazine and WebMD. Dr. Guarneri participated as a member of the writing committee for the American College of Cardiology Foundation. Dr. Guarneri also served on an advisory panel for the Institute of Medicine to explore the science and practice of integrative medicine for promoting the nation's health.

She is a fellow member of the American College of Cardiology, Alpha Omega Alpha, the American Medical Women's Association, and a diplomat of the American Board of Holistic Medicine.

ABOUT THE AUTHORS

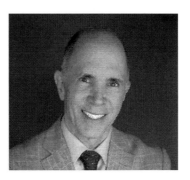

Mark J. Tager, MD.

Dr. Tager is CEO of San-Diego based ChangeWell Inc., (www.changewell.com) a training and consulting company that guides organizations and individuals to higher levels of health and performance. Dr. Tager brings a rich background to his work in leadership, organizational development and personal wellbeing. As an entrepreneur, he has built successful businesses and managed high performance teams. As a consultant and change agent, he has worked with a broad spectrum of organizations, from Fortune 100 companies to small non-profits. As a physician, he understands the unique dynamic that is at the center of health and wellbeing.

Dr. Tager's business career was founded on a passion for health promotion and disease prevention. As a medical student at Duke University Medical Center, he created one of the first training programs for medical students in nutrition. During medical school, he also spent time training promotores de salud (barefoot doctors) in the mountains of Guatemala. During his tenure in Portland Oregon, he founded one of the first integrative medicine centers in the US, the Institute of Preventive Medicine, in 1977. He also served as corporate Medical Director for Electroscientific Industries (NASDAQ: ESIO) and as Director of Health Promotion for Kaiser Permanente Oregon. Early in his career he wrote a syndicated newspaper column on wellness, produced videos and films, and authored books on health promotion.

In the mid 1980s, Dr. Tager founded a consumer health and medical publishing company that he ran for ten years before it was acquired by Mosby Yearbook, a Times Mirror Company. As VP of

Business Development for Mosby Consumer Health, he oversaw the acquisition of five companies as well as the design and deployment of wellness programs for major corporations, hospitals, HMOs, and non-profits.

Dr. Tager has served as the founding Vice President of Marketing for Reliant Technologies (NASDAQ: SLTM), where he launched the Fraxel® laser and introduced the science of fractional photothermolysis to physicians around the world. He then served as Chief Marketing Officer for Syneron (NASDAQ: ELOS) where he was responsible for corporate positioning, public and luminary relations, and new product launches.

Most recently he has been involved in training and consulting projects in aesthetics, stem cells, medical malpractice prevention, skincare, and advanced cardiac biomarkers. In addition to *Total Engagement*, Dr. Tager is the author of eight books on health promotion, aesthetics, leadership, stress and change management. He received his undergraduate and medical degrees from Duke University and trained in Family Practice at the University of Oregon Health Sciences Center